Corticosteroids

Editor

MARCY B. BOLSTER

RHEUMATIC DISEASE CLINICS OF NORTH AMERICA

www.rheumatic.theclinics.com

Consulting Editor
MICHAEL H. WEISMAN

February 2016 • Volume 42 • Number 1

ELSEVIER

1600 John F. Kennedy Boulevard • Suite 1800 • Philadelphia, Pennsylvania, 19103-2899
http://www.theclinics.com

RHEUMATIC DISEASE CLINICS OF NORTH AMERICA Volume 42, Number 1
February 2016 ISSN 0889-857X, ISBN 13: 978-0-323-41712-9

Editor: Jennifer Flynn-Briggs
Developmental Editor: Casey Jackson

Rheumatic Disease Clinics of North America (ISSN 0889-857X) is published quarterly by Elsevier Inc., 360 Park Avenue South, New York, NY 10010-1710. Months of issue are February, May, August, and November. Business and editorial offices: 1600 John F. Kennedy Boulevard, Suite 1800, Philadelphia, PA 19103-2899. Periodicals postage paid at New York, NY and additional mailing offices. Subscription prices are USD 335.00 per year for US individuals, USD 634.00 per year for US institutions, USD 100.00 per year for US students and residents, USD 395.00 per year for Canadian individuals, USD 791.00 per year for Canadian institutions, USD 465.00 per year for international individuals, USD 791.00 per year for international institutions, and USD 230.00 per year for Canadian and foreign students/residents. To receive student/resident rate, orders must be accompanied by name of affiliated institution, date of term, and the *signature* of program/residency coordinator on institution letterhead. Orders will be billed at individual rate until proof of status received. Foreign air speed delivery is included in all *Clinics* subscription prices. All prices are subject to change without notice. **POSTMASTER:** Send address changes to *Rheumatic Disease Clinics of North America,* Elsevier Health Sciences Division, Subscription Customer Service, 3251 Riverport Lane, Maryland Heights, MO 63043. **Customer Service: 1-800-654-2452 (US and Canada). From outside of the US and Canada: 314-447-8871. Fax: 314-447-8029. For print support, e-mail: JournalsCustomerService-usa@elsevier.com. For online support, e-mail: JournalsOnline Support-usa@elsevier.com.**

Reprints. For copies of 100 or more of articles in this publication, please contact the Commercial Reprints Department, Elsevier Inc., 360 Park Avenue South, New York, New York, 10010-1710; Tel.: +1-212-633-3874, Fax: +1-212-633-3820, and E-mail: reprints@elsevier.com.

Rheumatic Disease Clinics of North America is covered in *MEDLINE/PubMed (Index Medicus), Current Contents/Clinical Medicine, Science Citation Index, ISI/BIOMED,* and *EMBASE/Excerpta Medica.*

Contributors

CONSULTING EDITOR

MICHAEL H. WEISMAN, MD
Cedars-Sinai Chair in Rheumatology, Director, Division of Rheumatology, Professor of Medicine, Cedars-Sinai Medical Center, Distinguished Professor, David Geffen School of Medicine at UCLA, Los Angeles, California

EDITOR

MARCY B. BOLSTER, MD
Director, Rheumatology Fellowship Training Program, Massachusetts General Hospital; Associate Professor of Medicine, Harvard Medical School, Boston, Massachusetts

AUTHORS

CHRISTOPHER M. BURNS, MD
Associate Professor of Medicine, Section of Rheumatology, Department of Medicine, Dartmouth-Hitchcock Medical Center, Geisel School of Medicine at Dartmouth, Lebanon, New Hampshire

FRANK BUTTGEREIT, MD
Professor of Medicine, Department of Rheumatology and Clinical Immunology, Charité University Medicine, Berlin, Germany

JENNIFER K. CHEN, MD
Clinical Assistant Professor, Department of Dermatology, Stanford Hospital and Clinics, Redwood City, California

LORINDA CHUNG, MD, MS
Associate Professor, Division of Rheumatology and Immunology, Stanford University School of Medicine, Stanford, California; Division of Rheumatology, VA Palo Alto Health Care System, Palo Alto, California

JOHN A. CIDLOWSKI, PhD
Signal Transduction Laboratory, Department of Health and Human Services, National Institute of Environmental Health Sciences, National Institutes of Health, Research Triangular Park, North Carolina

BHASKAR DASGUPTA, MD
Professor of Medicine, Department of Rheumatology, Southend University Hospital, Westcliff, Essex, United Kingdom

CHRISTIAN DEJACO, MD, PhD, MBA
Associate Professor of Medicine, Departments of Rheumatology and Immunology, Medical University Graz, Graz, Austria

PAUL EMERY, MA, MD, FRCP, FRCPE, FMedSci
Professor, Leeds Institute of Rheumatic and Musculoskeletal Medicine,
University of Leeds, Chapel Allerton Hospital; NIHR Leeds Musculoskeletal Biomedical
Research Unit, Leeds Teaching Hospitals NHS Trust, Leeds, United Kingdom

JOANA FONSECA FERREIRA, MD
Hospitais da Universidade de Coimbra, Rheumatology Unit, Centro Hospitalar e
Universitário de Coimbra, Coimbra, Portugal; Leeds Institute of Rheumatic and
Musculoskeletal Medicine, University of Leeds, Leeds, United Kingdom

MARC A. JUDSON, MD
Division of Pulmonary and Critical Care Medicine, Albany Medical College, Albany,
New York

DIANE L. KAMEN, MD, MSCR
Associate Professor of Medicine, Division of Rheumatology and Immunology, Medical
University of South Carolina, Charleston, South Carolina

SHANTHINI KASTURI, MD
Division of Rheumatology, Hospital for Special Surgery, New York, New York

SARAH F. KELLER, MD
Resident in Internal Medicine, Department of Medicine, Massachusetts General Hospital,
Boston, Massachusetts

JOHN D. MARKMAN, MD
Department of Neurosurgery, Translational Pain Research Program, University of
Rochester School of Medicine and Dentistry, Rochester, New York

ERIC L. MATTESON, MD, MPH
Professor of Medicine, Division of Rheumatology, Department of Internal Medicine;
Division of Epidemiology, Department of Health Sciences Research, Mayo Clinic College
of Medicine, Rochester, Minnesota

ELI M. MILOSLAVSKY, MD
Division of Rheumatology, Department of Medicine, Yawkey Center for Outpatient Care,
Massachusetts General Hospital, Instructor, Harvard Medical School, Boston,
Massachusetts

ALAA ABDELKHALIK AHMED MOHAMED, MD
Leeds Institute of Rheumatic and Musculoskeletal Medicine, University of Leeds, Leeds,
United Kingdom; Rheumatology, Physical Medicine and Rehabilitation Department,
Assiut University Hospitals, Assiut, Egypt

SHANNON A. NOVOSAD, MD
Oregon Health and Science University, Portland, Oregon

ANNA POSTOLOVA, MD, MPH
Clinical Postdoctoral Fellow, Division of Rheumatology and Immunology, Stanford
University School of Medicine, Stanford, California

SIVAPRIYA RAMAMOORTHY, PhD
Signal Transduction Laboratory, Department of Health and Human Services, National
Institute of Environmental Health Sciences, National Institutes of Health, Research
Triangular Park, North Carolina

KENNETH G. SAAG, MD, MSc
Jane Knight Lowe Professor, Division of Clinical Immunology and Rheumatology; Vice Chair, Department of Medicine; Director, Center for Education and Research on Therapeutics (CERTs), Center for Outcomes, Effectiveness Research and Education (COERE), Center of Research Translation (CORT) in Gout and Hyperuricemia, University of Alabama at Birmingham, Birmingham, Alabama

LISA R. SAMMARITANO, MD
Division of Rheumatology, Hospital for Special Surgery, New York, New York

LOUISA S. SCHILLING, BSc
Department of Neuroscience, University of Toronto, Toronto, Ontario, Canada; Senior Fellow, Translational Pain Research Program, University of Rochester School of Medicine and Dentistry, Rochester, New York

XENA WHITTIER, MD
Rheumatology Fellow, Division of Clinical Immunology and Rheumatology, Birmingham, Alabama

KEVIN L. WINTHROP, MD, MPH
Oregon Health and Science University, Portland, Oregon

JAMEEL YOUSSEF, MD
Oregon Health and Science University, Portland, Oregon

ERIC S. ZOLLARS, MD, PhD
Assistant Professor of Medicine, Division of Rheumatology and Immunology, Medical University of South Carolina, Charleston, South Carolina

Contents

> Philip Hench, Edward Kendall, and Tadeus Reichstein received the Nobel Prize in medicine and physiology in 1950 for their "investigations of the hormones of the adrenal cortex." Hench and Kendall took compound E from the laboratory to the clinic to the Nobel Prize in a span of 2 years. This article examines the paths that led to the day when the first rheumatoid arthritis patient received cortisone, and from there to the 1950 Nobel Prize ceremony. The aftermath of this achievement is also discussed. Although there have been significant advances in corticosteroid preparations and use since 1950, the side effects remain daunting.

> Glucocorticoids are primary stress hormones that regulate a variety of physiologic processes and are essential for life. The actions of glucocorticoids are predominantly mediated through the classic glucocorticoid receptor (GR). GRs are expressed throughout the body, but there is considerable heterogeneity in glucocorticoid sensitivity and biologic responses across tissues. The conventional belief that glucocorticoids act through a single GR protein has changed dramatically with the discovery of a diverse collection of receptor isoforms. This article provides an overview of the molecular mechanisms that regulate glucocorticoid actions, highlights the dynamic nature of hormone signaling, and discusses the molecular properties of the GR isoforms.

> Glucocorticoids (GCs) were discovered in the 1940s and were administered for the first time to patients with rheumatoid arthritis in 1948. However, side effects were subsequently reported. In the last 7 decades, the mechanisms of action for both therapeutic properties and side effects have been elucidated. Mechanisms for minimizing side effects were also developed. GCs are the most frequently used class of drugs in the treatment of rheumatoid arthritis because of their efficacy in relieving symptoms and their low cost. A review of clinical applications, side effects, and drug interactions is presented.

Idiopathic inflammatory myopathies (IIMs) involve inflammation of the muscles and are classified by the patterns of presentation and immunohistopathologic features on skin and muscle biopsy into 4 categories: dermatomyositis, polymyositis, inclusion body myositis, and immune-mediated necrotizing myopathy. Systemic corticosteroid (CS) treatment is the standard of care for IIM with muscle and organ involvement. The extracutaneous features of systemic sclerosis are frequently treated with CS; however, high doses have been associated with scleroderma renal crisis in high-risk patients. Although CS can be effective first-line agents, their significant side effect profile encourages concomitant treatment with other immunosuppressive medications to enable timely tapering.

Corticosteroids are the drug of choice for the treatment of sarcoidosis. Because the natural course of sarcoidosis may be self-limiting and/or cause no long-term harm, treatment is not mandatory. Corticosteroids are usually effective for all forms of sarcoidosis, and they work quickly. However, because of the potential toxicities of corticosteroids, alternative medications often need to be considered. Efforts should be made to minimize the corticosteroid dose while keeping the risk of toxicity as low as possible. This article outlines the indications for corticosteroid therapy for sarcoidosis, discusses various dosing regimens, and suggests when alternative corticosteroid agents should be considered.

Targeted interventional delivery of corticosteroids remains a mainstay of treatment for spinal pain syndromes because this approach has a wider therapeutic index than other approaches. The best evidence for analgesic efficacy is in subacute radicular syndromes associated with new-onset or recurrent lumbar radiculitis. Complications often relate to drug delivery technique as much as actions of the steroid itself and require careful consideration and vigilance by the administering physician. Considerable uncertainty persists concerning which patients with chronic pain are most likely to benefit from corticosteroid injections. Matching this treatment option with specific spinal pain syndromes remains a major challenge.

Corticosteroids are frequently used to treat rheumatic diseases. Their use comes with several well-established risks, including osteoporosis, avascular necrosis, glaucoma, and diabetes. The risk of infection is of utmost concern and is well documented, although randomized controlled trials of short-term and lower-dose steroids have generally shown little or no increased risk. Observational studies from the real world, however, have consistently shown dose-dependent increases in risk for serious infections as well as certain opportunistic infections. In patients who begin chronic steroid therapy, vaccination and screening strategies should be used in an attempt to mitigate this risk.

Glucocorticoid-induced osteoporosis (GIOP) is one of the most common and serious adverse effects associated with glucocorticoid use. This article highlights GIOP pathophysiology, epidemiologic associations, effective treatment, and lifestyle modifications that can reduce fracture risk for long-term glucocorticoid users and additionally emphasizes the importance of early intervention.

RHEUMATIC DISEASE CLINICS
OF NORTH AMERICA

THE CLINICS ARE AVAILABLE ONLINE!
Access your subscription at:
www.theclinics.com

Foreword
Corticosteroids

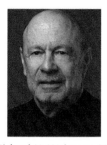

Michael H. Weisman, MD
Consulting Editor

Nowhere is there more controversy in rheumatic diseases than the role of corticosteroids, and that is the reason for the development of this issue. Marcy Bolster has done a magnificent job in creating a list of topics and expert reviews that address the individual pieces of the controversy, including the much maligned role of steroids in rheumatoid arthritis to the important role they play in the management of diseases where other options are few, such as vasculitis and myositis. Their acute versus chronic use is emphasized in articles on toxicity and mechanism of action, and we now have information about steroids on the molecular level that informs us about the variations we see clinically regarding risks and benefits. The history of corticosteroid discovery and its relationship to the war effort is a fascinating story that needed to be brought forward in this issue since many of our colleagues forget the influences of societal factors on discovery. With the almost explosive use of injectable steroids for localized conditions come the risks and dangers that are carefully laid out in this issue. As Dr Bolster indicates, it is time to acknowledge and reassess our use of these powerful tools.

Michael H. Weisman, MD
Division of Rheumatology
Cedars-Sinai Medical Center
David Geffen School of Medicine at UCLA
8700 Beverly Boulevard
Los Angeles, CA 90048, USA

E-mail address:
Michael.Weisman@cshs.org

Rheum Dis Clin N Am 42 (2016) xiii
http://dx.doi.org/10.1016/j.rdc.2015.10.002
0889-857X/16/$ – see front matter © 2016 Published by Elsevier Inc.

rheumatic.theclinics.com

Preface

Corticosteroids: Friends and Foes

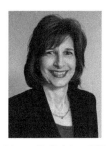

Marcy B. Bolster, MD
Editor

Corticosteroids have been a mainstay of treatment employed by rheumatologists since the Nobel Prize–winning discovery of cortisone in 1950 by Drs Hench, Kendall, and Reichstein. The history of cortisone discovery is eloquently described in the first article of this issue, as written by Christopher Burns, MD, and sets the stage for recognition of value in efficacy offered by this pharmacologic innovation as well as the quickly appreciated potential for toxicities. In the past 65 years, many of our patients have benefited from the rapid anti-inflammatory and immune-suppressing effects of these potent medications. Much continues to be learned about the varying biologic effects at the tissue level as mediated by the glucocorticoid receptor and its multiple isoforms. The mechanism of action is elegantly described by Drs Ramamoorthy and Cidlowski, distinguishing the recognized heterogeneity of glucocorticoid responsiveness among individuals. The other articles in this issue comprehensively address the impressive role played by corticosteroids in autoimmune and inflammatory diseases, such as rheumatoid arthritis, systemic lupus erythematosus, inflammatory myopathy, systemic sclerosis, polymyalgia rheumatica, giant cell arteritis, other systemic vasculitides, and sarcoidosis. In addition to these inflammatory conditions, Dr Markman reports on the utility of corticosteroid injections for spinal pain conditions. In contrast to the valued efficacy of corticosteroids for this multitude of conditions, it is essential that we acknowledge the inherent risks with particular emphasis placed on bone health and infection associated with corticosteroid use, as discussed by Drs Whittier and Saag and Drs Youssef, Novosad, and Winthrop, respectively. A fine balance exists between the good and the evil played by these powerful medications while tempering the immune response in rheumatic disease. We, as physicians, as well as our patients, must appreciate the "friendship" of corticosteroids in providing healing. It is essential

Rheum Dis Clin N Am 42 (2016) xv–xvi
http://dx.doi.org/10.1016/j.rdc.2015.10.001
0889-857X/16/$ – see front matter © 2016 Published by Elsevier Inc.

rheumatic.theclinics.com

that we, however, also acknowledge the intercalation of potential toxicities with the prospect of this therapeutic advantage.

Marcy B. Bolster, MD
Harvard Medical School
Rheumatology Fellowship Training Program
Massachusetts General Hospital
55 Fruit Street
Bulfinch 165
Boston, MA 02114, USA

E-mail address:
mbolster@mgh.harvard.edu

The History of Cortisone Discovery and Development

Christopher M. Burns, MD

KEYWORDS

- Cortisone • Hench • Kendall • Nobel Prize • Rheumatoid arthritis

KEY POINTS

- Hench, Kendall, and Reichstein won the Nobel Prize in Medicine 65 years ago for their "investigations of the hormones of the adrenal cortex."
- The discovery of cortisone is a fascinating tale of good science, perseverance, and luck that might not be possible in today's regulatory environment.
- Although advances in corticosteroid preparations and their use have occurred since 1950, the side effects observed by Hench and his colleagues within weeks after the first patient's dosing still haunt us today.
- Despite these issues, corticosteroids remain a critical and often life-saving component of treatment of many inflammatory diseases.

INTRODUCTION

Most rheumatologists are aware of the discovery of cortisone by Philip Hench and Edward Kendall for which they, along with the Polish chemist Tadeus Riechstein, received the Nobel Prize in medicine and physiology in 1950.[1,2] Hench, the gregarious, consummate clinician in the new field of rheumatology, and Kendall, the dedicated, sometimes stubborn hormone chemist, formed the nucleus of a team that produced this remarkable breakthrough (**Fig. 1**). In a fashion that is inconceivable today, they took the newly purified compound E from the laboratory to the clinic to the Nobel Prize in a span of 2 years. The reader is referred to the recent book by Rooke for a revealing page-turner on the subject.[3] This article examines the paths that led Hench and Kendall to that fateful day, September 21, 1948, when "Mrs G." became the first patient

Disclosure Statement: The author has nothing to disclose.
Section of Rheumatology, Department of Medicine, Dartmouth-Hitchcock Medical Center, Geisel School of Medicine at Dartmouth, Rheumatology 5C, One Medical Center Drive, Lebanon, NH 03756, USA
E-mail address: Christopher.M.Burns@Hitchcock.ORG

Rheum Dis Clin N Am 42 (2016) 1–14
http://dx.doi.org/10.1016/j.rdc.2015.08.001
0889-857X/16/$ – see front matter © 2016 Elsevier Inc. All rights reserved.
rheumatic.theclinics.com

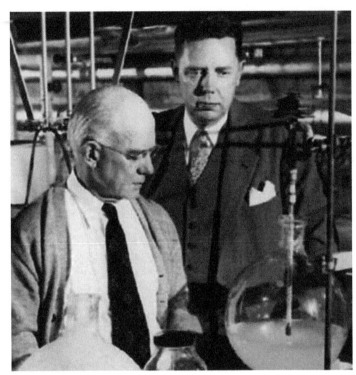

Fig. 1. Philip S. Hench, MD (*right*) and Edward C. Kendall, PhD. (*From* Lloyd M. Philip Showalter Hench, 1896–1965. Rheumatology (Oxford) 2002;41(5):583; with permission.)

with rheumatoid arthritis (RA) to receive cortisone, and from there to the 1950 Nobel Prize. We also look at the aftermath of this achievement for our heroes and their patients, a bittersweet legacy that we still live with today. The article also provides glimpses of others who played cameo roles in this poignant story, inseparable from the time of global upheaval in which it occurred.

PHILIP SHOWALTER HENCH

Philip Hench was born in Pittsburgh, Pennsylvania on February 2, 1896 with a severe cleft palate, but overcame his speech impediment to become a fine speaker. He attended Lafayette College, to which he remained loyal for life, and enlisted in the US Army Medical Corps after graduation in 1916. He graduated from Pittsburgh University Medical School in 1920, and from there began an uncanny string of firsts in medicine and rheumatology.[4] In 1922, he became the first medical resident to train at St. Mary's Hospital in Rochester, Minnesota, a hospital that rose from the ashes of the city after a devastating tornado in 1883. Through the dedicated efforts of Mother Alfred Moes of the Sisters of Saint Francis and Dr William W. Mayo, the 27-bed St. Mary's opened in 1889.[5] By the time Hench arrived, with William Mayo's sons, Will and Charlie, as driving forces, St. Mary's and the Mayo Clinic were becoming world leaders in medicine by adhering to the principles of patient care, research, and education. Hench subsequently became the first rheumatology fellow and then the head of the new rheumatic disease service at Mayo, established in 1926 (**Fig. 2**).[6]

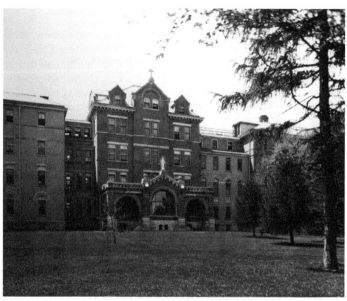

Fig. 2. Saint Mary's hospital in the 1920s. The rheumatology service was located on third floor center between 1925 and 1941. (*From* Hunder GG, Matteson EL. Rheumatology practice at Mayo Clinic: the first 40 years-1920 to 1960. Mayo Clin Proc 2010;85(4):e18; with permission.)

In April of 1929, Hench observed that a 65-year-old doctor experienced relief from his inflammatory arthritis with the onset of jaundice. That quiescence lasted for months after the jaundice had resolved. In 1933, he published on seven such cases.[7] By 1938, he had collected more than 30 cases, noting that the severity of the jaundice correlated with the benefit on inflammation.[8] Pregnancy, infection, and surgery could have similar effects. He postulated that a "substance X" was naturally produced under these conditions, the source unclear. Deliberate induction of jaundice in some patients had benefit.[9] The reasons for Hench's leap to considering the adrenal glands as the potential source of substance X are speculative, but it was already well-known that surgery led to an adrenal hormone response, and in some ways, Hench believed the profound fatigue of RA to be similar to that of Addison disease.

In 1935 he began collaborating with Edward Kendall, a professor of physiologic chemistry at Mayo, and already an accomplished scientist.[10] Kendall was involved in the highly competitive area of isolation of physiologically active adrenal hormones, of which he had identified four by 1940: compounds A (11-dehydorcoticosterone), B (corticosterone), E (dehydrocorticosterone), and F (17-hydroxycorticosterone).[4] In an animal model, adrenal extracts could rescue adrenalectomized subjects from death. The putative life-saving hormone therein was generically known as cortin. Compound E seemed to be the most potent in this capacity, and therefore a lead candidate. But Kendall's biggest competitor, Reichstein, working in Switzerland, had also identified the same hormone, designating it compound Fa. By 1941, Hench and Kendall were considering the possibility that compound E might not just be cortin, but in fact "substance X," the mysterious humor that improved RA.[4] The entrance of the United States into World War II was about to give their work an unexpected boost.[11,12]

EDWARD CHARLES KENDALL

Edward Kendall was born on March 8, 1886 in South Norwalk, Connecticut. He graduated from Columbia University in 1908, and remained for his doctorate in chemistry in 1910.[1,13,14] He briefly worked on the isolation of thyroid hormones at Parke-Davis, before moving onto St. Luke's Hospital in New York, a Columbia affiliate, in 1911. Feeling unappreciated, he left St. Luke's in 1914 for the Mayo Clinic Medical School, becoming director of biochemistry in 1915, and subsequently professor of physiologic chemistry. There, at the age of 28, on Christmas Day, 1914, he became the first to crystallize the hormone thyroxine, starting from 6500 pounds of hog thyroids.[15,16] A great disappointment of his career was his inability to then synthesize thyroxine. He also successfully studied glutathione and oxidative stress, but his biggest achievement was yet to come.[14]

Kendall began studying adrenal hormones in 1930. By 1940, a total of 28 compounds had been identified by several laboratories. In those times, success in the tedious purification processes hung on a reliable supply of glands with which to work. Kendall, using 3000 pounds of animal adrenal glands, was only able to produce 1 g of compound A.[4] Subsequently, with help from Merck & Company and Reichstein's modified technique, hundreds of pounds of ox bile were used to produce 100 g of compound A. Unfortunately, once adequate material was available, it was found to be ineffective in the adrenalectomy bioassay.[13,14] Compound A was clearly not cortin. Compound E differed from A by only one oxygen atom. Despite that, Hench and Kendall remained optimistic that compound E was the elusive cortin and substance X.

WORLD WAR II

With America's entry into World War II on the horizon, rumors were rampant that the Nazis were secretly importing bovine adrenal glands from Argentina via submarine to produce extracts for military use.[11,12] It was long known that adrenalectomized animals would quickly succumb when exposed to even minimal stress, based on the work of Addison and Brown-Sequard in the 1880s.[17,18] It seemed natural to postulate that adrenal extracts could protect against stress. The fear surfaced that Luftwaffe pilots were being given such a drug to allow them to tolerate hypoxia and fly at altitudes of 40,000 feet or more.[11-13] Although these rumors were undoubtedly untrue, the specter of a steroid-enhanced enemy grabbed the attention of the US government. In 1941, the National Research Council set three major priorities for government-funded research, all influenced by impending war. Number three was the development of antimalarials for potential tropical warfare. Number two was the development of penicillin, whose utility for battlefield infections was obvious. Remarkably, the number one priority was the isolation and production of cortin![14] A committee of 14 chemists was assembled, including Kendall. From a practical perspective, the most important outcomes were the flow of money into adrenal hormone research and the resultant partnering with industry. Kendall now had a consistent supply (900 pounds per week) of adrenal glands from Parke-Davis and Wilson Laboratories. But the process of purification of compound E, by this point the lead candidate for the elusive cortin, remained laborious and low-yield.[3]

Enter Lewis Sarett. Born in Champlain, Illinois in 1917, he received his bachelors of science degree in chemistry from Northwestern in 1939 and continued his work at Princeton, where his focus turned toward steroid synthesis.[19] After graduation, Sarett moved to Merck Pharmaceuticals, principally because of their involvement in the government-sponsored cortin project. In early 1942, Sarett went to Kendall's laboratory at Mayo for a 3-month sabbatical and discovered a key intermediary in the synthesis of compound E. He also became a close friend of Kendall before moving back to Merck headquarters in Rahway, New Jersey. By December 1944, Sarett, at the age of 26, was able to synthesize compound E from ox bile.[20] By November of 1948, with help from Kendall, he had perfected a complex, but commercially practical, 37-step process for synthesizing compound E.[21,22] The stage was now set.

Mrs G

Despite successes in the synthetic process, by 1948 Merck had invested more than $13 million in compound E without a clinical indication and with none on the horizon. At an investigator's meeting in New York on April 29, Kendall sensed waning interest and feared the plug would soon be pulled on the project.[14] In the meantime, Hench was continuing to induce jaundice, now using lactophenin as his preferred hepato-toxin.[9] Two patients with severe RA arrived at Mayo in July of 1948 for trials of lacto-phenin. One patient, Mrs G., a 29-year-old woman from Kokomo, Indiana did not respond.[23] In a fortuitous comingling of chutzpah and serendipity, she refused to leave until she felt better.[24] Hench consulted Kendall about using compound E, and he agreed. On September 4, 1948, after an initially lukewarm response, the Mayo team sent a painstakingly written letter to Merck outlining their rationale. Merck acquiesced and sent 5 g of compound E.[24]

On September 21, 1948, Mrs G. received her first of twice daily intramuscular injections of 50 mg of compound E at the hands of Dr Charles H. Slocumb, the hospital service junior rheumatologist.[14,24] The next day, she felt no better. But throughout Day 3, she had progressive improvement, and by Day 4, her pain and stiffness were gone and she was visiting other patients to show off her progress.[24] By September 28, she was pain-free and went shopping in downtown Rochester. "I have never felt better in my life."[14] Apparently, a miracle was happening at Mayo. We have all seen this miracle since, and we all know what usually happens next, but at the dawn of the cortisone era, all was well in Rochester, Minnesota.

THE STORY BREAKS

After the success with Mrs G., the team's mission became one of treating more patients to confirm their initial observations while keeping the discovery under wraps. At Merck's insistence, in February of 1949 Hench invited five master clinicians in rheumatology to Mayo where they witnessed first-hand the effects of compound E on two additional patients with RA.[25] They were convinced and so was Merck. Two months later, Hench was ready to formally present his findings, first at the weekly staff meeting, the custom at Mayo. On the evening of April 20, Hench described the outcomes in 14 treated patients, including films of all the patients before and after treatment (**Fig. 3**).[23] The packed house was stunned, including William Laurence, the *New York Times* science editor, who had been tipped off that something big was happening.[3] Hench's presentation was followed by Kendall's explanation of the basic science involved. That was followed by a raucous round of applause.[14] Laurence subsequently received the 1949 Lasker Foundation Award for medical journalism for his series on cortizone and corticotropin (ACTH) in the *Times*.[26,27] Hench also was awarded a 1949 Lasker, presented in 1950 by the American Public Health Association.[27] The seminal publication on the work appeared just months later, and included 16 patients treated with cortisone and 2 with ACTH, all responders (**Fig. 4**).[23]

Not surprisingly, the news led to a clamor for compound E, by then renamed cortisone by Kendall and Hench. Limited access to the miracle cure led to a black market of fake cortisone.[28] Five companies had various patent claims on cortisone. Kendall's

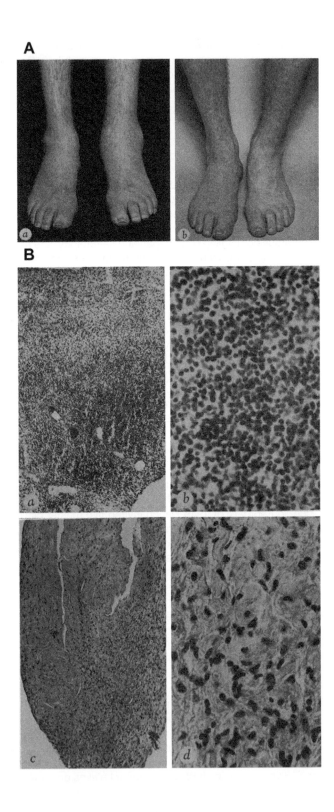

solution was to have the entities each agree to pay a royalty fee for a license from the Research Corporation of New York to use any of the patents for production. Amazingly, Kendall gave all his patents to Mayo Clinic, who in turn gave them to the Research Corporation, in compliance with Mayo's doctrine at the time, from William Mayo himself, that no physician should profit from a discovery developed to benefit the patient.[14,29] By 1952, a technique for manufacturing cortisone more rapidly using *Rhizopus nigricans* was discovered.[21] Cortisone became readily available for all the good and bad that it could do.

THE NOBEL PRIZE

On October 26 1950, just over 2 years after Mrs G. received her first injection, Kendall, Hench, and Reichstein were named the recipients of the Nobel Prize in physiology or medicine for "investigations of the hormones of the adrenal cortex."[1] Because this was the 50th anniversary of the awards, all 100 living laureates were invited and 25 attended, including the antibiotic pioneers Alexander Fleming and Gerhard Domagk. Hench brought his entire family by ocean liner to the festivities in Stockholm in December, including his wife, Mary, four children, and Mary's mother. Edward Kendall came with his wife, Rebecca.[2] Other recipients that year included C. F. Powell for physics, Otto Diels and Kurt Alder for chemistry, Bertrand Russell for literature and Ralph Bunche for peace (the first African American to receive a Nobel). William Faulkner accepted the 1949 Nobel for literature at the 1950 ceremony. A video of the ceremony is available online.[30] Other resources include the presentation speech by Professor G. Liljestrand, and the lectures and banquet speeches by Kendall, Hench, and Reichstein.[1] Hench shared his prize money with his Mayo colleagues, Slocumb and Howard Polley, but also used some of the proceeds to send his ward nurse, Sister Mary Pantaleon, to Rome for an audience with the Pope.[3,31]

AFTERMATH

Mrs G.'s protocol called for her to receive 50 mg intramuscularly of cortisone twice daily for 6 months. But after her miraculous improvement in the first 2 weeks, problems arose. Over a period of a month, she became grossly cushingoid. Her mood became erratic, with periods of depression, euphoria, hypomania, and psychosis, eventually leading to her transfer to a locked psychiatric ward at St. Mary's. Her dose was slowly reduced and she was discharged. Disenchanted with the Mayo, she never returned and eventually stopped cortisone and refused to take it again. She died in 1954 from complications of ACTH treatment.[3] Over time, all of the original patients began to experience the dreaded side effects of prolonged high-dose corticosteroids, so familiar to us now. The near-hysteria for cortisone in the general public was replaced by a healthy, albeit sometimes extreme, fear. In the 1956 movie "Bigger Than Life" James Mason portrayed a man with what sounds like cranial arteritis who suffers

---

Fig. 3. (*A*) Case 2: feet and ankles (*a*) before cortisone was given, (*b*) reduction of swelling by cortisone. (*B*) Case 10: synovia of right knee before cortisone was given (*a, b*) compared with synovia from same knee taken after 39 days of use of cortisone (*c, d*) (hematoxylin-eosin, original magnification ×70 in *a* and *c*, ×400 in *b* and *d*). (*Adapted from* Hench PS, Kendall EC, Slocumb CH, et al. Effects of cortisone acetate and pituitary ACTH on rheumatoid arthritis, rheumatic fever and certain other conditions. Arch Intern Med 1950;85(4):590; with permission.)

Proceedings of the

STAFF MEETINGS OF THE MAYO CLINIC

Published Fortnightly for the Information of the Members of the Staff and the Fellows of the Mayo Foundation for Medical Education and Research

Volume 24   ROCHESTER, MINNESOTA, WEDNESDAY, APRIL 13, 1949   Number 8

CONTENTS

THE EFFECT OF A HORMONE OF THE ADRENAL CORTEX
(17-HYDROXY-11-DEHYDROCORTICOSTERONE:
COMPOUND E) AND OF PITUITARY
ADRENOCORTICOTROPIC HORMONE ON
RHEUMATOID ARTHRITIS

Preliminary Report

Philip S. Hench, M.D., Sc.D., Division of Medicine, Edward C. Kendall, Ph.D., D.Sc., Division of Biochemistry, Mayo Foundation, Charles H. Slocumb, M.D., M.S. and Howard F. Polley, M.D., M.S. in Medicine, Division of Medicine: The adrenal cortical hormone 17-hydroxy-11-dehydrocorticosterone, hereinafter called "compound E,"[1,2] has been administered to 14 patients with severe or moderately severe rheumatoid arthritis. In each case improvement in clinical features and in sedimentation rates began to occur within a few days.

1. Mason, H. L., Hoehn, W. M. and Kendall, E. C.: Chemical Studies of the Suprarenal Cortex. IV. Structures of Compounds C, D, E, F and G. J. Biol. Chem. 124:459-474 (July) 1938.
2. Reichstein, T. and Shoppee, C. W.: The Hormones of the Adrenal Cortex. In Harris, R. S. and Thimann, K. V.: Vitamins and Hormones. New York, Academic Press, Inc., 1943, vol. 1, pp. 345-413.

Fig. 4. Original publication in 1949. (*Adapted from* Hench PS, Kendall EC, Slocumb CH, et al. The effect of a hormone of the adrenal cortex (17-hydroxy-11-dehydrocorticosterone; compound E) and of pituitary adrenocorticotropic hormone on rheumatoid arthritis. Proc Staff Meet Mayo Clin 1949;24(8):181; with permission)

the ravages of the life-saving cortisone and becomes a "drug addict." Clearly, the gild was off the lily, and cortisone was not going to be the solution for RA.

THE EMPIRE STRIKES BACK

Patients were not the only ones to suffer personality changes from cortisone. It is generally accepted that Hench's demeanor changed over time after receiving the Nobel Prize. Early on, Hench had emphasized that cortisone was not primarily a treatment of RA, but an experimental drug that might allow us to better understand disease pathogenesis. Yet as its use spread and the dangers of the drug were appreciated, he became defensive. In 1954, a British study compared cortisone and ACTH with aspirin in 61 patients with early RA, and found no difference in outcome.[32] Yearly follow-up studies bore out those observations. Hench (probably correctly) did not believe the results. There were other skeptics, including the rheumatologist, Dr John Glyn, who helped conduct the trials but believed they were poorly designed.[33] Partly because of surprise with these findings, the EMPIRE Rheumatism Council Research Subcommittee, chaired by Dr Eric Bywaters, conducted a trial in patients with RA of longer duration, but found similar results.[34] In 1956, a *Lancet* editorial urged caution: "Before adopting a policy of 'safe' maintenance therapy we must try to establish whether we are, in fact, using an expensive drug to any good purpose."[35] Hench considered many of the authors on these papers colleagues and friends, including Bywaters (**Fig. 5**). At some deep level, Hench felt betrayed. In turn, others began to notice the change in Hench's normally affable nature.[3]

But in 1957, a study appeared showing that patients with RA who switched from cortisone to prednisone, a more potent corticosteroid with less mineralocorticoid effects than cortisone (**Fig. 6**), had better outcomes.[36] In 1959, 2-year data showing superiority of prednisolone to aspirin in RA, including radiograph erosion data, was published.[37] Three-year results confirmed those findings. But unfortunately for Hench, the vindicating data came too late.[3] In 1998, John Glyn recalled the metamorphosis: "He remained deeply offended by his old friends and was even heard to refer to them as traitors. He refused to meet or even to talk to them, much to their mystification and distress. Toward the end of his life he fell out not only with his British friends but also with many American colleagues."[38] Despite that, Glyn concluded, as many did, that "Philip Showalter Hench was the most remarkable man I have ever met."

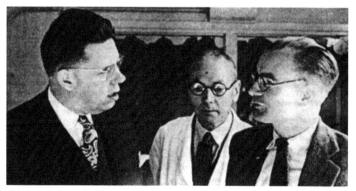

Fig. 5. Philip Hench, Reggie Lightwood (*center*), and Eric Bywaters (*right*). (*From* Lloyd M. Philip Showalter Hench, 1896-1965. Rheumatology (Oxford) 2002;41(5):583; with permission.)

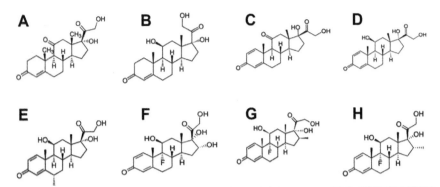

Fig. 6. The chemical structures and properties of common corticosteroid preparations. (*Adapted from* Chang C. Unmet needs in the treatment of autoimmunity: From aspirin to stem cells. Autoimmun Rev 2014;13(4–5):331–46; with permission.)

Compound	Glucocorticoid Potency	Mineralocorticoid Potency	Duration of Action (t 1/2)
A. Cortisone (Compound E)	0.8	0.8	8 h
B. Cortisol (Compound F)	1.0	1.0	8 h
C. Prednisone	3.5–5.0	0.8	16–36 h
D. Prednisolone	4.0	1.0	16–36 h
E. Methylprednisolone	5.0–7.5	0.5	18–40 h
F. Triamcinolone	5.0	0.8	12–36 h
G. Betamethasone	25–80	0	36–54 h
H. Dexamethasone	25–80	0	36–54 h

EPILOGUE

As a Nobel laureate, Hench spent more time traveling and lecturing overseas and focusing on his two avocations: the Sherlock Holmes stories by Sir Arthur Conan Doyle and the history of Walter Reed's conquest of yellow fever. In June 1957, Hench took early retirement at the age of just 61 (**Fig. 7**).[3] By the 1960s, his psychological issues were joined by physical decline, including the development of diabetes. Incredibly, Hench refused to take insulin to control the disease.[39] Philip Showalter Hench died of pneumonia at the age of 69 on March 30, 1965 while on vacation in Ochos Rios, Jamaica.

Remarkably, just 3 years after Mrs G.'s first dose of cortisone, and just a year after receiving the Nobel Prize, Edward Kendall was forced to retire from Mayo in 1951, having hit the no-exception retirement age of 65. He moved to Princeton University, which had a program for former Nobel laureates, and he continued his research for another 20 years.[3] He never was able to duplicate the extraordinary impact of his earlier work, but that was a tall order. At the age of 86, on a consulting visit at Merck, he developed chest pain while having lunch with some old friends. He died 3 days later on May 4, 1972.

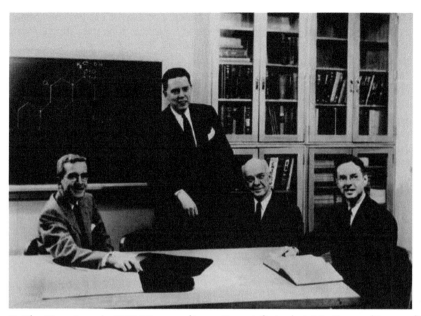

Fig. 7. The Mayo team in 1958, 10 years after cortisone's first administration and 1 year after Hench's retirement. From left to right, Drs Charles H. Slocumb, Phillip S. Hench, Edward C. Kendall, and Howard F. Polley. (*From* Hunder GG, Matteson EL. Rheumatology practice at Mayo Clinic: the first 40 years—1920 to 1960. Mayo Clin Proc 2010;85(4):e24; with permission.)

THE LEGACY OF CORTICOSTEROIDS

In many ways, all rheumatologists have experienced the Shakespearian trials and tribulations of Philip Hench in taking us from before cortisone to the modern era of rheumatology, albeit on a less grand and glorious stage. We go from initial awe at the effectiveness of corticosteroids to disillusionment with their sometimes dramatic, usually insidious, but seemingly inevitable side effects. In fact, it is striking how little things have changed in that regard over 65 years. Prednisone and prednisolone, developed in 1954 at the Schering Corporation, have three to five times the potency of cortisone, and less mineralocorticoid effect, and are the usual drugs of choice (see **Fig. 6**).[40] A large body of evidence over the years has confirmed that low-doses of corticosteroids do have an ameliorative effect on erosive disease in RA, and are not just more potent anti-inflammatories (reviewed in Ref.[41]). A delayed-release formulation of prednisone designed to take effect in the early morning to coincide with peak cortisol release and maximum inflammatory cytokine production in RA is now available and may modestly improve outcome and reduce side effects.[42,43] But the ideal way to use corticosteroids in RA remains elusive.[41,44] For other diseases, high-dose steroids remain the mainstay of treatment.

This edition of *Rheumatic Disease Clinics* delves into the use of corticosteroids in many rheumatologic diseases. Other medical specialties also rely heavily on the use of these drugs. Envision a world without corticosteroids, and one sees many patients dying from acute and chronic inflammatory conditions that are now routinely shut down, or at least controlled, by corticosteroids. The massive efforts over time to pharmacologically modify corticosteroids to maintain their benefits and reduce side effects have largely failed, with rare exceptions, such as budesonide in inflammatory bowel disease (reviewed in Ref.[45]). Intra-articular, inhaled, and topical steroids are preferred and useful in many situations, but their roles are limited or none in systemic rheumatologic processes. Clinicians are better at prophylaxis against some side effects, such as osteoporosis and pneumocystis pneumonia, but most remain unpreventable. And so, the love-hate relationship with corticosteroids continues.[44]

Consider whether cortisone would be approved for use if it was just discovered now. Certainly the way in which Kendall and Hench first gave cortisone would never be allowed in the twenty-first century. If the drug, following the current path to approval, were shown to cause side effects in virtually 100% of subjects in preliminary studies, would its commercial development continue? If the dose were reduced to avoid such side effects, would it appear ineffective in the life-threatening diseases for which the Food and Drug Administration would allow trials? Be thankful that the descendants of compound E are already in the armamentarium. As our mentors and patients have taught us over the last 65 years, use corticosteroids judiciously and with great humility.

REFERENCES

1. The Nobel Prize in physiology or medicine 1950. Nobelprize.org. Nobel Media AB; 2014. Available at: http://www.nobelprize.org/nobel_prizes/medicine/laureates/1950/. Accessed June 1, 2015.
2. Hench PS. Reminiscences of the Nobel Festival, 1950. Proc Staff Meet Mayo Clin 1951;26(23):424–37.
3. Rooke T. The quest for cortisone. East Lansing (MI): Michigan State University Press; 2012.
4. Lloyd M. Philip Showalter Hench, 1896-1965. Rheumatology (Oxford) 2002;41(5):582–4.
5. Clapesattle H. The doctors Mayo. New York: Pocket Books; 1954.
6. Hunder GG, Matteson EL. Rheumatology practice at Mayo Clinic: the first 40 years-1920 to 1960. Mayo Clin Proc 2010;85(4):e17–30.
7. Hench PS. Analgesia accompanying hepatitis and jaundice in cases of chronic arthritis, fibrositis, and sciatic pain. Proc Staff Meet Mayo Clin 1933;8:430–7.
8. Hench PS. Effect of jaundice on rheumatoid arthritis. Br Med J 1938;2(4050):394–8.
9. Hench PS. Potential reversibility of rheumatoid arthritis. Ann Rheum Dis 1949;8(2):90–6.
10. Hench PS. A reminiscence of certain events before, during and after the discovery of cortisone. Minn Med 1953;36(7):705–10.
11. Le Fanu J. The rise and fall of modern medicine. New York: Little, Brown; 1999.
12. Beamish R, Ritchie I. The spectre of steroids: Nazi propaganda, cold war anxiety and patriarchal paternalism. Int J Hist Sport 2005;22(5):777–95.
13. Ingle DJ. Edward C. Kendall. Biogr Mem Natl Acad Sci 1974;47:249–90.
14. Kendall EC. Cortisone: memoirs of a hormone hunter. New York: Scribner; 1971.
15. Kendall EC. Reminiscences on the isolation of thyroxine. Mayo Clin Proc 1964;39:548–52.
16. Simoni RD, Hill RI, Vaughan M. The isolation of thyroxine and cortisone: the work of Edward C. Kendall. J Biol Chem 2002;277(21):21–2.
17. Jeffcoate W. Thomas Addison: one of the three "giants" of Guy's Hospital. Lancet 2005;365(9476):1989–90.
18. Lovas K, Husebye ES. Addison's disease. Lancet 2005;365(9476):2058–61.

19. Patchett AA. Lewis Hastings Sarett, December 22, 1917-November 29, 1999. Biogr Mem Natl Acad Sci 2002;81:278–92.
20. Sarett LH. Partial synthesis of pregnene-4-triol-17(beta), 20(beta), 21-dione-3,11 and pregnene-4-diol-17(beta), 21-trione-3,11,20 monoacetate. J Biol Chem 1946; 162:601–31.
21. Hetenyi G Jr, Karsh J. Cortisone therapy: a challenge to academic medicine in 1949-1952. Perspect Biol Med 1997;40(3):426–39.
22. Kendall EC. Cortisone. Ann Intern Med 1950;33(4):787–96.
23. Hench PS, Kendall EC, Slocumb CH, et al. The effect of a hormone of the adrenal cortex (17-hydroxy-11-dehydrocorticosterone; compound E) and of pituitary adrenocorticotropic hormone on rheumatoid arthritis. Proc Staff Meet Mayo Clin 1949;24(8):181–97.
24. Polley HF, Slocumb CH. Behind the scenes with cortisone and ACTH. Mayo Clin Proc 1976;51(8):471–7.
25. Freyberg R. Witness to a miracle: the initial cortisone trial: an interview with Richard Freyberg, MD. Interview by Mary Ellen Warner. Mayo Clin Proc 2001; 76(5):529–32.
26. Laurence WL. Aid in rheumatoid arthritis is promised by new hormone. New York Times 1949;1:4.
27. Lasker Foundation prior awards. Laskerfoundation.org. Lasker Foundation; 2014. Available at: www.laskerfoundation.org/awards/formaward.htm. Accessed June 3, 2015.
28. Marks HM. Cortisone, 1949: a year in the political life of a drug. Bull Hist Med 1992;66(3):419–39.
29. Burnett JC Jr. Biomedical research at Mayo Clinic: a tradition of collaboration and a vision for year 2000 and beyond. Mayo Clin Proc 2000;75(4):337–9.
30. Video player. Nobelprize.org. Nobel Media AB; 2014. Available at: http://www. nobelprize.org/mediaplayer/index.php?id=634. Accessed June 1, 2015.
31. O'Hanlon C, Williams T. Remembering a medical milestone: Mayo Clinic celebrates 50th anniversary of Nobel Prize for cortisone. Mayo Alumni 2001;37:2–6.
32. A comparison of cortisone and aspirin in the treatment of early cases of rheumatoid arthritis; a report by the Joint Committee of the Medical Research Council and Nuffield Foundation on Clinical Trials of Cortisone, A.C.T.H., and Other Therapeutic Measures in Chronic Rheumatic Diseases. Br Med J 1954;1(4873): 1223–7.
33. Glyn JH. Cortisone and aspirin in rheumatoid arthritis. Br Med J 1954;1(4875): 1376.
34. EMPIRE Rheumatism Council; multi-centre controlled trial comparing cortisone acetate and acetyl salicylic acid in the long-term treatment of rheumatoid arthritis; results up to one year. Ann Rheum Dis 1955;14(4):353–70.
35. Cortisone versus aspirin. Lancet 1956;270(6916):325–6.
36. A comparison of cortisone and prednisone in treatment of rheumatoid arthritis; a report by the Joint Committee of the Medical Research Council and Nuffield Foundation on Clinical Trials of Cortisone, ACTH and other therapeutic measures in chronic rheumatic diseases. Br Med J 1957;2(5038):199–202.
37. A comparison of prednisolone with aspirin on other analgesics in the treatment of rheumatoid arthritis. Ann Rheum Dis 1959;18:173–88.
38. Glyn J. The discovery and early use of cortisone. J R Soc Med 1998;91(10): 513–7.
39. Nickeson RW. Philip Showalter Hench, Nobel Laureate. Alumni News University of Pittsburgh Medical Center. Spring ed; 1993. p. 14–6.

40. Herzog H, Oliveto EP. A history of significant steroid discoveries and developments originating at the Schering Corporation (USA) since 1948. Steroids 1992;57(12):617–23.
41. Kavanaugh A, Wells AF. Benefits and risks of low-dose glucocorticoid treatment in the patient with rheumatoid arthritis. Rheumatology (Oxford) 2014;53(10): 1742–51.
42. Buttgereit F, Doering G, Schaeffler A, et al. Efficacy of modified-release versus standard prednisone to reduce duration of morning stiffness of the joints in rheumatoid arthritis (CAPRA-1): a double-blind, randomised controlled trial. Lancet 2008;371(9608):205–14.
43. Buttgereit F, Mehta D, Kirwan J, et al. Low-dose prednisone chronotherapy for rheumatoid arthritis: a randomised clinical trial (CAPRA-2). Ann Rheum Dis 2013;72(2):204–10.
44. Krasselt M, Baerwald C. The current relevance and use of prednisone in rheumatoid arthritis. Expert Rev Clin Immunol 2014;10(5):557–71.
45. Prantera C, Marconi S. Glucocorticosteroids in the treatment of inflammatory bowel disease and approaches to minimizing systemic activity. Therap Adv Gastroenterol 2013;6(2):137–56.

Corticosteroids
Mechanisms of Action in Health and Disease

 CrossMark

Sivapriya Ramamoorthy, PhD, John A. Cidlowski, PhD*

KEYWORDS

- Glucocorticoid • Glucocorticoid receptor • Glucocorticoid signaling
- Hypothalamic-pituitary-adrenal axis • Isoforms • Phosphorylation • Polymorphism

KEY POINTS

- An important challenge in the clinical application of glucocorticoids is the heterogeneity in glucocorticoid responsiveness among individuals with a significant portion of the population exhibiting some degree of glucocorticoid resistance.
- Glucocorticoid sensitivity and specificity is influenced by GR isoform expression profile. Inflammatory and pathologic processes modulate cellular GR isoform profiles.
- Assessing glucocorticoid sensitivity in individual patients is important for an optimal glucocorticoid treatment plan in the clinic.
- Understanding the heterogeneity of GR signaling in health and disease aids in the development of safer and more effective glucocorticoid therapies with improved benefit/risk ratios for patients.

INTRODUCTION

Corticosteroids are a class of steroid hormones released by the adrenal cortex, which includes glucocorticoids and mineralocorticoids.[1] However, the term "corticosteroids" is generally used to refer to glucocorticoids. Named for their effect in carbohydrate metabolism, glucocorticoids regulate diverse cellular functions including development, homeostasis, metabolism, cognition, and inflammation.[2] Because of

---

Disclosure: None.
Support provided by the Intramural Research Program of the National Institutes of Health/National Institute of Environmental Health Sciences.
Conflict of Interest Statement: The authors declare that they have no relevant conflicts of interest.
Signal Transduction Laboratory, Department of Health and Human Services, National Institute of Environmental Health Sciences, National Institutes of Health, Research Triangular Park, 111 T. W. Alexander Drive, NC 27709, USA
* Corresponding author. National Institute of Environmental Health Sciences, PO Box 12233, MD F3-07, Research Triangle Park, NC 27709.
E-mail address: cidlows1@niehs.nih.gov

Rheum Dis Clin N Am 42 (2016) 15–31
http://dx.doi.org/10.1016/j.rdc.2015.08.002
0889-857X/16/$ – see front matter Published by Elsevier Inc.

their profound immunomodulatory actions, glucocorticoids are one of the most widely prescribed drugs in the world and the worldwide market for glucocorticoids is estimated to be worth more than $10 billion per year.[3] Glucocorticoids have become a clinical mainstay for the treatment of numerous inflammatory and autoimmune diseases, such as asthma, allergy, septic shock rheumatoid arthritis, inflammatory bowel disease, and multiple sclerosis. Unfortunately, the therapeutic benefits of glucocorticoids are limited by the adverse side effects that are associated with high dose (used in the treatment of systemic vasculitis and systemic lupus erythematosus) and long-term use. These side effects include osteoporosis, skin atrophy, diabetes, abdominal obesity, glaucoma, cataracts, avascular necrosis and infection, growth retardation, and hypertension.[3]

Furthermore, patients on long-term glucocorticoid therapy also develop tissue-specific glucocorticoid resistance.[4] Understanding the molecular mechanisms underlying the physiologic and pharmacologic actions of glucocorticoids is of great importance because it may aid in developing synthetic glucocorticoids with increased tissue selectivity, which can thereby minimize the side effects by dissociating the desired anti-inflammatory functions from undesirable adverse outcomes. This article summarizes the recent advances and molecular processes involved in glucocorticoid action and function and discusses in detail the potential role of the glucocorticoid receptor (GR) in determining cellular responsiveness to glucocorticoids.

GLUCOCORTICOID SYNTHESIS, SECRETION, AND BIOAVAILABILITY

Glucocorticoids (cortisol in humans and corticosterone in rodents) are steroid hormones synthesized and released by the adrenal glands in a circadian manner, in response to physiologic cues and stress.[5] The circadian profile of glucocorticoid release from the adrenal glands is regulated by the hypothalamic-pituitary-adrenal (HPA) axis. Inputs from the suprachiasmatic nucleus stimulate the paraventricular nucleus of the hypothalamus to release corticotrophin-releasing hormone and arginine vasopressin. These hormones act on the anterior pituitary where they activate corticotroph cells to secrete adrenocorticotrophin hormone (ACTH) into the general circulation. Subsequently, ACTH acts on the adrenal cortex to stimulate the synthesis and release of glucocorticoids (**Fig. 1**A).[6] Once released from the adrenal glands into the blood circulation, glucocorticoids access target tissues to regulate a myriad of physiologic processes, including metabolism, immune function, skeletal growth, cardiovascular function, reproduction, and cognition. Because of its lipophilic nature, glucocorticoids cannot be presynthesized and stored in adrenal glands, but have to be rapidly synthesized (using several enzymatic reactions) on ACTH stimulation. This feed-forward mechanism within the HPA system is balanced by negative feedback of glucocorticoids acting at the anterior pituitary and within the hypothalamus to inhibit further release of ACTH and corticotrophin-releasing hormone, respectively (see **Fig. 1**A).[7]

Biologically active glucocorticoids are synthesized from cholesterol through a multi-enzyme process termed steroidogenesis.[5,7] ACTH increases adrenal gland activity via protein kinase A activation leading to nongenomic regulation of steroidogenic proteins. This includes phosphorylation of hormone-sensitive lipase, a protein that increases the levels of intracellular cholesterol, and phosphorylation of steroidogenic acute regulatory protein, which promotes the transport of cholesterol into the mitochondria, where cholesterol is converted into pregnenolone by the enzyme side-chain cleavage cytochrome P-450. This process is followed by several enzymatic reactions within the mitochondria and the endoplasmic reticulum that ultimately leads

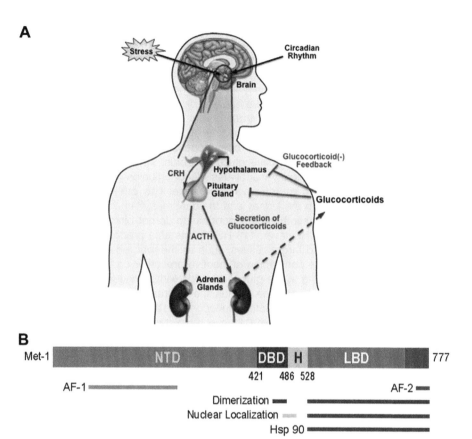

Fig. 1. (*A*) Regulation of glucocorticoid secretion by the HPA axis. Stress induces the release of corticotropin releasing hormone (CRH) from the hypothalamus, which is transported to the anterior pituitary, where it triggers the release of ACTH into the bloodstream. ACTH stimulates the adrenal cortex to synthesize and release the glucocorticoids (cortisol in humans or corticosterone in rodents). Subsequently, the glucocorticoids act on the hypothalamus and pituitary to dampen excess activation of the HPA axis ("negative feedback system"). (*B*) Domain structure of hGR-α. GR contains three major functional regions: the N-terminal transactivation domain (NTD), the central DNA binding domain (DBD), and the C-terminal ligand-binding domain (LBD). The region located between the DBD and LBD is known as the hinge region (H). Regions involved in transcriptional activation (AF1 and AF2), dimerization, nuclear localization, and chaperone hsp90 binding are indicated. CRH, corticotrophin-releasing hormone. (*Adapted from* Ramamoorthy S, Cidlowski JA. Exploring the molecular mechanisms of glucocorticoid receptor action from sensitivity to resistance. Endocr Dev 2013;24:44; with permission.)

to glucocorticoid synthesis within the cells, which in turn is released into the general blood circulation.[7]

The HPA axis has been shown to exhibit a circadian oscillation, thus coupling glucocorticoid synthesis to diurnal patterns. Consequently in humans, serum cortisol concentrations peak in the mornings and are lowest at night. HPA axis is the central stress response system responsible for the adaptation component of the stress response, which attempts to restore homeostasis.[8] Inappropriate regulation of the stress response has been linked to a wide array of pathologies including autoimmune disease, hypertension, affective disorders, and major depression. Systemic serum glucocorticoid level is maintained by adrenal glucocorticoid synthesis, but glucocorticoid availability is further regulated at a tissue or cellular level. In humans, 80% to 90% of circulating glucocorticoids are bound to corticosteroid-binding globulin (CBG) and 5% to 15% are bound to albumin to maintain most glucocorticoids in an inactive form. Only 5% of systemic glucocorticoids are free and bioactive.[9] Hence, the accessibility of cortisol is regulated by CBG concentration.

Glucocorticoid availability at the cellular level is sustained by tissue-specific metabolic enzymes 11β-hydroxysteroid dehydrogenases (11β-HSDs).[10] 11β-HSDs catalyze the interconversion of active glucocorticoids. 11β-HSD2 functions as a potent dehydrogenase that rapidly inactivates glucocorticoids (converts cortisol to cortisone), thus allowing aldosterone selective access to otherwise nonselective mineralocorticoid receptor in the kidney and the pancreas.[10] In contrast to endogenous glucocorticoids, most synthetic glucocorticoids do not bind CBG and are not metabolized by 11β-HSD2. However, 11β-HSD1 acts as a predominant 11β-reductase in all the glucocorticoid target tissues, such as the liver, adipose tissue, brain, and lung, and facilitates the conversion of inactive precursor cortisone to bioactive cortisol, thereby regenerating active glucocorticoids within tissues by exploiting the circulating high levels of inert cortisone.[11] Thus, the contrasting functions of the isoenzymes 11β-HSD1 and 11β-HSD2 maintain glucocorticoid availability and activity at the cellular level and inhibitors of 11β-HSD1 have been designed to limit the adverse metabolic side effects of increased endogenous glucocorticoids in such conditions as Cushing syndrome. In fact, impaired hepatic 11b-HSD1 occurs in patients with polycystic ovary syndrome and primary obesity.[11]

GLUCOCORTICOID RECEPTOR

The physiologic and pharmacologic functions of glucocorticoids are mediated by the intracellular GR, a member of the nuclear receptor family of ligand-activated transcription factors. The GR is a modular protein comprised of three functional domains: an N-terminal transactivation domain (NTD), a central DNA binding domain (DBD), and a C-terminal ligand-binding domain (LBD).[12] Two nuclear localization signals are situated within the LBD and at the DBD-hinge region, respectively (**Fig. 1**B). The NTD, covering amino acids 1 to 420 of the GR, is least conserved and is thus the most variable domain among all the nuclear receptors. The NTD contains transcription activation function (AF1) that activates target genes in a ligand-independent fashion and is the primary site for all the posttranslational modifications. The central DBD is the most conserved domain across all the nuclear receptor proteins and harbors two zinc finger motifs that bind target DNA sequences called glucocorticoid response elements (GREs). The LBD houses the hydrophobic ligand-binding pocket formed by 12 α-helices and 4 β-sheets. A second AF domain (AF2) is located within this carboxy-terminal region along with sequences essential for ligand-dependent coregulator interactions.[13]

MECHANISMS OF GLUCOCORTICOID ACTION
Genomic Actions of Glucocorticoids

Glucocorticoids signal through genomic and nongenomic pathways. The classic, genomic actions of glucocorticoids are mediated through GR. In the absence of hormone, GR predominantly resides in the cytoplasm of cells as part of a large multiprotein complex that includes chaperone proteins (hsp90, hsp70, and p23) and immunophilins (FKBP51 and FKBP52).[14] The multiprotein complex maintains GR in a conformation that favors high-affinity ligand binding.[15] On binding ligand GR undergoes a conformational change, resulting in the dissociation of the multiprotein complex. This leads to a structural reorganization of the GR protein exposing the two nuclear localization signals, and the ligand-bound GR is rapidly translocated into the nucleus through nuclear pores (**Fig. 2**). Once inside the nucleus, GR binds directly to GREs and stimulates target gene expression. The consensus GRE is a palindromic sequence comprised of two half sites (GGAACAnnnTGTTCT) separated by a three-nucleotide spacer.[16] GR binds GRE as a dimer and each half site is occupied by one receptor and thus the three-nucleotide spacer between the two half sites is strictly required for GR:DNA interaction (see **Fig. 2**).[17] Binding of GR to GRE induces conformational changes in GR leading to coordinated recruitment of coregulator and chromatin-remodeling complexes that influence the activity of RNA polymerase II and activates gene transcription and repression. A recent study has identified a negative GRE (nGRE) that mediates glucocorticoid-dependent repression of target genes by recruiting corepressors (NCoR1 and SMRT) and histone deacetlyases (see **Fig. 2**).[18] The consensus nGRE is palindromic (CTCC(n)0-2GGAGA), but differs from the classic GRE in having a variable spacer that ranges from zero to two nucleotides and is occupied by two GR monomers.[19]

Genome-wide GR recruitment studies have shown that only a small proportion of GREs are occupied by GR and specific GR binding sites vary between tissues because of differences in chromatin landscape, which influences GRE accessibility.[20,21] Comprehensive GR binding analyses revealed that many GR-binding sites identified are located far from the promoter proximal region of target genes and showed an unexpected difference between the activation and repressive functions of the GR.[22] For example, glucocorticoid induction of b-arrestin 1 and repression of b-arrestin 2 occurs through an intron 1 GRE and an intron 11 nGRE, respectively.[23] Another example of a GR-binding site located a great distance from the transcription start site is the intragenic nGRE recently identified in exon 6 of the GR gene that mediates homologous downregulation of GR expression.[24] A significant proportion of the GR-binding sites lack a consensus GRE element, which suggests that binding of GR to the chromatin may in many cases occur by tethering to other transcription factors. What remains to be established, however, is the functionality of these distant GR-binding sites in relation to the transcription of genes or other undiscovered functions encoded in the GR protein.

Additionally, GR can physically interact with the members of the signal transducer and activator of transcription family, either in conjunction with binding a GRE or apart, to enhance transcription of certain target genes (see **Fig. 2**).[25] Most of the anti-inflammatory effects of glucocorticoids seem to result from an important negative regulatory mechanism called transrepression,[26] in which ligand-bound GR is recruited to chromatin by protein-protein interactions with DNA-bound transcription factors, particularly nuclear factor (NF)-κB and activator protein-1 (AP1). GR directly binds the Jun subunit of AP1 and the p65 subunit of NF-kB and interferes with the transcriptional activation of these two proteins (see **Fig. 2**). For certain genes, transrepression is accomplished by the GR tethering itself to these DNA-bound transcription factors without itself directly interacting with the DNA.[27,28] However, for some genes, GR functions in a composite manner, binding directly to a GRE and physically associating with AP1 or NF-kB bound to a neighboring site on the DNA (see **Fig. 2**).

Glucocorticoid-induced gene expression is frequently cell type–specific and only a small proportion of genes are commonly activated between different tissues.[29] Tissue-specific target gene activation by glucocorticoids has been shown to be dependent on accessibility of the GR-binding site, which in turn is determined by DNA methylation

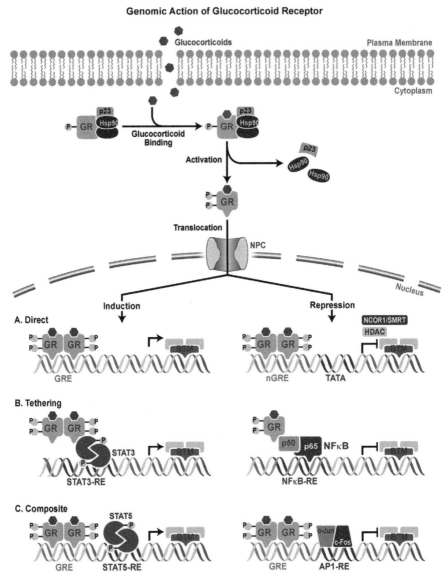

Fig. 2. Genomic action of GR. On binding glucocorticoids, cytoplasmic GR undergoes a conformation change (activation), becomes hyperphosphorylated (P), dissociates from multiprotein complex, and translocates into the nucleus, where it regulates gene expression. GR activates or represses transcription of target genes by direct GRE binding, by tethering itself to other transcription factors apart from DNA binding, or in a composite manner by both direct GRE binding and interactions with transcription factors bound to neighboring sites. AP1, activator protein-1; BTM, basal transcription machinery; nGRE, negative GRE; NF-κB, nuclear factor κB; NPC, nuclear pore complex; RE, response element; STAT, signal transducer and activator of transcription; TBP, TATA-binding protein. (*Modified from* Ramamoorthy S, Cidlowski JA. Exploring the molecular mechanisms of glucocorticoid receptor action from sensitivity to resistance. Endocr Dev 2013;24:41–56.)

and higher order chromatin structures, such as long-range chromatin loops. Thus, tissue-specific target gene activation may be determined by the tissue-specific chromatin landscape, which influences binding of GR to the cognate DNA elements.[20,30] Transcriptional regulation by GR is also modulated by recruitment of coactivators, which mediate posttranslational modifications of histones (acetylation and methylation).[31,32] This property aids in altering the chromatin structure and recruiting other cofactors, thus making the chromatin more accessible for the assembly of general transcription factors and the RNA polymerase complex at the target gene promoter.[33,34] The identity of coregulators that contribute to GR transactivation has grown in the recent years to numbers in the hundreds. Some of the well-studied GR coregulators are the SRC family proteins, mediator complex, and SWI/SNF complexes, NCoR1 and SMRT.[35]

Nongenomic Actions of Glucocorticoids

Rapid, nongenomic glucocorticoid actions are mediated through physiochemical interactions with cytosolic GR or membrane-bound GR. Unlike genomic effects, nongenomic effects of glucocorticoids do not require protein synthesis, and occur within seconds to minutes of GR activation.[36] A growing body of evidence suggests that the rapid nongenomic functions of GR use the activity of various kinases, such as phosphoinositide 3-kinase, AKT, and mitogen-activated protein kinases.[37] Binding of glucocorticoids to GR not only activates the receptor, but also liberates accessory proteins that participate in secondary signaling cascades. For example, when released from the inactive GR protein complex, c-Src activates signaling cascades that inhibit phospholipase A_2 activity, phosphorylate annexin 1, and impair the release of arachidonic acid.[38,39] In thymocytes, activated GR translocates to mitochondria and regulates apoptosis.[40] GR has also been reported to localize in caveolae and glucocorticoid-mediated activation of this membrane-associated GR regulates gap junction intercellular communication and neural progenitor cell proliferation.[41,42] Thus, rapid nongenomic GR signaling adds greater complexity and diversity to glucocorticoid-dependent biologic actions.

GLUCOCORTICOID RECEPTOR HETEROGENEITY
Glucocorticoid Receptor Splice Variants

The GR protein is encoded by the Nr3c1 gene and consists of nine exons; exon 1 forms the 5'-untranslated region, whereas exons 2 to 9 code for the GR protein. Exon 2 forms the N-terminal domain of GR, exons 3 to 4 constitute the central DBD, whereas exons 5 to 9 code for the hinge and LBD. Alternative splicing at exon 9 of primary GR transcript generates two highly homologous mRNA transcripts that result in the production of two GR isoforms termed GRα and GRβ (**Fig. 3A**).[43,44] The two isoforms are identical up to amino acid 727, but vary beyond this position. GRα, the predominant form of GR, is composed of an additional 50 amino acids, whereas GRβ contains an additional 15 nonhomologous amino acids (see **Fig. 3A**).[44] The distinct carboxy-terminal residues in GRβ confer unique properties to this GR isoform. GRβ does not bind ligand (because of the lack of helix 12), resides predominantly in the nucleus, and is inactive on glucocorticoid-responsive reporter genes.[45,46] Conversely, in the presence of GRα, GRβ functions as a dominant negative inhibitor and antagonizes GRα activity on many glucocorticoid-responsive target genes. Recent studies from multiple laboratories suggest that GRβ can function as a bona fide transcription factor by directly inducing and repressing a large number of genes independent of its dominant negative activity on GRα. Indeed, GRβ has

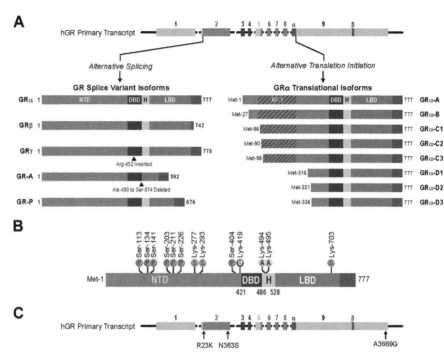

Fig. 3. (*A*) Alternative splicing and translation initiation of hGR primary transcript. The hGR primary transcript is composed of nine exons, with exon 2 encoding most of the NTD, exons 3 and 4 encoding the DBD, and exons 5 to 9 encoding the hinge region (H) and LBD. GR splice variant isoform: the classic GRα protein results from splicing of exon 8 to the beginning of exon 9. GRβ is produced from an alternative splice acceptor site that links the end of exon 8 to downstream sequences in exon 9, encoding a variant with a unique 15 amino acid at C terminus (positions 728–742). GRγ is generated from an alternative splice donor site in the intronic sequence separating exons 3 and 4, resulting in a protein with an arginine insertion (Arg-452) between the two zinc fingers of the DBD. GR-A is produced from alternative splicing that joins exon 4 to exon 8, deleting the proximal 185 amino acids of the LBD (Ala-490-Ser-674) encoded by exons 5 to 7. GR-P is formed by a failure to splice exon 7 to exon 8. The retained intronic sequence introduces a stop codon, resulting in a truncated receptor mutant missing the distal half of the LBD. GRα translational isoforms: Domain organization of the GRα translational isoforms. Initiation of translation from eight different AUG start codons in a single GR-mRNA generates receptor isoforms with progressively shorter NTDs. This generates the GRα translational isoforms GRα-A, B, C1, C2, C3, D1, D2, and D3. (*B*) Domain structure and posttranslational modifications of hGR-α. Sites of posttranslational modifications, such as phosphorylation (P), sumoylation (S), ubiquitination (U), and acetylation (A), are indicated. (*C*) hGR polymorphisms. Arrows indicate polymorphisms that result in amino acid changes and A3669G, which leads to GR stability. (*Modified from* Ramamoorthy S, Cidlowski JA. Exploring the molecular mechanisms of glucocorticoid receptor action from sensitivity to resistance. Endocr Dev 2013;24:41–56.)

been shown to recruit histone deacetylases and repress certain genes, such as interleukin-5 and -13.[47,48] Although GRβ does not bind glucocorticoids, it actively binds GR antagonist mifepristone (RU486),[49] and the endogenous ligand for GRβ is currently unknown.

GRβ is expressed in different tissues but generally at lower levels than GRα. However, GRβ is abundant in certain cell types, such as neutrophils and epithelial cells.[50]

The molecular factors that control GRβ expression are poorly understood, but several studies have implicated the involvement of the splicing factor, SRp30c.[51,52] Besides, the expression of GRβ can be increased by proinflammatory cytokines and other immune activators and lead to reduced GRα/GRβ ratio and glucocorticoid resistance. Reduced GRα/GRβ ratio has been associated with mood disorders, such as schizophrenia, bipolar, and major depressive disorders. Elevated GRβ levels have been associated with glucocorticoid resistance in several inflammatory diseases, including asthma, rheumatoid arthritis, ulcerative colitis, nasal polyposis, systemic lupus erythematosus, sepsis, acute lymphoblastic leukemia, and chronic lymphocytic leukemia.[46] Thus, manipulating GRα/GRβ expression ratios may provide a means to modulate glucocorticoid sensitivity. Another significant finding has been the discovery of GRβ in mice, rat, and zebra fish. These isoforms arise from a distinct splicing mechanism that uses alternative splice donor sites in the intron separating exons 8 and 9, resulting in a GRβ isoform similar in structure and function to human GRβ.[53–55]

The additional splice variants of GR, GRγ, GR-A, and GR-P were discovered in glucocorticoid-resistant cancer cells, and later in healthy tissues. Initially identified in cancer cells and blood mononuclear cells, GRγ is a splice variant in which exon 4 is alternatively spliced to exon 3, thereby including 3 bp of the intron region resulting in an additional arginine residue between the zinc fingers of the DBD (see **Fig. 3**A).[56] GRγ exhibits approximately 50% of the activity of GRα for canonical glucocorticoid target genes, and GRγ expression in childhood acute lymphoblastic leukemia has been shown to correlate with resistance to glucocorticoid treatment.[57] Glucocorticoid resistance in small cell lung carcinoma and corticotroph adenomas is also associated with GRγ expression in these cancers.[58] The GR-A variant is generated by splicing of exon 4 to exon 8, resulting in a transcript lacking exon 5 to 7, which encoded the amino-terminal half of the LBD (see **Fig. 3**A). Failure to splice at exon 7/8 boundary yields GR-P isoform, which lacks the carboxy-terminal half of the LBD (see **Fig. 3**A). Because of defective LBD, GR-A and GR-P do not bind glucocorticoids. Little is known about the biologic functions of GR-A; however, GR-P has been shown to modulate the transcriptional activity of GRα in a cell type–specific manner.[59,60] The GR-P variant is expressed in normal tissue and has been reported to be up-regulated in many glucocorticoid-resistant hematologic malignancies (acute lymphoblastic leukemia, non-Hodgkin lymphoma, and multiple myeloma).[61]

Glucocorticoid Receptor Translational Isoforms

Apart from GR splice variants, alternative translation initiation from the single GRα mRNA produces an additional cohort of diverse GR proteins, adding to GR heterogeneity.[62,63] Eight highly conserved AUG start codons in exon 2 of the GR transcript give rise to eight GRα variant with progressively shorter N-terminus. These receptor isoforms are designated GRα-A, -B, -C1, -C2, -C3, -D1, -D2, and -D3 (see **Fig. 3**A). The GRα-A isoform is the classical full-length receptor containing amino acids 1–777. Ribosomal leaky scanning and ribosomal shunting mechanisms are involved in the generation of the GRα subtypes. Each of the GR splice variants (GRβ, GRγ, GR-A, and GR-P) would also be predicted to give rise to a similar complement of N-terminal isoforms. The GRα translational isoforms, distinguished only by the length of the NTD, have similar affinity for glucocorticoids and similar GRE binding capability following ligand-dependent activation. However, the subcellular localization of the isoforms differs, with GRα-D isoforms residing constitutively in the nucleus. In contrast, GRα-A, GRα-B, and GRα-C isoforms are localized in the cytoplasm of cells in the absence of hormone and translocate to the nucleus on glucocorticoid binding.[62]

An interesting difference among the GRα isoforms is that each GR variant possesses a distinct transcription profile. When individual isoforms are expressed in U2OS osteosarcoma or Jurkat T-lymphoblastic leukemia cells, they each regulate a unique set of genes, with less than 10% being commonly regulated by all the isoforms.[64,65] The isoform-specific gene-regulatory profile produced functional differences in glucocorticoid-induced apoptosis in these cells. Cells expressing GRα-C3 exhibited highest sensitivity to glucocorticoid-induced apoptosis, whereas the GRα-D3-expressing cells were the most resistant.[66] The GRα-C3 is the most active and the heightened activity has been linked to an N-terminal motif (residues 98–115) that is sterically hindered in the larger GR isoforms. The unobstructed AF1 domain of GRα-C3 effectively recruits various coregulators and enhances the transcriptional activity of GRα-C3.[67] However, the lack of AF1 domain might be responsible for diminished transcriptional activity in GRα-D3. Unlike the other receptor isoforms, GRα-D3 does not repress the transcription of antiapoptotic genes Bcl-xL, cellular inhibitor of apoptosis protein 1, and survivin. The inability of GRα-D to downregulate the expression of these genes is associated with a weak interaction between GRα-D and NF-κB.[66]

The translational isoforms exhibit extensive tissue distribution, although their relative levels vary between and within cells. In rodents, the GRα-A and GRα-B isoforms are the most abundant GR proteins in many tissues.[62] The highest GRα-C expression is found in pancreas, lung, and colon. The GRα-D variants are prevalent in the spleen and bladder but are expressed at low levels, whereas GRα-B is more abundant in thymus and colon. Recent studies have also demonstrated changes in the cellular complement of GRα translational isoforms in response to various cellular stimuli.[68] Moreover, the relative levels of the GRα subtypes expressed in the human brain were found to change during development and the aging process.[69,70] The molecular mechanisms governing the expressed complement of translational isoforms are poorly understood. Therefore, genetic manipulation of the GR translational isoforms in animal models may shed new light on the biologic importance of these intriguing GR variants, and it is important to determine the contributions of a single GR isoform in a whole animal. Furthermore, it is critical to verify if glucocorticoid-resistant cells exhibit an altered pattern of GR isoform expression.

Posttranslational Modifications of Glucocorticoid Receptor

Posttranslational modifications of GR further modulate the transcriptional landscape of the receptor. The most extensively studied covalent modification of GR is phosphorylation and at least seven serine residues (Ser-113, Ser-134, Ser-141, Ser-203, Ser-211, Ser-226, and Ser-404) that are phosphorylated in hGR, and all these sites are also conserved in mouse and rat (**Fig. 3B**). Other phosphorylation sites include Ser-45 and -267. The receptor displays a basal level of phosphorylation and becomes hyperphosphorylated on binding glucocorticoids; however, the structure of the ligand determines the pattern and extent of GR phosphorylation. Different kinases are involved in the phosphorylation of GR, which includes mitogen-activated protein kinases, cyclin-dependent kinases, casein kinase II, and glycogen synthase kinase 3β. Phosphorylation of GRα changes its transcriptional activity, often in a gene-specific manner.[71,72] Ligand-dependent phosphorylation of GR at Ser-211 correlates with elevated transcriptional activity, whereas phosphorylation at Ser-226 decreases GR transcriptional activity. Impaired Ser-211 phosphorylation might lead to glucocorticoid resistance in malignant lymphoid cells; in contrast, hyperphosphorylation at Ser-226 might account for decreased GR signaling in the pathology of depression.[72,73] Ligand-induced phosphorylation at Ser-404 has been shown to impact transcriptional activity of GR by impairing activation and repression of target genes.[74] Ser-134 is exclusive in that it is phosphorylated in a glucocorticoid-independent manner by stress stimuli including glucose starvation, oxidative stress, UV irradiation, and osmotic shock.[75]

Phosphorylation of GR also modifies other properties of GR that affect GR signaling.[76] The cellular compartmentalization of GR is altered by phosphorylation, GR phosphorylation at Ser-203, Ser-226, or Ser-404 enhances cytoplasmic retention thus reducing transcriptional activity. Degradation of the GR protein is enhanced by glucocorticoid-dependent phosphorylation at Ser-404 because phosphorylation-deficient mutants are stabilized in the presence of glucocorticoids.[77]

GR protein is also subject to a variety of other posttranslational modifications that regulate the function of the receptor. Ubiquitin is a 76-amino-acid protein that, when attached to specific lysine residues, marks proteins for proteasomal degradation. GR is ubiquitinated at a conserved lysine residue located at position 419 (Lys-419), and this modification targets the receptor for degradation by the 26S proteasome (see **Fig. 3**B).[78,79] Mutation of this conserved Lys residue enhances the glucocorticoid-induced transcriptional activity of GR and blocks ligand-dependent downregulation of GR.[80] Another important posttranslational modification of GR is the covalent addition of a small ubiquitin-related modifier-1 termed sumoylation. GR is sumoylated at residues Lys-277, Lys-293, and Lys-703 (see **Fig. 3**B). Sumoylation of GRα has been shown to promote its degradation and inhibits the transcriptional activity of GR in a promoter-specific manner by recruiting corepressors.[81] It has been suggested that GR can be acetylated at lysine residues 494 and 495 and acetylation of GR alters the inhibitory actions of glucocorticoids on NF-κB (see **Fig. 3**B). Recent studies have shown that acetylation of GR by clock transcription factor reduces GR transcriptional activity.[82,83] In summary, posttranslational modification of GR regulates multiple aspects of GR function and adds to receptor heterogeneity.

Glucocorticoid Receptor Polymorphisms

A polymorphism is defined as an inheritable genetic germ line variant of a single locus (most frequently a single nucleotide variation) that is present in at least 1% of the population. Polymorphisms in the GR gene that alter the amino acid sequence are linked to impaired GR function as a transcriptional activator or repressor. The N363S polymorphism, located within exon 2 (**Fig. 3**C), occurs in approximately 4% of the population, results in modest increases in GR transcriptional activity, and is associated with generalized increases in glucocorticoid sensitivity. N363S carriers have been reported to have an increased body mass index, coronary artery disease, and decreased bone mineral density.[84] The ER22/23EK polymorphism that occurs in approximately 3% of the individuals results in an arginine (R) to lysine (K) change at position 23 (R23K) within the N terminus (see **Fig. 3**C). ER22/23EK is associated with decreased GR transcriptional activity. The ER22/23EK polymorphism has been shown to increase the ratio of GRα-A to GRα-B and the carriers of ER22/23EK polymorphism have a lower tendency to develop impaired glucose tolerance, type-2 diabetes, and cardiovascular disease.[85]

The A3669G polymorphism in GRβ 3′ untranslated region results in an increase of both GRβ mRNA and protein (see **Fig. 3**C). Moreover, carriers of A3669G polymorphism have a higher incidence of rheumatoid arthritis and cardiovascular disease. Individuals homozygous for A3669G polymorphism were associated with a proinflammatory phenotype with an increased risk for myocardial infarction and coronary heart disease.[86]

SUMMARY AND FUTURE CONSIDERATIONS

Glucocorticoids are primary stress hormones that regulate a vast array of physiologic processes, and synthetic derivatives of these molecules are widely used in the clinic for treating inflammatory disorders, autoimmune diseases, and hematologic cancers. Despite the efficacy of glucocorticoids in the treatment of inflammatory and immune disorders, their use is limited by harmful side effects of chronic and/or high-dose treatment. These side effects include diabetes, impaired wound healing, skin atrophy, muscle atrophy, HPA dysfunction, cataracts, peptic ulcers, hypertension, metabolic syndrome, osteoporosis, and water/electrolyte imbalance. Considerable effort has been dedicated over the last several decades to enhance glucocorticoid potency while minimizing adverse side effects by modifying the chemical structure of the natural glucocorticoids.[87] The discovery that multiple GR isoforms with unique expression, gene-regulatory, and functional profiles are generated by alternative splicing, alternative translation initiation of the mature mRNA, and posttranslational modifications has advanced the understanding of molecular basis for the diversity in glucocorticoid sensitivity (hyposensitivity or hypersensitivity). Genome-wide GR recruitment studies have shown that tissue-specific chromatin landscape also exhibits profound differences in glucocorticoid sensitivity.

An important challenge in the clinical application of glucocorticoids is the heterogeneity in glucocorticoid responsiveness among individuals, with a significant portion of the population (up to 30%) exhibiting some degree of glucocorticoid resistance. Progress in the understanding of glucocorticoid expression patterns has uncovered a variety of mechanisms that contribute to reduced glucocorticoid responsiveness, including increased expression of the GRβ and GRα-D isoforms, changes in GR phosphorylation, and homologous downregulation of GR. Dissecting the molecular mechanisms of resistance permits not only the prediction of patient responsiveness to glucocorticoids but also the design of novel therapeutic strategies for combating glucocorticoid insensitivity. In summary, understanding the heterogeneity of GR signaling in health and disease will aid in the development of safer and more effective glucocorticoid therapies with improved benefit/risk ratios for patients.

REFERENCES

1. Van Staa TP, Leufkens HG, Abenhaim L, et al. Use of oral corticosteroids in the United Kingdom. QJM 2000;93:105–11.
2. Rhen T, Cidlowski JA. Antiinflammatory action of glucocorticoids: new mechanisms for old drugs. N Engl J Med 2005;353:1711–23.
3. Schacke H, Docke WD, Asadullah K. Mechanisms involved in the side effects of glucocorticoids. Pharmacol Ther 2002;96:23–4.
4. Barnes PJ. Mechanisms and resistance in glucocorticoid control of inflammation. J Steroid Biochem Mol Biol 2010;120:76–85.
5. Miller WL, Auchus RJ. The molecular biology, biochemistry, and physiology of human steroidogenesis and its disorders. Endocr Rev 2011;32:81–151.
6. Webster JI, Tonelli L, Sternberg EM. Neuroendocrine regulation of immunity. Annu Rev Immunol 2002;20:125–63.
7. John CD, Buckingham JC. Cytokines: regulation of the hypothalamo-pituitary-adrenocortical axis. Curr Opin Pharmacol 2003;3:78–84.
8. Walker JJ, Spiga F, Gupta R, et al. Rapid intra-adrenal feedback regulation of glucocorticoid synthesis. J R Soc Interface 2015;12:20140875.

9. Breuner CW, Orchinik M. Plasma binding proteins as mediators of corticosteroid action invertebrates. J Endocrinol 2002;175:99–112.
10. Seckl JR. 11beta-hydroxysteroid dehydrogenases: changing glucocorticoid action. Curr Opin Pharmacol 2004;4:597–602.
11. Cooper MS, Stewart PM. 11Beta-hydroxysteroid dehydrogenase type 1 and its role in the hypothalamus-pituitary-adrenal axis, metabolic syndrome, and inflammation. J Clin Endocrinol Metab 2009;94:4645–54.
12. Kumar R, Thompson EB. Gene regulation by the glucocorticoid receptor: structure:function relationship. J Steroid Biochem Mol Biol 2005;94:383–94.
13. Bledsoe RK, Montana VG, Stanley TB, et al. Crystal structure of the glucocorticoid receptor ligand binding domain reveals a novel mode of receptor dimerization and coactivator recognition. Cell 2002;110:93–105.
14. Grad I, Picard D. The glucocorticoid responses are shaped by molecular chaperones. Mol Cell Endocrinol 2007;275:2–12.
15. Pratt WB, Toft DO. Steroid receptor interactions with heat shock protein and immunophilin chaperones. Endocr Rev 1997;18:306–60.
16. Beato M. Gene regulation by steroid hormones. Cell 1989;56:335–44.
17. Freedman LP. Anatomy of the steroid receptor zinc finger region. Endocr Rev 1992;13:129–45.
18. Surjit M, Ganti KP, Mukherji A, et al. Widespread negative response elements mediate direct repression by agonist-liganded glucocorticoid receptor. Cell 2011;145:224–41.
19. Hudson WH, Youn C, Ortlund EA. The structural basis of direct glucocorticoid-mediated transrepression. Nat Struct Mol Biol 2013;20:53–8.
20. John S, Sabo PJ, Thurman RE, et al. Chromatin accessibility predetermines glucocorticoid receptor binding patterns. Nat Genet 2011;43:264–8.
21. Burd CJ, Archer TK. Chromatin architecture defines the glucocorticoid response. Mol Cell Endocrinol 2013;380(1–2):25–31.
22. Reddy TE, Pauli F, Sprouse RO, et al. Genomic determination of the glucocorticoid response reveals unexpected mechanisms of gene regulation. Genome Res 2009;19:2163–71.
23. Oakley RH, Revollo J, Cidlowski JA. Glucocorticoids regulate arrestin gene expression and redirect the signaling profile of G protein-coupled receptors. Proc Natl Acad Sci U S A 2012;109:17591–6.
24. Ramamoorthy S, Cidlowski JA. Ligand-induced repression of the glucocorticoid receptor gene is mediated by an NCoR1 repression complex formed by long-range chromatin interactions with intragenic glucocorticoid response elements. Mol Cell Biol 2013;33:1711–22.
25. Uhlenhaut NH, Barish GD, Yu RT, et al. Insights into negative regulation by the glucocorticoid receptor from genome-wide profiling of inflammatory cistromes. Mol Cell 2013;49:158–71.
26. Rogatsky I, Ivashkiv LB. Glucocorticoid modulation of cytokine signaling. Tissue Antigens 2006;68:1–12.
27. Nissen RM, Yamamoto KR. The glucocorticoid receptor inhibits NFkappaB by interfering with serine-2 phosphorylation of the RNA polymerase II carboxy-terminal domain. Genes Dev 2000;14:2314–29.
28. Yang-Yen HF, Chambard JC, Sun YL, et al. Transcriptional interference between c-Jun and the glucocorticoid receptor: mutual inhibition of DNA binding due to direct protein-protein interaction. Cell 1990;62:1205–15.
29. Lamberts SW, Huizenga AT, de Lange P, et al. Clinical aspects of glucocorticoid sensitivity. Steroids 1996;61:157–60.

30. Reddy TE, Gertz J, Crawford GE, et al. The hypersensitive glucocorticoid response specifically regulates period 1 and expression of circadian genes. Mol Cell Biol 2012;32:3756–67.

31. Jenkins BD, Pullen CB, Darimont BD. Novel glucocorticoid receptor coactivator effector mechanisms. Trends Endocrinol Metab 2001;12:122–6.

32. Lonard DM, O'Malley BW. Expanding functional diversity of the coactivators. Trends Biochem Sci 2005;30:126–32.

33. Rosenfeld MG, Glass CK. Coregulator codes of transcriptional regulation by nuclear receptors. J Biol Chem 2001;276:36865–8.

34. Meijsing SH, Pufall MA, So AY, et al. DNA binding site sequence directs glucocorticoid receptor structure and activity. Science 2009;324:407–10.

35. Ronacher K, Hadley K, Avenant C, et al. Ligand-selective transactivation and transrepression via the glucocorticoid receptor: role of cofactor interaction. Mol Cell Endocrinol 2009;299:219–31.

36. Groeneweg FL, Karst H, de Kloet ER, et al. Mineralocorticoid and glucocorticoid receptors at the neuronal membrane, regulators of nongenomic corticosteroid signaling. Mol Cell Endocrinol 2012;350:299–309.

37. Samarasinghe RA, Witchell SF, DeFranco DB. Cooperativity and complemenarity: synergies in non-classical and classical glucocorticoid signaling. Cell Cycle 2012;11:2819–27.

38. Croxtall JD, Choudhury Q, Flower RJ. Glucocorticoids act within minutes to inhibit recruitment of signaling factors to activated EGF receptors through a receptor-dependent, transcription-independent mechanism. Br J Pharmacol 2000;130:289–98.

39. Solito E, Mulla A, Morris JF, et al. Dexamethasone induces rapid serine-phosphorylation and membrane translocation of annexin 1 in a human folliculostellate cell line via a novel nongenomic mechanism involving the glucocorticoid receptor, protein kinase C, phosphatidylinositol 3-kinase, and mitogen-activated protein kinase. Endocrinology 2003;144:1164–74.

40. Boldizsar F, Talaber G, Szabo M, et al. Emerging pathways of non-genomic glucocorticoid (GC) signalling in T cells. Immunobiology 2010;215:521–6.

41. Matthews L, Berry A, Ohanian V, et al. Caveolin mediates rapid glucocorticoid effects and couples glucocorticoid action to the antiproliferative program. Mol Endocrinol 2008;22:1320–30.

42. Samarasinghe RA, Di Maio R, Volonte D, et al. Nongenomic glucocorticoid receptor action regulates gap junction intercellular communication and neural progenitor cell proliferation. Proc Natl Acad Sci U S A 2011;108:16657–62.

43. Bamberger CM, Bamberger AM, de Castro M, et al. Glucocorticoid receptor beta, a potential endogenous inhibitor of glucocorticoid action in humans. J Clin Invest 1995;95:2435–41.

44. Oakley RH, Sar M, Cidlowski JA. The human glucocorticoid receptor beta isoform. Expression, biochemical properties, and putative function. J Biol Chem 1996;271:9550–9.

45. Kino T, Su YA, Chrousos GP. Human glucocorticoid receptor isoform beta: recent understanding of its potential implications in physiology and pathophysiology. Cell Mol Life Sci 2009;66:3435–48.

46. Lewis-Tuffin LJ, Cidlowski JA. The physiology of human glucocorticoid receptor beta (hGRbeta) and glucocorticoid resistance. Ann N Y Acad Sci 2006;1069:1–9.

47. Kelly A, Bowen H, Jee YK, et al. The glucocorticoid receptor beta isoform can mediate transcriptional repression by recruiting histone deacetylases. J Allergy Clin Immunol 2008;121:203–8.e1.

48. Kim SH, Kim DH, Lavender P, et al. Repression of TNF-alpha-induced IL-8 expression by the glucocorticoid receptor-beta involves inhibition of histone H4 acetylation. Exp Mol Med 2009;41:297–306.

49. Lewis-Tuffin LJ, Jewell CM, Bienstock RJ, et al. The Human glucocorticoid receptor b (hGRb) binds RU-486 and is transcriptionally active. Mol Cell Biol 2007;27: 2266–82.

50. Hauk PJ, Hamid QA, Chrousos GP, et al. Induction of corticosteroid insensitivity in human PBMCs by microbial superantigens. J Allergy Clin Immunol 2000;105:782–7.

51. Jain A, Wordinger RJ, Yorio T, et al. Spliceosome protein (SRp) regulation of glucocorticoid receptor isoforms and glucocorticoid response in human trabecular meshwork cells. Invest Ophthalmol Vis Sci 2012;53:857–66.

52. Zhu J, Gong JY, Goodman OB Jr, et al. Bombesin attenuates pre-mRNA splicing of glucocorticoid receptor by regulating the expression of serine-arginine protein p30c (SRp30c) in prostate cancer cells. Biochim Biophys Acta 2007; 1773:1087–94.

53. DuBois DC, Sukumaran S, Jusko WJ, et al. Evidence for a glucocorticoid receptor beta splice variant in the rat and its physiological regulation in liver. Steroids 2013;78:312–20.

54. Hinds TD Jr, Ramakrishnan S, Cash HA, et al. Discovery of glucocorticoid receptor-beta in mice with a role in metabolism. Mol Endocrinol 2010;24:1715–27.

55. Schaaf MJ, Champagne D, van Laanen IH, et al. Discovery of a functional glucocorticoid receptor beta-isoform in zebrafish. Endocrinology 2008;149:1591–9.

56. Ray DW, Davis JR, White A, et al. Glucocorticoid receptor structure and function in glucocorticoid-resistant small cell lung carcinoma cells. Cancer Res 1996;56: 3276–80.

57. Beger C, Gerdes K, Lauten M, et al. Expression and structural analysis of glucocorticoid receptor isoform gamma in human leukaemia cells using an isoform-specific real-time polymerase chain reaction approach. Br J Haematol 2003; 122:245–52.

58. Rivers C, Levy A, Hancock J, et al. Insertion of an amino acid in the DNA-binding domain of the glucocorticoid receptor as a result of alternative splicing. J Clin Endocrinol Metab 1999;84:4283–6.

59. de Lange P, Segeren CM, Koper JW, et al. Expression in hematological malignancies of a glucocorticoid receptor splice variant that augments glucocorticoid receptor-mediated effects in transfected cells. Cancer Res 2001;61:3937–41.

60. Gaitan D, DeBold CR, Turney MK, et al. Glucocorticoid receptor structure and function in an adrenocorticotropin-secreting small cell lung cancer. Mol Endocrinol 1995;9:1193–201.

61. Krett NL, Pillay S, Moalli PA, et al. A variant glucocorticoid receptor messenger RNA is expressed in multiple myeloma patients. Cancer Res 1995;55:2727–9.

62. Lu NZ, Cidlowski JA. Translational regulatory mechanisms generate N-terminal glucocorticoid receptor isoforms with unique transcriptional target genes. Mol Cell 2005;18:331–42.

63. Oakley RH, Cidlowski JA. Cellular processing of the glucocorticoid receptor gene and protein: new mechanisms for generating tissue-specific actions of glucocorticoids. J Biol Chem 2011;286:3177–84.

64. Lu NZ, Collins JB, Grissom SF, et al. Selective regulation of bone cell apoptosis by translational isoforms of the glucocorticoid receptor. Mol Cell Biol 2007;27:7143–60.

65. Wu I, Shin SC, Cao Y, et al. Selective glucocorticoid receptor translational isoforms reveal glucocorticoid-induced apoptotic transcriptomes. Cell Death Dis 2013;4:e453.

66. Gross KL, Oakley RH, Scoltock AB, et al. Glucocorticoid receptor a isoform-selective regulation of antiapoptotic genes in osteosarcoma cells: a new mechanism for glucocorticoid resistance. Mol Endocrinol 2011;25: 1087–99.
67. Bender IK, Cao Y, Lu NZ. Determinants of the heightened activity of glucocorticoid receptor translational isoforms. Mol Endocrinol 2013;27:1577–87.
68. Cao Y, Bender IK, Konstantinidis AK, et al. Glucocorticoid receptor translational isoforms underlie maturational stage-specific glucocorticoid sensitivities of dendritic cells in mice and humans. Blood 2013;121:1553–62.
69. Sinclair D, Webster MJ, Wong J, et al. Dynamic molecular and anatomical changes in the glucocorticoid receptor in human cortical development. Mol Psychiatry 2011;16:504–15.
70. Sinclair D, Webster MJ, Fullerton JM, et al. Glucocorticoid receptor mRNA and protein isoform alterations in the orbitofrontal cortex in schizophrenia and bipolar disorder. BMC Psychiatry 2012;12:84.
71. Beck IM, Vanden Berghe W, Vermeulen L, et al. Crosstalk in inflammation: the interplay of glucocorticoid receptor-based mechanisms and kinases and phosphatases. Endocr Rev 2009;30:830–82.
72. Wang Z, Frederick J, Garabedian MJ. Deciphering the phosphorylation "code" of the glucocorticoid receptor in vivo. J Biol Chem 2002;277:26573–80.
73. Avenant C, Ronacher K, Stubsrud E, et al. Role of ligand-dependent GR phosphorylation and half-life in determination of ligand-specific transcriptional activity. Mol Cell Endocrinol 2010;327:72–88.
74. Galliher-Beckley AJ, Williams JG, Collins JB, et al. Glycogen synthase kinase 3beta-mediated serine phosphorylation of the human glucocorticoid receptor redirects gene expression profiles. Mol Cell Biol 2008;28:7309–22.
75. Galliher-Beckley AJ, Williams JG, Cidlowski JA. Ligand-independent phosphorylation of the glucocorticoid receptor integrates cellular stress pathways with nuclear receptor signaling. Mol Cell Biol 2011;31:4663–75.
76. Webster JC, Jewell CM, Bodwell JE, et al. Mouse glucocorticoid receptor phosphorylation status influences multiple functions of the receptor protein. J Biol Chem 1997;272:9287–93.
77. Chen W, Dang T, Blind RD, et al. Glucocorticoid receptor phosphorylation differentially affects target gene expression. Mol Endocrinol 2008;22:1754–66.
78. Deroo BJ, Rentsch C, Sampath S, et al. Proteasomal inhibition enhances glucocorticoid receptor transactivation and alters its subnuclear trafficking. Mol Cell Biol 2002;22:4113–23.
79. Wallace AD, Cidlowski JA. Proteasome-mediated glucocorticoid receptor degradation restricts transcriptional signaling by glucocorticoids. J Biol Chem 2001; 276:42714–21.
80. Wang X, DeFranco DB. Alternative effects of the ubiquitin-proteasome mediated by CHIP, an E3 ligase. Mol Endocrinol 2005;19:1474–82.
81. Le Drean Y, Mincheneau N, Le Goff P, et al. Potentiation of glucocorticoid receptor transcriptional activity by sumoylation. Endocrinology 2002;143: 3482–9.
82. Ito K, Yamamura S, Essilfie-Quaye S, et al. Histone deacetylase 2-mediated deacetylation of the glucocorticoid receptor enables NF-kappaB suppression. J Exp Med 2006;203:7–13.
83. Charmandari E, Chrousos GP, Lambrou GI, et al. Peripheral CLOCK regulates target-tissue glucocorticoid receptor transcriptional activity in a circadian fashion in man. PLoS One 2011;6:e25612.

84. Jewell CM, Cidlowski JA. Molecular evidence for a link between the N363S gluco-corticoid receptor polymorphism and altered gene expression. J Clin Endocrinol Metab 2007;92:3268–77.
85. van Rossum EF, Lamberts SW. Polymorphisms in the glucocorticoid receptor gene and their associations with metabolic parameters and body composition. Recent Prog Horm Res 2004;59:333–57.
86. Derijk RH, Schaaf MJ, Turner G, et al. A human glucocorticoid receptor gene variant that increases the stability of the glucocorticoid receptor beta-isoform mRNA is associated with rheumatoid arthritis. J Rheumatol 2001;28:2383–8.
87. Clark AR, Belvisi MG. Maps and legends: the quest for dissociated ligands of the glucocorticoid receptor. Pharmacol Ther 2012;134:54–67.

Glucocorticoids and Rheumatoid Arthritis

Joana Fonseca Ferreira, MD[a], Alaa Abdelkhalik Ahmed Mohamed, MD[b],
Paul Emery, MA, MD, FRCP, FRCPE, FMedSci[c],*

KEYWORDS

- Rheumatoid arthritis • Glucocorticoids • Prednisolone • Dose • Side effect
- Drug-drug interactions

KEY POINTS

- Endogenous glucocorticoids (GCs) are produced in the adrenal cortex.
- GCs exert their effect by genomic and nongenomic mechanisms.
- GCs improve pain, morning stiffness, and fatigue.
- In early rheumatoid arthritis (RA), low-dose to medium-dose GCs can prevent joint damage.
- In clinical practice, low doses of GCs can be used in RA as a maintenance therapy. Medium and high doses are used initially as a bridge therapy. Very high doses or pulse therapy are reserved for acute life-threatening or organ-threatening complications.

INTRODUCTION

Glucocorticoids (GCs) were discovered in the 1940s by Kendal and Hench and were administered for the first time to patients with rheumatoid arthritis (RA) in 1948. Two years later, Drs Kendal and Hench won the Nobel Prize.

This was the first time a medication had ever brought relief to patients with arthritis. However, in the following years, side effects were reported.[1]

In the last 7 decades, the mechanism of action has been elucidated. There are 2 fundamental modes of actions: genomic and nongenomic action. The genomic mechanism starts with diffusion of the free plasmatic hormone through the membrane lipids.

[a] Rheumatology Unit, Hospitais da Universidade de Coimbra, Centro Hospitalar e Universitário de Coimbra, Praceta Prof. Mota Pinto, 3000-075 Coimbra, Portugal; [b] Rheumatology, Physical medicine and Rehabilitation Department, Assiut University Hospitals, Assiut 71515, Egypt; [c] Musculoskeletal Biomedical Research Unit, Leeds Teaching Hospital NHS Trust and Leeds Institute of Rheumatic and Musculoskeletal Medicine, University of Leeds, Chapel Allerton Hospital, Chapeltown Road, Leeds LS7 4SA, UK
* Corresponding author.
E-mail address: p.emery@leeds.ac.uk

Rheum Dis Clin N Am 42 (2016) 33–46
http://dx.doi.org/10.1016/j.rdc.2015.08.006   rheumatic.theclinics.com
0889-857X/16/$ – see front matter © 2016 Elsevier Inc. All rights reserved.

A binding site for the hormone is situated on cytoplasmic and nuclear receptors. The GC receptor (GCR) complex enters through nuclear pores and binds to the DNA, resulting in modification of gene transcription and messenger RNA production, and the subsequent translation and protein synthesis. The GCR complex also affects post-transcription events, resulting in alteration of cellular structure and activity, such as leukocytosis with neutrophil increase and reduction of all other leukocyte subsets.[2,3]

Nongenomic effects are complex; they occur more rapidly and involve membrane-bound receptors. This mechanism needs further clarification but it is hoped that doing so will lead to new therapeutic targets.[3]

CLINICAL APPLICATIONS IN RHEUMATOID ARTHRITIS
Inflammation Under Control

Administration of GCs results in diminished activation, proliferation, differentiation, and survival of various inflammatory cells.[4] The higher the dose, the stronger is the effect. In RA, low doses are effective; however, in life-threatening events, high doses are often used. Although, the absolute number of inflammatory cell subsets is decreased, the total blood leukocyte count increases. This increase could be explained by reduction of the adhesion molecules, which subsequently prevents migration of neutrophils from the circulation to the tissues and increases their levels in plasma. Leukocyte subsets all decrease except B cells, which remain stable. GCs inhibit T-helper 1 (Th1) cells, resulting in a reduction of proinflammatory cytokine levels, such as interleukin (IL)-1β, IL-2, IL-3, IL-6, tumor necrosis factor alpha, interferon gamma, and IL-17 and explaining their antiinflammatory effect.[2]

Pain Relief and Structural Progression

Relief of arthritis symptoms, including pain and swelling, is the predominant effect of GCs. New therapeutic strategies target rapid relief of symptoms but also aim to change the course of the disease (ie, preventing joint damage).[5] A high-quality Cochrane Review identified 15 studies with 1414 patients and confirmed that treatment with GCs provided not only symptom relief but also reduction of radiographic progression with low doses of GCs in patients with early arthritis (RA<2 years). All these studies chose low doses of GCs (<7.5 mg/day) to minimize side effects.[6]

This Cochrane Review provides support that GCs behave as disease-modifying antirheumatic drugs (DMARDs) and should be included as the first line of therapy in early arthritis.[6]

Fatigue, Anxiety, and Depression

Other debilitating RA symptoms are fatigue, anxiety, and depression. In contrast with pain and morning stiffness, which correlate with the presence of proinflammatory cytokines, the pathophysiology of these symptoms is unclear.[5]

An analysis of 388 patients with early arthritis suggested an association between morning stiffness and fatigue.[7] Both symptoms improved after taking GCs, underscoring a potential common pathway. Consistent with these results, modified-release prednisone treatment for 12 weeks significantly reduces fatigue scores compared with placebo circadian administration of prednisone in rheumatoid arthritis (CAPRA-2).[8]

Depression and anxiety are sometimes related to disease activity and pain; amelioration of the disease activity and pain improves these symptoms. However, GCs can also have a psychological side effect that paradoxically results in increased anxiety (Table 1).

DOSING IN RHEUMATOID ARTHRITIS

There are very different doses of GC's used in RA, depending of clinical manifestations, treatment objectives and duration of therapy. In order to standardized nomenclature for GC dosages and GC treatment regimens a set of definitions was proposed, summarized in **Table 1**.

Table 1	
Glucocorticoid dosage and treatment regiments is RA	
Dose	**Definition**
Low dose	≤7.5 mg prednisone equivalent per day
Medium dose	>7.5 but ≤30 mg prednisone equivalent per day
High dose	>30 mg but ≤100 mg prednisone equivalent per day
Very high dose	>100 mg prednisone equivalent per day
Pulse therapy	≥250 mg prednisone equivalent per day for 1 d or a few days

Data from Buttgereit F, da Silva JA, Boers M, et al. Standardised nomenclature for glucocorticoid dosages and glucocorticoid treatment regimens: current questions and tentative answers in rheumatology. Ann Rheum Dis 2002;61(8):720.

Equivalents of Prednisone

Steroid hormones, including sex hormones, mineralocorticoids, and GCs, are all derived from cholesterol. Mineralocorticoids (mainly aldosterone) and GCs (mainly cortisol) are synthesized in the adrenal cortex. Sex hormones are produced in the adrenal cortex but are predominantly produced in the gonads.[9]

Classification of mineralocorticoids and GCs depends on the main effect of the hormones. There is an overlap in function between the naturally produced hormones; however, the synthetic drugs are more restricted to a GC effect.[9]

GCs, as alcohols, are insoluble in water. They can be taken as oral tablets and are absorbed in 30 minutes with high bioavailability. GCs, as esters, are lipid soluble and can be used for intramuscular, intra-articular, and peritendinous administrations. GC salts are water soluble and can be administered intravenously.[3]

Circulating GCs are bound to proteins, mostly to corticosteroid-binding globulin or transcortin, but they also can be bound to albumin. The free form, which represents 5% to 10%, is the active form. Therefore, all patients with low levels of plasma proteins are more susceptible to GC effects, both adverse and therapeutic, and should be considered for a dose reduction. Cortisone and prednisone are inactive forms; they are metabolized in the liver to active hormones, cortisol and prednisolone, which have high affinity to GCR. The active forms are recommended when severe liver insufficiency exists. In all other situations the prohormones are preferred.[3]

Prednisolone has a plasma half-life of 2.5 to 5 hours, depending on transcortin-binding body distribution, affinity to GCR, and rate of metabolism. It can be administered once daily, with a maximum effect after peak serum concentration. In the normal circadian rhythm, natural GC levels start to increase after 6 AM and reach the highest peak in the morning. They tend to gradually decline throughout the day and increase again, to a smaller peak, around 6 PM. This small peak is followed by a gradual decline, reaching a plateau around 11 PM, concurrent with normal sleep time. The CAPRA study, with modified-release prednisone, showed that the administration of prednisone at night resulted in an earlier peak with subsequent pain and morning stiffness relief, allowing a better outcome with even low doses and thus fewer side effects.

Nevertheless, further studies are needed to verify whether this regimen is equally effective in preventing joint damage in early RA.[3] (**Table 2**).

ADMINISTRATION IN RHEUMATOID ARTHRITIS

In patients with RA, the recommended plan of treatment is based on the current disease manifestations, the desired therapeutic effect, and the potential side effects. The prescribed GCs should include the recommended type, dose, route, administration time, frequency, and the duration of therapy.[10]

Systemic

Oral

Oral GCs are frequently used in early RA as a bridge therapy for other DMARDs but they can also be used in low doses, as a maintenance therapy, concurrent with other DMARDs.[11] It is preferable for oral GCs to be administered once daily in intermediate-acting or short-acting forms.[12] The rationale for initiation and maintenance of low-dose GCs as additional therapy is the probable relative adrenal insufficiency in patients with active RA.[1] As previously described, the role of low-dose GCs administered for 2 years in delaying the radiographic progression of RA has been highlighted in the last 2 decades and was thought to be superior to the use of DMARDs alone.[11,13] Current practice is to use GCs as bridging therapy until stable state, ideally remission, is reached, then to taper ideally to no therapy. Modifications of the daily oral regimens have been devised to alternate-day regimens in an attempt to reduce the hypothalamic-pituitary-adrenal (HPA) suppression. However, these regimens proved unsuccessful in controlling the symptoms. In practice, they are used in juvenile idiopathic arthritis, in which the alternate-day regimen causes less inhibition of growth.[14]

Parenteral

Parenteral administration is usually by the intramuscular route to control flares or as a bridge therapy in early RA, providing a symptom-free period until other DMARDs

Table 2
Equivalents of prednisone

	Equivalent to Hydrocortisone Dose (mg)	Relative GC Activity	Protein Binding	Plasmatic Half-life (h)	Biological Half-life (h)
Short Acting					
Cortisone	25	0.8	–	0.5	8–12
Cortisol	20	1	++++	1.5–2	8–12
Intermediate Acting					
Methylprednisolone	4	5	–	>3.5	18–36
Prednisolone	5	4	++	2.1–3.5	18–36
Prednisone	5	4	+++	3.4–3.8	18–36
Deflazacort	6	6	++	–	12–36
Triamcinolone	4	5	++	2 to >5	18–36
Long Acting					
Dexamethasone	0.75	20–30	++	3–4.5	36–54
Betamethasone	0.6	20–30	++	3–5	36–54

Adapted from Jacobs JVdGM, Buttgereit F. Glucocorticoid in rheumatic diseases. In: WJ Bijlsma J, editor. EULAR textbook on rheumatic diseases. 1: BMJ Group; 2012. p. 1224.

become efficacious when patient compliance with the oral regimens is questionable. Note that the long-acting lipid-soluble forms of GCs may be efficacious for 3 to 4 months. It is recommended not to repeat more than 3 to 4 times a year to avoid side effects.[15]

Intravenous administration, as pulse therapy, is another form of parenteral use, reserved for induction of remission in major flares, particularly with initiation of new DMARDs strategy or for serious disease manifestations such as vasculitis with specific regimens.[16] The soluble form, given in a very high dose, is administered once daily (it is sometimes given on 3 successive days but without good evidence for efficacy) followed by oral GCs. The duration of action of intravenous methylprednisolone is variable but it normally lasts for up to 6 weeks. Pulse therapy can be used as a bridge therapy for symptoms relief with reduced risks of side effects because many side effects depend more on the cumulative dose.[16]

Intra-articular

The intra-articular administration of GCs in patients with RA is often used, particularly when the disease is active in a limited number of joints. The outcome of the intra-articular treatment is variable depending on several factors: the size of the joint, the amount of weight bearing on the joint, the degree of activity in the joint in terms of synovial fluid volume or presence of synovial hypertrophy, and history of previous joint aspiration. The more of these factors that are present, the less favorable an outcome is anticipated. It also depends on the type and dose of the administered GCs, injection technique, and on the duration of rest permitted after the injection. Rest is always recommended and the period of rest should be longer in weight-bearing joints. There is no evidence-based recommendation for the duration of rest; however, it is usually recommended to rest for 24 hours after injection and avoid overuse of the joint, even when it becomes pain free, for 3 to 6 weeks.[17,18]

Concurrent administration of GCs with local anesthetics is usually preferred because the latter helps to relieve pain immediately. Soluble forms have the advantages of reduced risk of subcutaneous tissue atrophy and rapid onset of action, albeit the duration of symptoms relief is shorter. Lipid-soluble forms have a delayed onset of action but a more prolonged effect. A mixture of both forms of GCs can be used, combining the advantages of each.[17,18]

The frequency of injection should not be more than once every 3 to 4 weeks with a total of 3 to 4 injections per year to minimize GC-induced cartilage injury.[17,18]

Infection, as a cause of synovitis, should be excluded before the administration of intra-articular GCs. Infection can be a potential complication of the injection, but is rare when the procedure is done with stringent aseptic technique. Other local complications include subcutaneous fat atrophy, local skin depigmentation, tendon slip or rupture, and injury of other local structures such as nerves. Systemic effects also can occur, similar to other forms of GCs, but are rare.

SIDE EFFECTS
Patient Education

Patients should be educated about the beneficial and adverse effects of GCs. Adjusting the dose or taking some preventive measures can minimize most of the side effects. This information should be conveyed to the patients with written forms. It is hoped that patient education will lead to early recognition of hazardous side effects and improve compliance.[19]

Minimizing glucocorticoid side effects

GC-induced osteoporosis is a risk for all patients starting GC therapy at medium to high dose. Measures to prevent and treat GC-induced osteoporosis should be considered when initiating or continuing GC therapy for patients with RA.[20,21]

Concomitant administration of nonsteroidal antiinflammatory drugs (NSAIDs) with GC therapy warrants the addition of a gastroprotective medication; otherwise, selective cyclooxygenase-2 inhibitors should be given, depending on the gastrointestinal and cardiovascular risk profile of individual patients. Patients receiving only GCs do not necessarily require gastroprotective treatment.[21,22]

Monitoring disease activity and side effects is essential. The need for continuing GC treatment should be under constant review, and the dose should be titrated against therapeutic response, risk of undertreatment, and development of side effects. Dose monitoring requires collection of baseline parameters, such as body weight, blood pressure, blood glycemia, edema, intraocular pressure, and bone mineral density, that could be used to help direct future management decisions. Some side effects are asymptomatic and, if detected early, their progression could be halted.[21,23]

Osteoporosis and Fractures

GC-induced osteoporosis is a potentially serious complication of prolonged GC therapy. GCs cause accelerated reduction of bone mineral density with most of the bone loss occurring in the first 6 to 12 months of treatment.[24] Trabecular bone is the first affected, but, with continuation of treatment, cortical bone loss also occurs. The precise mechanisms that lead to bone loss are not yet fully understood. GCs decrease calcium absorption and increase renal calcium loss. They also modulate the osteoclast crosstalk, increasing bone resorption, and inhibit osteoblast production, leading to osteoblast apoptosis and prevention of bone formation.[24] In addition, GCs cause osteocyte apoptosis.[24]

A recent meta-analysis included 4 randomized controlled studies that evaluated bone mineral density in patients taking low doses of GCs. None of these studies found statistically significant effects of prednisone on bone mineral density compared with placebo, potentially confirming a dose-related effect.[25] However, measuring the bone mineral density at the baseline, modifying the risk factors for osteoporosis, and the initiation of calcium and vitamin D intake are considered prerequisites to GC therapy. Commencing oral or parenteral bisphosphonates or teriparatide is recommended based on the duration and dose of GC therapy, risk assessment, and the age group of the patients.[20,21]

Other Musculoskeletal Adverse Events

Osteonecrosis is a potential serious side effect of GCs. It rarely occurs in RA and is more common in systemic lupus erythematosus (SLE) and in patients receiving high-dose GC treatment for prolonged periods. No preventive measures can be undertaken apart from minimizing the doses. Awareness is an important factor for early detection and management.[23,25]

Myopathy rarely occurs in patients taking low-dose GCs. It is normally associated with higher doses of GCs for long durations (>3 months).[26]

Endocrine and Metabolic Adverse Events

Glucose metabolism and diabetes

Development of de novo diabetes in previously normoglycemic patients is uncommon. However, in patients with diabetes or glucose intolerance, the fasting and postprandial blood glucose levels may be increased and difficult to control in a dose-dependent manner, and improve noticeably with GC dose reduction.[27]

Risk factors for new-onset hyperglycemia during GC therapy are the same as for other patients, including a family history of diabetes, age, obesity, and a history of gestational diabetes.[27]

GCs cause hyperglycemia by a multifactorial mechanism that includes increased hepatic gluconeogenesis, inhibition of glucose uptake in adipose tissue, and alteration of receptor and postreceptor functions. Nevertheless, GCs present glycogenic effects, explaining why ketoacidosis, a severe diabetes complication, rarely occurs.[27]

Weight gain

Most patients receiving long-term GCs report an increased appetite. The higher intake may contribute to increased body and truncal fat, causing truncal obesity with centripetal fat accumulation and thin extremities. Development of a moon face is uncommon in therapy with subphysiologic doses. The incidence of iatrogenic Cushing syndrome depends on dose and duration of therapy.[28]

Hypothalamic-pituitary-adrenal axis suppression

Administration of GCs results in negative feedback on the hypothalamus and pituitary glands, causing reduced secretion of a corticotropin-releasing hormone and adrenocorticotropic hormone (ACTH), respectively (**Fig. 1**). A sustained negative feedback results in diminished cortisol secretory capacity of the adrenal cortex because the inner cortical zone depends on adrenocorticotropic hormone for structure and function.[29]

HPA axis suppression with tertiary insufficiency is hard to predict but the prevalence increases with GC dose and treatment duration. Potential adrenal insufficiency is

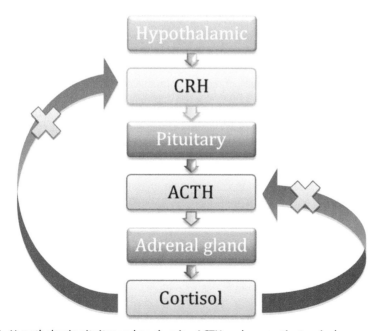

Fig. 1. Hypothalamic-pituitary-adrenal axis. ACTH, adrenocorticotropic hormone; CRH, corticotropin-releasing hormone.

anticipated in patients who receive 7.5 mg of prednisone or equivalent per day. In this case, gradual tapering of GCs dose is preferred rather than rapid withdrawal.[21]

Ordinarily, when an individual is subjected to acute injury and stress, the normal reaction of the body is to increase the endogenous production of cortisol. Similar stresses precipitate adrenal insufficiency if HPA axis suppression exists; therefore, GC dose modification is essential in situations of stress to the body. Often a temporary increase of the dose to 15 mg of prednisone equivalent per day is sufficient for minor surgery.[30]

The ACTH stimulation test is used to evaluate adrenal insufficiency. Synthetic ACTH is administered in the morning. In healthy individuals, cortisol responses are greatest in the morning but, in patients with adrenal insufficiency, the response to synthetic ACTH is the same in the morning and afternoon. A subnormal response confirms the diagnosis of adrenal insufficiency.[21]

Cardiovascular Risk Factors and Atherosclerosis

Long-term use of prednisone in patients with RA may be associated with a higher risk of hypertension. Baseline blood pressure and age are more important for the development of significant hypertension than are low-dose GCs.[31]

Atherosclerosis seems to be accelerated in patients with RA taking GC therapy. Patients with RA without medications are still at a higher risk of advanced atherosclerosis than the normal population, which suggests that atherosclerosis can be disease related and medication related.[32]

The lipid profile is also influenced by GCs, with an increase in total plasma cholesterol, low-density lipoprotein cholesterol, high-density lipoprotein cholesterol, and triglyceride levels, in a dose-dependent effect. In low doses, the antiinflammatory effect of GCs results in a favorable lipid profile.[31,33]

The cardiovascular risk in patients with RA is related to the GC dose, disease activity, comorbidities, and cotherapies.[31,33]

Infections

Cohort and case-control studies report a higher incidence of infections in patients with RA taking GCs, and the risk of infection is increased particularly in patients receiving GCs in high doses combined with immune suppressive treatment.[34]

Patients on GC therapy should be evaluated carefully for typical and atypical microorganisms, including *Pneumocystis* and herpes virus, taking into consideration that GCs can mask infection, resulting in delayed diagnosis and treatment.[34]

Specific screening tests for infection, such as the tuberculin skin test and interferon gamma release assay, should be performed before initiation of GC therapy because these tests are suppressed by GCs, giving false-negative results. Vaccination is an ideal method to diminish infection risk because immunization capacity is preserved before and during treatment. Specific recommendations for vaccination in patients with inflammatory diseases have been developed.[35,36] Short-acting GCs and alternate-day GC therapy are considered other measures to reduce risk of infection.[37]

Renal Dysfunction

Although synthetic GCs have low mineralocorticoid effect, in high doses they can cause fluid retention with a potential risk to patients with underlying heart or kidney disease.

Kaliuresis occurs early with GC therapy and the risk of hypokalemia and metabolic alkalosis is increased with pulse GC therapy. However, clinically significant hypokalemia is uncommon.[38]

Dermatologic Side Effects

Easy bruising, ecchymosis, skin atrophy, striae, delayed wound healing, acne, hirsutism, and thinning of genital and scalp hair are dermatologic side effects that can occur even with low-dose GCs. They are attributed to changes in vascular structure and also to catabolic effects on keratinocytes and fibroblasts of the skin.[25]

Ophthalmologic Side Effects

Posterior subcapsular cataract is a common side effect of GC therapy, without apparent relation to cumulative doses. Cortical cataracts can also be related to GC use but are uncommon.[37]

Mild increased intraocular pressure, causing minor visual disturbances, can occur in GC-treated patients. Glaucoma, threatening eyesight, is rare in low-dose therapy and tends to occur in patients who present with other risk factors, such as a family history of glaucoma, high myopia, and diabetes.[37]

It is recommended for patients possessing high risk factors for glaucoma to be consulted by ophthalmologists before initiation of therapy, even low-dose therapy.[23]

Gastrointestinal Side Effects

GCs, on their own, have a low risk of gastrointestinal adverse effects such as gastritis, ulcers, and bleeding; however, their risk increases dramatically when combined with NSAIDs, showing synergy between both drugs. Measures should be undertaken as described previously if GCs are given with NSAIDs.[22,26]

Table 3
Medications that affect the bioavailability of GCs

	Effect	Class	Sample Agents
Medications that are inducers of CYP 3A	Decrease GC exposure and efficacy	Anticonvulsants	Carbamazepine, fosphenytoin, oxcarbazepine, pentobarbital, phenobarbital, phenytoin, primidone
		Antiinfectives	Efavirenz, etravirine, nafcillin, nevirapine, rifampin, rifabutin, rifapentine
		Others	Bosentan
Medications that are strong inhibitors of CYP 3A and/or P-gp	Increase GC exposure and toxicity	Antibiotics	Clarithromycin, telithromycin
		Antifungals	Itraconazole, ketoconazole, posaconazole, voriconazole
		Antimycobacterial	Isoniazid
		Antivirals (including HIV and HCV)	Atazanavir, boceprevir, darunavir, delavirdine, fosamprenavir, indinavir, lopinavir, nelfinavir, ritonavir, saquinavir, telaprevir
		Estrogens	Estrogen-containing oral contraceptives, conjugated estrogens, esterified estrogens, others
		Immunosuppressants	Cyclosporine, tacrolimus, everolimus

Abbreviations: HCV, hepatitis C virus; HIV, human immunodeficiency virus; P-gp, P-glycoprotein, a drug-transporting protein that also result in change in bioavailability of GCs.

Other complications can occur, such as hepatic steatosis (fatty liver), visceral perforation, and pancreatitis, but the mechanisms are unclear. GCs may mask the symptoms of serious gastrointestinal complications, resulting in delay in diagnosis.[22]

Neuropsychological Side Effects

An increase in well-being, not related to improvement in disease activity, is reported in patients starting GC therapy. Symptoms of mental restlessness, insomnia, and depression have also been recorded. Sleep disturbances occur more commonly in split daily dose because the night dose can change the circadian rhythm. This effect can be avoided by a single morning dose. Memory impairment is also reported, particularly in older patients.[21]

True psychosis is rare in patients with RA and seems to be a more frequent side effect of pulse therapy in patients with SLE.[26]

DRUG-DRUG INTERACTIONS

Active forms of GCs are metabolized in the liver by cytochrome P (CYP)-450 and drug interactions depend on induction and inhibition of CYP enzymes.

Table 4
Multiple drug interactions in which GCs administration results in a change in drug efficacy

Drug Class	Drug	Effect	Comment
Anticoagulants, oral	Warfarin	GCs may increase anticoagulant effect of warfarin	Most patients require a warfarin dose alteration after initiating GCs (3–7 d). INR should be monitored closely
Diuretics, potassium wasting	Furosemide, hydrochlorothiazide, others	GCs may enhance potassium depletion	Monitor serum potassium and if necessary adjust diuretic dose or supplement with oral potassium
Fluoroquinolone antiinfectives	Ciprofloxacin, gemifloxacin, levofloxacin, moxifloxacin, ofloxacin, sparfloxacin, others	Increased risk of developing tendonitis and rupture	Monitor for new onset of tendon/joint pain
Hypoglycemic agents (oral and insulin)	Acarbose, glipizide, glyburide, insulins, metformin, pioglitazone, sitagliptin, others	Starting GCs treatment may result in glucose dysregulation	Blood sugar should be closely monitored and medication should be adjusted according to glycemic profile
NSAIDs	Ibuprofen, indomethacin, ketorolac, ketoprofen, naproxen, others	Combination of GCs and NSAIDs results in an increased risk of peptic ulcer compared with the use of either alone	PPIs should be used when NSAIDs or aspirin are administered with GCs

Abbreviations: INR, International Normalized Ratio; PPIs, proton pump inhibitors.

Oral antacids can cause change in oral GCs absorption and decrease bioavailability. To minimize this effect, the administration of these medications should be 2 or more hours apart (**Table 3**).

There are other multiple drug interactions in which GCs administration results in a change in drug efficacy. These interactions are listed in **Table 4**.

FUTURE CONSIDERATIONS

An increased understanding of the pathophysiology of RA and different GCs mechanisms will potentially lead to an optimization of therapy. The most recent example is the modified-release prednisone tablet. This preparation, tested recently, showed amelioration of the duration of morning stiffness when received at night compared with the same dose of prednisolone taken in the morning. However, the long-term benefits and risks of this preparation have not been investigated yet.[39]

The antiinflammatory effect seems to be related to transrepression mechanisms and most of the side effects seem to be linked to gene transactivation, therefore research is focused on creation of GC ligands that selectively activate the genetic transrepression mechanism. The new class, known as SEGRAs (selective GC receptor agonists), has exciting potential but is still experimental and warrants further investigation.[40]

Other research is being done for the combination of GCs with other drugs, such as nitric oxide. When released, nitric oxide can enhance antiinflammatory effects, but more studies are needed to confirm clinical efficacy.[41]

SUMMARY

GCs are the most effective drugs in relieving symptoms of RA and should be used in association with other DMARDs. Recently, it was shown that GCs also prevent radiographic progression in patients with early RA.

New formulations are being developed to improve clinical efficacy and minimize adverse effects. Until these are available, monitoring for side effects and constant reviewing of treatment adequacy and drug interactions are appropriate to prevent adverse events.

REFERENCES

1. Neeck G. Fifty years of experience with cortisone therapy in the study and treatment of rheumatoid arthritis. Ann N Y Acad Sci 2002;966:28–38.
2. Buttgereit F, Straub RH, Wehling M, et al. Glucocorticoids in the treatment of rheumatic diseases: an update on the mechanisms of action. Arthritis Rheum 2004; 50(11):3408–17.
3. Spies CM, Bijlsma JW, Burmester GR, et al. Pharmacology of glucocorticoids in rheumatoid arthritis. Curr Opin Pharmacol 2010;10(3):302–7.
4. Gotzsche PC, Johansen HK. Meta-analysis of short-term low dose prednisolone versus placebo and non-steroidal anti-inflammatory drugs in rheumatoid arthritis. BMJ 1998;316(7134):811–8.
5. Kirwan JR, Buttgereit F. Symptom control with low-dose glucocorticoid therapy for rheumatoid arthritis. Rheumatology (Oxford) 2012;51(Suppl 4):iv14–20.
6. Kirwan JR, Bijlsma JW, Boers M, et al. Effects of glucocorticoids on radiological progression in rheumatoid arthritis. Cochrane database Syst Rev 2007;(1):CD006356.

7. Buttgereit F, Doering G, Schaeffler A, et al. Efficacy of modified-release versus standard prednisone to reduce duration of morning stiffness of the joints in rheumatoid arthritis (CAPRA-1): a double-blind, randomised controlled trial. Lancet (London) 2008;371(9608):205–14.
8. Buttgereit F, Mehta D, Kirwan J, et al. Low-dose prednisone chronotherapy for rheumatoid arthritis: a randomised clinical trial (CAPRA-2). Ann Rheum Dis 2013;72(2):204–10.
9. Buttgereit F, Burmester GR, Straub RH, et al. Exogenous and endogenous glucocorticoids in rheumatic diseases. Arthritis Rheum 2011;63(1):1–9.
10. Dernis E, Ruyssen-Witrand A, Mouterde G, et al. Use of glucocorticoids in rheumatoid arthritis - practical modalities of glucocorticoid therapy: recommendations for clinical practice based on data from the literature and expert opinion. Jt Bone Spine 2010;77(5):451–7.
11. Boers M, Verhoeven AC, Markusse HM, et al. Randomised comparison of combined step-down prednisolone, methotrexate and sulphasalazine with sulphasalazine alone in early rheumatoid arthritis. Lancet (London) 1997;350(9074): 309–18.
12. Criswell LA, Saag KG, Sems KM, et al. Moderate-term, low-dose corticosteroids for rheumatoid arthritis. Cochrane database Syst Rev 2000;(2): CD001158.
13. Svensson B, Boonen A, Albertsson K, et al. Low-dose prednisolone in addition to the initial disease-modifying antirheumatic drug in patients with early active rheumatoid arthritis reduces joint destruction and increases the remission rate: a two-year randomized trial. Arthritis Rheum 2005;52(11):3360–70.
14. Avioli LV. Glucocorticoid effects on statural growth. Br J Rheumatol 1993; 32(Suppl 2):27–30.
15. Choy EH, Kingsley GH, Khoshaba B, et al. A two year randomised controlled trial of intramuscular depot steroids in patients with established rheumatoid arthritis who have shown an incomplete response to disease modifying antirheumatic drugs. Ann Rheum Dis 2005;64(9):1288–93.
16. Weusten BL, Jacobs JW, Bijlsma JW. Corticosteroid pulse therapy in active rheumatoid arthritis. Semin Arthritis Rheum 1993;23(3):183–92.
17. Gray RG, Tenenbaum J, Gottlieb NL. Local corticosteroid injection treatment in rheumatic disorders. Semin Arthritis Rheum 1981;10(4):231–54.
18. Jones A, Regan M, Ledingham J, et al. Importance of placement of intra-articular steroid injections. BMJ 1993;307(6915):1329–30.
19. van der Goes MC, Jacobs JW, Boers M, et al. Patient and rheumatologist perspectives on glucocorticoids: an exercise to improve the implementation of the European League Against Rheumatism (EULAR) recommendations on the management of systemic glucocorticoid therapy in rheumatic diseases. Ann Rheum Dis 2010;69(6):1015–21.
20. Grossman JM, Gordon R, Ranganath VK, et al. American College of Rheumatology 2010 recommendations for the prevention and treatment of glucocorticoid-induced osteoporosis. Arthritis Care Res 2010;62(11):1515–26.
21. van der Goes MC, Jacobs JW, Boers M, et al. Monitoring adverse events of low-dose glucocorticoid therapy: EULAR recommendations for clinical trials and daily practice. Ann Rheum Dis 2010;69(11):1913–9.
22. Piper JM, Ray WA, Daugherty JR, et al. Corticosteroid use and peptic ulcer disease: role of nonsteroidal anti-inflammatory drugs. Ann Intern Med 1991;114(9): 735–40.

23. Da Silva JA, Jacobs JW, Kirwan JR, et al. Safety of low dose glucocorticoid treatment in rheumatoid arthritis: published evidence and prospective trial data. Ann Rheum Dis 2006;65(3):285–93.

24. O'Brien CA, Jia D, Plotkin LI, et al. Glucocorticoids act directly on osteoblasts and osteocytes to induce their apoptosis and reduce bone formation and strength. Endocrinology 2004;145(4):1835–41.

25. Santiago T, da Silva JA. Safety of glucocorticoids in rheumatoid arthritis: evidence from recent clinical trials. Neuroimmunomodulation 2015;22(1–2):57–65.

26. Jacobs JVdGM, Buttgereit F. Glucocorticoid in rheumatic diseases. In: Wj Bijlsma J, editor. EULAR textbook on rheumatic diseases. 1: BMJ Group; 2012. p. 1218–33.

27. Hoes JN, van der Goes MC, van Raalte DH, et al. Glucose tolerance, insulin sensitivity and beta-cell function in patients with rheumatoid arthritis treated with or without low-to-medium dose glucocorticoids. Ann Rheum Dis 2011; 70(11):1887–94.

28. Hoes JN, Jacobs JW, Boers M, et al. EULAR evidence-based recommendations on the management of systemic glucocorticoid therapy in rheumatic diseases. Ann Rheum Dis 2007;66(12):1560–7.

29. Straub RH, Cutolo M. Circadian rhythms in rheumatoid arthritis: implications for pathophysiology and therapeutic management. Arthritis Rheum 2007;56(2): 399–408.

30. van der Goes MC, Jacobs JW, Bijlsma JW. The value of glucocorticoid co-therapy in different rheumatic diseases–positive and adverse effects. Arthritis Res Ther 2014;16(Suppl 2):S2.

31. Naranjo A, Sokka T, Descalzo MA, et al. Cardiovascular disease in patients with rheumatoid arthritis: results from the QUEST-RA study. Arthritis Res Ther 2008; 10(2):R30.

32. Park YB, Ahn CW, Choi HK, et al. Atherosclerosis in rheumatoid arthritis: morphologic evidence obtained by carotid ultrasound. Arthritis Rheum 2002;46(7): 1714–9.

33. Sokka T, Toloza S, Cutolo M, et al. Women, men, and rheumatoid arthritis: analyses of disease activity, disease characteristics, and treatments in the QUEST-RA study. Arthritis Res Ther 2009;11(1):R7.

34. Dixon WG, Suissa S, Hudson M. The association between systemic glucocorticoid therapy and the risk of infection in patients with rheumatoid arthritis: systematic review and meta-analyses. Arthritis Res Ther 2011;13(4):R139.

35. Muller-Ladner C, Muller-Ladner U. Vaccinations in patients with autoimmune inflammatory rheumatic diseases–EULAR recommendations for pediatric and adult patients. Medizinische Monatsschrift fur Pharmazeuten 2012;35(10):353–64 [quiz: 65–6]. [in German].

36. van Assen S, Elkayam O, Agmon-Levin N, et al. Vaccination in adult patients with auto-immune inflammatory rheumatic diseases: a systematic literature review for the European League Against Rheumatism evidence-based recommendations for vaccination in adult patients with auto-immune inflammatory rheumatic diseases. Autoimmun Rev 2011;10(6):341–52.

37. Khanna DPH. Corticosteroids. rheumatoid arthritis. Philadelphia: Lippincott Williams & Wilkins; 2004.

38. Whitworth JA, Gordon D, Andrews J, et al. The hypertensive effect of synthetic glucocorticoids in man: role of sodium and volume. J Hypertens 1989;7(7): 537–49.

39. Bijlsma JW, Jacobs JW. Glucocorticoid chronotherapy in rheumatoid arthritis. Lancet (London) 2008;371(9608):183–4.
40. Schacke H, Berger M, Rehwinkel H, et al. Selective glucocorticoid receptor agonists (SEGRAs): novel ligands with an improved therapeutic index. Mol Cell Endocrinol 2007;275(1–2):109–17.
41. Buttgereit F. Current issues of basic and clinical glucocorticoid research. Clin Exp Rheumatol 2003;21(2):145–7.

Corticosteroids in Lupus

Shanthini Kasturi, MD*, Lisa R. Sammaritano, MD

KEYWORDS

- Systemic lupus erythematosus • Glucocorticoids • Corticosteroids • Prednisone
- Methylprednisolone

KEY POINTS

- Corticosteroids are the mainstay of therapy for patients with systemic lupus erythematosus but use is associated with numerous adverse effects.
- Treatment with corticosteroids should be tailored to control symptoms with the lowest possible dose for the shortest possible duration to minimize adverse effects.
- Comorbidities predisposing to adverse effects such as diabetes, cardiovascular disease, peptic ulcer disease, and osteoporosis should be evaluated and controlled when initiating corticosteroid therapy.

INTRODUCTION

Corticosteroids play a central role in the treatment of systemic lupus erythematosus (SLE), a complex autoimmune disease with multiorgan involvement. Corticosteroids were trialed in SLE in the late 1940s to early 1950s, soon after their successful use in rheumatoid arthritis, and quickly revolutionized the treatment of SLE by rapidly inducing remission.[1–3] It became clear early on that steroid therapy came with a price because cessation of symptoms gave way to the hazards of a cushingoid state.[2] The struggle to balance risks and benefits continues because steroids remain the cornerstone of SLE treatment. Long-term follow-up of SLE cohorts shows that up to 88% of patients are treated with steroids, with as many as 57% to 86% receiving continuous treatment.[4–6] Steroids have not only been credited with symptom relief but also with mortality reduction in SLE.[7] This article discusses the role of corticosteroids in SLE, describing clinical applications, dosing and administration, side effects, and drug interactions. Nomenclature for corticosteroid dosing ranges is adapted from Buttgereit and colleagues[8] (**Table 1**).

Disclosure: The authors have nothing to disclose.
Division of Rheumatology, Hospital for Special Surgery, 535 East 70th Street, New York, NY 10021, USA
* Corresponding author.
E-mail address: kasturis@hss.edu

Rheum Dis Clin N Am 42 (2016) 47–62
http://dx.doi.org/10.1016/j.rdc.2015.08.007
0889-857X/16/$ – see front matter © 2016 Elsevier Inc. All rights reserved.

Table 1	
Standardized nomenclature for glucocorticoid dosage	
EULAR Grading	**Dose; Prednisone Equivalent (mg)**
Low dose	≤7.5
Medium (moderate) dose	7.5–30
High dose	30–100
Very high dose	>100
Pulse therapy	≥250

Abbreviation: EULAR, European League Against Rheumatism.

Data from Buttgereit F, da Silva JA, Boers M, et al. Standardised nomenclature for glucocorticoid dosages and glucocorticoid treatment regimens: current questions and tentative answers in rheumatology. Ann Rheum Dis 2002;61(8):720.

CLINICAL APPLICATIONS

SLE is a condition with protean manifestations and a relapsing and remitting course. Corticosteroids can be used for nearly every manifestation of SLE, although evidence guiding dose and duration is limited and clinical practice is largely eminence based. A comprehensive review by Luijten and colleagues[9] details the available clinical evidence for steroid treatment in SLE (**Table 2**).

In general, corticosteroids are best used for acute treatment of exacerbations in SLE; in light of their serious long-term side effects, every effort should be made to implement steroid-sparing medications for ongoing chronic therapy. Hydroxychloroquine (HCQ) is indicated as baseline treatment for most patients with SLE unless a specific contraindication is present, and is often effective alone for mild systemic, mucocutaneous, and musculoskeletal symptoms. When HCQ is inadequate, when corticosteroids cannot be tapered, or when more serious inflammation is present, steroid-sparing immunosuppressive agents are used and include azathioprine (AZA), mycophenolate mofetil (MMF), and methotrexate. Cyclophosphamide (CYC) is generally reserved for renal and neurologic disease but may also be necessary for other less common life-threatening complications such as pulmonary hemorrhage or noncutaneous vasculitis.

General

General systemic manifestations of SLE include fever, fatigue, weight loss, and lymphadenopathy. Two cohort studies examining use of corticosteroids to treat SLE-related fever showed prednisone doses from 20 to 100 mg daily to be effective.[10,11] Similarly, a cohort study found that 20 mg daily was effective in treating lymphadenopathy.[12] Constitutional symptoms generally occur in conjunction with organ-specific manifestations of SLE, and, as a result, treatment is typically tailored toward the latter. However, when systemic symptoms occur in isolation, low-dose to medium-dose corticosteroids are often effective with the addition of HCQ. Immunosuppressive agents are often necessary if symptoms persistently recur with taper of steroid despite use of HCQ.

Mucocutaneous

Rashes, alopecia, and oral ulcers are common organ-specific manifestations of SLE but typically do not require treatment with systemic steroids. Topical and intralesional steroids are often used for rashes and alopecia in association with antimalarial medications. When rash is not controlled with HCQ, other agents, such as chloro-quine, dapsone, or thalidomide, may be used. Mucocutaneous manifestations for which systemic steroids and steroid-sparing immunosuppressive medications are often necessary include bullous lupus, lupus panniculitis, severe cutaneous vasculitis, erythema multiforme, and severe chronic discoid lupus: in these situations, medium to high dosages of steroids are usually necessary.

Musculoskeletal

Arthritis, arthralgias, and myalgias are a common reason for steroid treatment. There are no formal studies, but doses of up to 20 mg daily of prednisone are usual, and ongoing low-dose steroid may be required. Methotrexate is often preferred as the initial steroid-sparing agent for lupus arthritis. Myositis, a less common manifestation, generally requires higher dose corticosteroid, especially in the initial treatment phase, with the addition of steroid-sparing medications when severe or persistent.

Hematologic

Mild SLE-related cytopenias generally require only careful monitoring. More severe manifestations of leukopenia, thrombocytopenia, antibody-mediated hemolytic ane-mia, or aplastic anemia are typically treated with high-dose or pulse corticosteroid therapy and immunosuppressive medication. In addition to traditional immunosup-pressives such as AZA or MMF, severe immune-mediated cytopenias are often treated with intravenous immunoglobulin or rituximab when life threatening or when initial therapy does not induce a lasting response.

Cardiac

Pericarditis generally responds to moderate-dose steroid; myocarditis is uncommon but requires high doses for effective control with concomitant aggressive immunosup-pressive therapy. Libman-Sacks endocarditis, often clinically silent, is not treated with steroids.

Pulmonary

Pulmonary manifestations include pulmonary hemorrhage, pleural effusions, pleurisy, interstitial lung disease, pulmonary hypertension, and shrinking lung disease. CYC is often administered along with pulse steroid for severe pulmonary manifestations, such as pulmonary hemorrhage, whereas serositis is generally controlled with low to mod-erate dosing of corticosteroids. Shrinking lung disease, a rare complication, typically responds well to moderate-dose to high-dose steroids, whereas pulmonary hyperten-sion and interstitial lung disease are less likely to be steroid responsive.

Gastrointestinal

Gastrointestinal manifestations include lupus enteritis, hepatitis, pancreatitis, perito-nitis, and protein-losing enteropathy; diagnosis may be difficult and is often one of exclusion. Uncommon but potentially severe gastrointestinal indications respond well to high-dose or pulse-dose steroid after other causes are excluded, such as infec-tion. Longer term therapy may require addition of immunosuppressive agents.

Ophthalmologic

Serious conditions involving the eye are rare, but may include uveitis, episcleritis or scleritis, retinal vasculitis, and neuromyelitis optica. When mild, local ophthalmologic steroid solutions are adequate; severe conditions such as retinal vasculitis or

Table 2
Corticosteroid dosing per SLE manifestation

	Indication	Number of References	Total Number of Patients	Pulse	Range, Oral Prednisone	Mean Dose	Combination	Level of Evidence
General	Fever	4	283	None	10–100 mg	40–100 mg	—	2b
	Lymphadenopathy	2	24	None	20–30 mg	20–30 mg	—	4
Mucocutaneous	Bullous	6	6	None	30–90 mg	30–40 mg	Dapsone	4
	Erythema multiforme	4	5	None	20–60 mg	20–30 mg	None	4
	Discoid	2	4	None	10 mg–1 mg/kg	10–30 mg	None	4
	Subacute cutaneous lupus erythematosus	2	2	None	40 mg–1 mg/kg	20–40 mg	None	4
	Lupus panniculitis	3	4	Not necessary	32–40 mg	40 mg	None	4
	Necrotizing vasculitis	4	24	Possibly MP 3 × 500 mg	0.5–1 mg/kg	1 mg/kg (max 60 mg)	Possibly icw CYC	2b
Hematologic	Thrombocytopenia	9	45	None	25 mg–1 mg/kg	0.5–1 mg/kg	Possibly icw IVIG	2b
	Autoimmune anemia	12	86	MP 3 × 500 mg	10 mg–2 mg/kg	1 mg/kg (max 60 mg)	Possibly icw IVIG, MMF, danazol, CYC	2b
	Pure red cell aplasia	6	7	MP 3 × 500 mg	0–1 mg/kg	1 mg/kg (max 60 mg)	—	4
	Hemophagocytosis syndrome	8	24	MP 3 × 1000 mg	60–100 mg (1–2 mg/kg)	1 mg/kg (max 60 mg)	Possibly icw IVIG, cyclosporine, CYC	4
	TTP/ITP	7	13	MP 3 × 1000 mg	0–100 mg	1 mg/kg (max 60 mg)	Possibly icw plasma exchange, CYC	4

Gastrointestinal	Pancreatitis	10	44	MP 3 × 500 mg	10 mg–1 mg/kg	0.5–1 mg/kg	Possibly icw plasma exchange, CYC	4
	Autoimmune hepatitis	7	13	None	20–60 mg	40 mg	—	4
	Lupus enteritis	2	50	None	10 mg–1 mg/kg	1 mg/kg (max 60 mg)	Possibly icw CYC, rituximab	2b
	Gastrointestinal vasculitis	2	3	MP 3 × 1000 mg	40–100 mg	1 mg/kg (max 60 mg)	icw CYC	4
	Protein-losing enteropathy	5	34	MP 3 × 1000 mg	40–60 mg (0.8–1 mg/kg)	1 mg/kg (max 60 mg)	—	2a
	Lupus peritonitis	3	3	MP 3 × 1000 mg	40–100 mg	1 mg/kg (max 60 mg)	—	4
Ocular	Neuromyelitis optica	11	19	MP 3–5 × 1000 mg	25 mg–2 mg/kg	1 mg/kg (max 60 mg)	—	4
Genitourinary	Lupus cystitis	8	9	MP 3 × 1000 mg	20–60 mg	40 mg	—	4
Pulmonary	Pleuritis	4	40	None	33.6 mg–2 mg/kg	40–60 mg	Possibly icw CYC, AZA	2b
	Shrinking lung syndrome	3	13	MP 3 × 1000 mg	20–40 mg	40 mg	Possibly icw CYC, AZA	4
	Pulmonary hemorrhage	3	64	MP 3 × 1000 mg	40 mg–3 mg/kg	1 mg/kg (max 60 mg)	Possibly icw CYC	2b
Cardiovascular	Myocarditis	8	27	MP 3 × 1000 mg	30 mg–1 mg/kg	1 mg/kg	Possibly icw CYC	3a/4
	Pericarditis	4	47	None	30–60 mg	30–40 mg	Possibly icw CYC, AZA	2b
Musculoskeletal	Polyarthritis	3	3	None	Low dose–10 mg	<10 mg	—	4
	Myositis	1	1	None	60 mg	1 mg/kg (max 60 mg)	icw CYC	5

Levels of evidence: 1a, systematic review of randomized control trials; 1b, individual randomized control trial; 2a, systematic review of cohort studies; 2b, cohort study; 3a, systematic review of case-control studies; 3b, case-control studies; 4, case series; 5, expert opinion.

Abbreviations: AZA, azathioprine; CYC, cyclophosphamide; icw, in combination with; IVIG, intravenous immunoglobulin; max, maximum; MMF, mycophenolate mofetil; MP, methylprednisolone; TTP/ITP, thrombotic thrombocytopenic purpura/idiopathic thrombocytopenic purpura.

Adapted from Luijten RK, Fritsch-Stork RD, Bijlsma JW, et al. The use of glucocorticoids in systemic lupus erythematosus. After 60 years still more an art than science. Autoimmun Rev 2013;12(5):621; with permission.

neuromyelitis optica generally require systemic high-dose or pulse steroid in conjunction with aggressive immunosuppressive therapy including CYC.

Nephritis and Neuropsychiatric

Nephritis and neurologic involvement are potentially severe, debilitating manifestations of SLE and clinical evidence supports the use of high-dose or pulse steroid in conjunction with aggressive immunosuppressive therapy. Treatment of these serious manifestations are discussed in the article.[13]

Pregnancy and Lactation

The use of corticosteroids during pregnancy and lactation is a significant issue given the increased prevalence of lupus in women of childbearing age. Steroid use during pregnancy is common; patients may require continuous therapy or experience flares requiring initiation of or increase in dose of steroids. Although HCQ is generally continued throughout pregnancy and lactation, several common immunosuppressive therapies, such as MMF, are contraindicated in pregnancy, limiting therapeutic options. AZA is regarded as low risk for use throughout pregnancy and is usually the immunosuppressive of choice in this setting. When AZA is ineffective or not tolerated, cyclosporine or tacrolimus may be substituted.

Nonfluorinated steroids such as prednisone are largely metabolized to inactive forms by the placenta, in contrast with fluorinated steroids such as betamethasone or dexamethasone, which pass through the placenta easily.[14] As a result, when maternal steroid therapy during pregnancy is necessary, prednisone or methylprednisolone is preferable, with about 10% of active drug reaching the fetus.[15] Fluorinated steroids should be used only when the intention is to treat the fetus rather than the mother. Stress-dose hydrocortisone is recommended for patients during labor and delivery or at the time of cesarean section who have taken corticosteroids throughout pregnancy.[15]

Patients on corticosteroids may breastfeed with little risk to the newborn, because minimal amounts are excreted in breast milk. At doses up to 80 mg of prednisone daily, breast milk concentrations are reported to range from 5% to 25% of maternal serum levels.[16] Even at a dose of 80 mg/d, infant exposure is less than 10% of endogenous cortisol production. There is an initial equilibrium between serum and breast milk concentrations; as a result, patients on prednisone doses greater than 20 mg daily are recommended to delay feeding for 4 hours after taking medication to minimize infant exposure.[16]

Side effects of corticosteroid therapy during pregnancy for mother and fetus include general side effects as well as pregnancy-specific considerations. Maternal hypertension, infection, osteoporosis, avascular necrosis, and hyperglycemia/gestational diabetes are potential complications with special relevance in pregnancy. Increased risk of premature rupture of membranes has been associated with corticosteroid use. Fetal complications may include intrauterine growth restriction and increased incidence of oral clefts, although evidence is conflicting. One meta-analysis of studies evaluating prednisone exposure in 184 pregnant women showed a 3.4-times increased odds of cleft palate after first-trimester exposure; in contrast, another review of 1449 pregnancies with maternal inhaled or oral steroid use through the first trimester showed a rate lower than that in the control arm.[17,18] There have also been rare case reports of neonatal cataracts and adrenal suppression, but immunosuppression and increased incidence of infection have not been shown.[15]

DOSING
Systemic Lupus Erythematosus Pathogenesis

Autoimmunity in SLE is mediated by dysfunction of both the adaptive and innate immune systems. Polyclonal B-cell hyperreactivity is a central feature, leading to perpetuation of autoantibodies thought to be pathogenic.[19] These antibodies, such as anti–double-stranded DNA antibodies, are produced by class-switched B cells with the assistance of autoreactive T cells. Defects in CD8+ T and T-regulatory cells and aberrant cytokine signaling pathways, including decreased production of interleukin (IL)-2 and increased production of IL-17, lower the threshold for lymphocyte activation in SLE.[20]

Dysfunction of the innate immune system also contributes to the pathogenesis of SLE. Physiologic clearing of apoptotic debris by macrophages, neutrophils, and complement becomes a pathologic inflammatory process in patients with SLE. Neutrophils, including a subset referred to as low-density granulocytes, have also been implicated in the pathogenesis of SLE. Lupus neutrophils are predisposed toward cell death via NETosis, a process resulting in the creation of neutrophil extracellular traps (NETs) through the externalization of chromatin fibers and granule-derived antimicrobial peptides.[21] Patients with SLE are not only more likely to produce NETs but may also have an impaired ability to clear them.[22]

Mechanism of Corticosteroids

Corticosteroids are effective therapeutic agents in SLE because they target these multiple pathogenic pathways. As discussed elsewhere in this issue, these agents suppress production of proinflammatory cytokines and diminish numbers of circulating T cells, monocytes, and macrophages. They also inhibit leukocyte activity in areas of inflammation by decreasing endothelial cell permeability, adhesion molecule production, and fibroblast function, and exert their effects via genomic and nongenomic mechanisms.[23] In the genomic pathway, corticosteroids bind to cytosolic receptors and translocate into the nucleus, where they bind to glucocorticoid corticosteroid response elements and activate expression of antiinflammatory proteins (transactivation) and bind to and compete with transcription factors for nuclear coactivators, preventing expression of proinflammatory cytokines (transrepression).[24] Selective glucocorticoid corticosteroid receptor agonists that preferentially induce the clinically desirable transrepression genomic effects are currently under study, offering the potential for more targeted corticosteroid effect while limiting undesirable side effects.[25]

Patients with SLE have lower levels of corticosteroid receptors in peripheral blood mononuclear cells than healthy controls, suggesting a role for endogenous corticosteroids in the pathogenesis of SLE; receptor levels inversely correlate with disease activity and treatment.[26]

The rapid antiinflammatory effects of corticosteroids, particularly at high doses, are mediated by nongenomic mechanisms. Corticosteroids decrease immune cell function by altering mitochondrial and plasma membranes, and further reduce proinflammatory cytokines by inhibiting release of arachidonic acid and via membrane-bound receptors through processes independent of transcription.[24] The latter pathway may be of particular significance in SLE, because membrane-bound corticosteroid receptors are upregulated on monocytes in patients with SLE and are downregulated by corticosteroids in a dose-related manner.[27]

Dosing

Cytosolic corticosteroid receptors are saturated in a dose-dependent fashion: at high to pulse doses, 100% of receptors are filled; pharmacodynamics of receptor-mediated genomic activities are optimized; and, importantly, nongenomic effects emerge.[8]

The use of very-high-dose intravenous or pulse steroids for life-threatening SLE manifestations is standard practice with limited supporting evidence.[28] A double-blind placebo-controlled trial of 25 patients compared high-dose oral steroids (40–60 mg of prednisolone) versus pulse steroids (1 g daily × 3 days) plus high-dose oral steroids in patients with moderate to severe lupus and found a more rapid initial response but similar improvements in disease severity at 1 month.[29] The literature supporting pulse steroids in SLE is strongest for treatment of central nervous system (CNS) or renal disease, but even these studies do not compare dosages, durations, or routes, and suggest that pulse steroids in the absence of steroid-sparing immunosuppression are less effective in the long term.[30,31]

There are data suggesting that lower doses of pulse steroids may be as effective, and better tolerated, than higher doses. A double-blinded randomized controlled trial assigned 21 patients with active SLE (fevers, renal or CNS lupus, or failure to respond to oral steroids or chloroquine) to 3 daily infusions of 100 or 1000 mg of intravenous methylprednisolone and found no difference in outcomes at 3 months.[32] A retrospective study of 55 patients showed that less than or equal to 1500 mg of intravenous methylprednisolone over 3 days were as effective as 3 to 5 g over the same time period, but were associated with fewer serious infections.[33] Potential advantages of pulse therapy include decreased cumulative steroid exposure because of the ability to taper oral steroids more rapidly and reduced hypothalamic-pituitary-adrenal axis suppression compared with longer courses of oral steroids.[34]

High-dose oral steroids are often used following initial pulse therapy for renal or CNS disease, in conjunction with immunosuppressive therapies including AZA, MMF, or CYC. Pulmonary, cardiovascular, hematologic, and gastrointestinal manifestations are typically treated with high doses of oral steroids, whereas low-dose to medium-dose steroids usually suffice for musculoskeletal, mucocutaneous, and systemic symptoms (see **Table 2**). This pattern of therapy is largely eminence rather than evidence based, with support drawn from case reports, case series, or at best small cohort studies.[9] Addition of immunosuppressive agents is determined by severity of disease manifestation and, in some cases, resistance to corticosteroid therapy or taper attempts.

Given the significant toxicity of high doses and prolonged therapy, corticosteroids are commonly tapered as quickly as possible to minimize adverse effects. Taper protocols are largely based on physicians' personal experience. The nephritis literature serves as a reference in the initial stages of tapering, but does not delineate the long-term withdrawal of therapy.[35] Significant practice variation in the withdrawal of steroids after achievement of remission in SLE nephritis has been reported.[36] Although supporting data are limited, a common practice is to taper prednisone by 10 mg weekly until a dose of 20 mg, and then to taper by 2.5 to 5 mg weekly until reaching the lowest dose required to control symptoms.

Resistance to Corticosteroids

Individual responsiveness to therapy varies among patients with SLE, with some patients requiring dose escalation to achieve adequate clinical response, suggesting the existence of corticosteroid resistance. Several mechanisms for this have been hypothesized. First, changes in the expression of corticosteroid receptors have been associated with patterns of resistance.[37] In contrast, a small study showed increased levels of glucocorticoid corticosteroid receptor beta, an inhibitor of corticosteroid action, in patients with high (vs low) SLE disease activity.[38] Specific genetic polymorphisms that correlate with changes in receptor expression and responsiveness have also been identified.[39]

A second proposed mechanism for corticosteroid resistance in SLE is the transport of intracellular steroids outside of the cell by membrane transporters. Patients with SLE with high disease activity who are resistant to steroids show increased lymphocyte expression of the membrane-associated transporter P-glycoprotein.[40] The overproduction of nuclear factor kappa-B by activated plasmacytoid dendritic cells may be another source of steroid resistance in SLE.[41]

ADMINISTRATION

Steroids can be administered via oral, intravenous, intramuscular, intra-articular, intralesional, and topical routes. Oral and intravenous steroids are used most commonly for systemic manifestations, with intravenous steroids used for severe disease and faster onset of action. The intravenous (or intramuscular) route may also be preferable in patients with hypoalbuminemia and presumed bowel wall edema, or in patients with gastrointestinal disorders likely to interfere with oral absorption.

Prednisone, prednisolone, and methylprednisolone are most frequently given, although dexamethasone and triamcinolone are also occasionally used for CNS disease or per provider preference. Corticosteroids may be administered once daily or in divided doses, particularly at higher doses to optimize pharmacokinetics, and with the use of methylprednisolone, which has a shorter half-life than prednisone. Data do not clearly support a difference in efficacy for once-daily or divided doses, although, anecdotally, divided doses may be more effective in suppressing symptoms for occasional individual patients. However, a single morning daily dose is preferable because it seems less likely to induce suppression of circadian peak adrenal cortisol production.[42] Alternate-day dosing has been suggested to produce fewer side effects but may be less effective.[43]

There are limited data regarding the relative efficacy of different routes of steroid delivery: one randomized study found that intramuscular triamcinolone was equally effective and more rapid in onset than an oral 6-day methylprednisolone taper for mild to moderate flares.[44] Topical corticosteroids are frequently used for cutaneous lupus, although data consist of a limited number of studies, including 1 randomized trial that showed benefit of high-potency corticosteroids (fluocinonide 0.05%) compared with low-potency corticosteroids (hydrocortisone 1%) in treating discoid lupus.[45]

SIDE EFFECTS

The adverse effects associated with steroid therapy are numerous, occurring from time of initiation of therapy and increasing with dose and duration. Over long-term follow-up, patients with SLE most commonly experience musculoskeletal complications, including osteoporosis, avascular necrosis, and myopathy.[4] Early side effects of steroids include endocrine manifestations such as hyperglycemia and weight gain, which are reversible with tapering but may lead to diabetes mellitus, obesity, hypertension, hyperlipidemia, and atherosclerosis. Cardiovascular complications, including myocardial infarction and cerebrovascular disease, are frequent in SLE, with a complex interplay between underlying disease activity and steroid therapy contributing to pathogenesis.[46] Dermatologic effects, such as skin atrophy, striae, purpura, bruising, acne, and impaired wound healing, are common, as are infections, psychological disturbances, gastritis/peptic ulcer disease, cataracts, and glaucoma.[23]

Corticosteroids and Damage

Given the near-universal use of corticosteroids for disease activity, the long-term prognosis of SLE has been largely inextricable from the consequences of steroid therapy. Steroid-related side effects therefore weigh heavily in measurements of lupus disease–related damage. The Systemic Lupus International Collaborating Clinics/American College of Rheumatology Damage Index (SDI) measures irreversible organ damage that has occurred since onset of SLE on a scale of 0 to 46; half of the 12 domains included in the index relate at least in part to steroid therapy.[47]

Several studies have attempted to determine the association between lupus damage and steroid use. In one inception cohort of 73 patients followed for 15 years, damage increased over time (SDI scores increased from 0.9 at year 1 to 1.99 at year 15) with the attributable role of steroids increasing over time (58% at year 1 to 80% at year 15).[4] A study of 539 patients in the Hopkins Lupus Cohort found that cumulative prednisone dose was significantly associated with the development of osteoporotic fractures (relative risk [RR], 2.5 for every 10 mg/d of prednisone), symptomatic coronary artery disease (RR, 1.7), and cataracts (RR, 1.9). Intravenous pulse therapy was associated with small nonsignificant increases in osteoporotic fracture and avascular necrosis, and high-dose intervals of prednisone were associated with increased risk of avascular necrosis and stroke (RR, 1.2 for both).[5] The association of avascular necrosis with short intervals of high-dose steroids, but not with cumulative prednisone dosage, has been replicated in several studies.[23]

A subsequent Hopkins study further examined the relationship between prednisone dose and organ damage while accounting for underlying lupus activity, a significant confounder in prior studies. Five-hundred and twenty-five incident lupus cases were followed for an average of 4.8 years. After controlling for disease activity, damage increased with higher average cumulative doses of prednisone: doses between 6 and 12 mg/d were associated with a hazard ratio of 1.5, whereas the hazard ratio for doses averaging more than 18 mg/d was 2.5. Note that lower doses of prednisone (cumulative average <6 mg/d) did not increase the risk of irreversible organ damage (hazard ratio of 1.16).[48] These findings support the clinical practice of using steroid-sparing therapies and tapering steroids to a dose of less than 6 mg/d when possible.

Corticosteroids and Cardiovascular Disease

The increased incidence of cardiovascular disease in patients with SLE is well documented and multifactorial, with steroid use likely playing a role. Analyses of large cohorts have all shown an association between prednisone dose and duration and cardiovascular events.[49–51] However, it is unclear how much of the increased disease burden is caused by steroid treatment versus underlying lupus disease activity. One case-control study showed that patients with SLE and atherosclerosis had longer disease duration, higher damage scores, and were less likely to have been treated with prednisone and other immunosuppressive therapies than those without plaque, suggesting the importance of ongoing untreated lupus activity and proposing that the relative benefit of steroids in controlling lupus activity may outweigh typical harms.[52] However, multivariate analyses of large cohorts have shown a persistent association between steroid use and cardiovascular events even after controlling for disease activity.[51] As a result, it is especially important to address modifiable cardiovascular risk factors, such as obesity, hypertension, and hypercholesterolemia, in patients with SLE.

Corticosteroids and Infections

Infection is a well-known steroid side effect and a leading cause of mortality in SLE. In general, early death in lupus is associated with effects of the disease itself and infection, with later deaths more likely to be caused by cardiovascular disease and malignancy. The association of corticosteroid use and infection in SLE is well established, even for low doses. A nested case-control study in the Lupus-Cruces Cohort investigated risk factors for serious infection and found that steroid use was one of 2 predictors. Patients with major infections were on a median dose of 7.5 mg/d of prednisone, whereas those without were on a median dose of 2.5 mg/d; the logistic regression model showed the likelihood of a major infection to increase by 12% for each milligram of prednisone per day (odds ratio, 1.12).[53]

Corticosteroids and Fracture

Studies have shown a nearly 5-fold increase in fractures in women with SLE compared with the general population, with older age at diagnosis of SLE and longer duration of corticosteroid use as predictors of fracture risk in multivariate models.[54] Cumulative steroid dose has been associated with an increase in osteoporotic fractures in SLE. Bisphosphonate therapy has a protective effect against steroid-induced osteoporosis, and should be considered as concurrent therapy for patients on medium-dose or high-dose therapy for greater than 3 months, if no contraindications exist. Osteoporosis is of particular significance in patients with SLE because they are often premenopausal and of childbearing age. Use of bisphosphonates in women planning pregnancy, even several years in the future, is controversial given the long half-life of these medications and the theoretic risk of fetal skeletal anomalies. For women with significant steroid-induced osteoporosis who plan pregnancy in the near future, daily subcutaneous teriparatide may be a more desirable option to stabilize or increase bone density in the short term. Preventive strategies such as calcium supplementation, optimization of vitamin D, weight-bearing activity, and minimization of cumulative steroid exposure are critical to protecting bone health in every patient with SLE.

DRUG-DRUG INTERACTIONS

Prednisone and methylprednisolone are weak substrates of the cytochrome P450 3A4 (CYP3A4) enzyme and have potential for drug interactions with any medications that induce or inhibit this metabolic pathway. Despite many hypothetical interactions, the literature suggests that only a few drugs are of clinical significance in patients with rheumatic disease.[55] The coadministration of warfarin and steroids, common in patients with antiphospholipid syndrome, has been associated with a higher incidence of bleeding, possibly related to increased warfarin levels caused by competition for CYP3A4 or to a steroid-induced increase in serum pH.[56] Prophylactic dose adjustment of warfarin is not indicated, but close monitoring and use of proton pump inhibitors for gastric protection is recommended.

Corticosteroids and antibiotics are frequently coadministered, particularly given the increased incidence of infection in SLE. Data suggest that coadministration of steroids and fluoroquinolones increases the risk of tendon rupture and should be avoided when possible.[55] A second antibiotic interaction involves azoles, which are potent inhibitors of CYP3A4. Methylprednisolone has been reported to interact more strongly with itraconazole and ketoconazole than does prednisone.[57] When prescribed together, close monitoring for toxicity and potential dose reduction of steroids are recommended.

Patients with SLE are frequently treated with a variety of immunosuppressive agents that are metabolized through similar mechanisms to corticosteroids. MMF, cyclosporine, tacrolimus, and sirolimus are metabolized via CYP3A4 and transported by P-glycoprotein.[58] In theory, potential for drug interactions is present, but the literature on medication interactions is largely conflicting.[58] As with warfarin and antibiotics, close monitoring of drug levels and toxicities is warranted.

PRACTICAL TREATMENT CONSIDERATIONS

Although ongoing research efforts work toward specifically directed therapies for SLE, corticosteroids remain the first-line treatment of significant lupus manifestations, especially organ-threatening or life-threatening disease. Higher dosage and longer duration of therapy, which are common in SLE, result in greater risk of adverse effects. Recent efforts have formalized recommendations regarding management of medium-dose to high-dose corticosteroids with attempts to support these recommendations with evidence-based data.[59] Methods used for the recent European League Against Rheumatism (EULAR) recommendations included a systematic literature search with a Delphi consensus approach and evaluation of 10 initial propositions. Although supporting evidence was overall weak, 9 evidence-based and consensus-based recommendations were eventually suggested that address education and prevention, dosing and the risk/benefit ratio, and monitoring (**Box 1**).

FUTURE CONSIDERATIONS/SUMMARY

Corticosteroids are the mainstay of therapy for prompt control of acute disease-related inflammation in patients with SLE. Although guidelines for dosing for serious

---

Box 1
EULAR recommendations on management of medium-dose to high-dose glucocorticoid (GC) therapy

- Explain the aim of medium-dose/high-dose GC treatment and the potential risks associated with such therapy to both patients and caregivers (including other health care providers).
- Discuss measures to mitigate such risks, including diet, regular exercise, and appropriate wound care.
- Patients with, or at risk of, GC-induced osteoporosis should receive appropriate preventive/therapeutic interventions.
- Patients and the patients' treatment teams should receive appropriate, practical advice on how to manage with GC-induced hypothalamic-pituitary-adrenal axis suppression.
- Provide an accessible resource to promote best practice in the management of patients using medium-dose/high-dose GCs to general practitioners.
- Before starting medium-dose/high-dose GC treatment consider comorbidities predisposing to adverse events (AEs), including diabetes, glucose intolerance, cardiovascular disease, peptic ulcer disease, recurrent infections, immunosuppression, glaucoma, and osteoporosis. Patients with these comorbidities require tight control to manage the risk/benefit ratio.
- Select the appropriate starting dose to achieve therapeutic response, taking into account the risk of undertreatment.
- Keep the requirement for continuing GC treatment under constant review, and titrate the dose against therapeutic response, risk of undertreatment, and development of AEs.

Adapted from Duru N, Van der Goes M, Jacobs J, et al. EULAR evidence-based and consensus-based recommendations on the management of medium to high-dose glucocorticoid therapy in rheumatic diseases. Ann Rheum Dis 2013;72(12):1907; with permission, BMJ Publishing Group Limited.

manifestations such as nephritis or CNS involvement are based on clinical evidence, treatment of most other manifestations relies largely on general consensus. The basic tenets of steroid treatment of SLE include using the lowest possible dose to control inflammation, tapering as quickly as possible with the use of steroid-sparing immuno-suppressive therapy when necessary, and assessing and treating patients for comor-bidities that may contribute to the risk of side effects.

Newer methods for delivering prednisone as well as development of new corticoste-roid-like drugs may eventually limit adverse effects. A recently approved delayed-release prednisone preparation taken at bedtime releases active drug 4 hours later, when proinflammatory cytokine levels peak, suggesting it may be feasible to use a lower dose delivered at a better time for similar effect.[60]

New drugs with some but not all standard corticosteroid effects may also permit control of inflammation with fewer side effects. Selective corticosteroid receptor ago-nists that preferentially induce the clinically desirable transrepression genomic effects show early promising results in ongoing studies.[25] If successful, these drugs may pro-vide greater antiinflammatory effect with less adverse effects, favorably shifting the risk/benefit ratio for both patients and rheumatologists.

REFERENCES

1. Baehr G, Soffer LJ. Treatment of disseminated lupus erythematosus with corti-sone and adrenocorticotropin. Bull N Y Acad Med 1950;26:229–34.
2. Dubois EL, Commons RR, Starr P, et al. Corticotropin and cortisone treatment for systemic lupus erythematosus. J Am Med Assoc 1952;149:995–1002.
3. Dubois EL. Prednisone and prednisolone in the treatment of systemic lupus erythematous. J Am Med Assoc 1956;161:427–33.
4. Gladman DD, Urowitz MB, Rahman P, et al. Accrual of organ damage over time in patients with systemic lupus erythematosus. J Rheumatol 2003;30(9):1955–9.
5. Zonana-Nacach A, Barr SG, Magder LS, et al. Damage in systemic lupus erythe-matosus and its association with corticosteroids. Arthritis Rheum 2000;43(8): 1801–8.
6. Mosca M, Tani C, Carli L, et al. Glucocorticoids in systemic lupus erythematosus. Clin Exp Rheumatol 2011;29(6):S126–9.
7. Albert DA, Hadler NM, Ropes MW. Does corticosteroid therapy affect the survival of patients with systemic lupus erythematosus. Arthritis Rheum 1979;22(9): 945–53.
8. Buttgereit F, da Silva JA, Boers M, et al. Standardised nomenclature for glucocor-ticoid dosages and glucocorticoid treatment regimens: current questions and tentative answers in rheumatology. Ann Rheum Dis 2002;61(8):718–22.
9. Luijten RK, Fritsch-Stork RD, Bijlsma JWJ, et al. The use of glucocorticoids in sys-temic lupus erythematosus. After 60 years still more an art than science. Autoim-mun Rev 2013;12(5):617–28.
10. Zhou W, Yang C. The causes and clinical significance of fever in systemic lupus erythematosus: a retrospective study of 487 hospitalised patients. Lupus 2009; 18(9):807–12.
11. Rovin B, Tang Y, Sun J, et al. Clinical significance of fever in the systemic lupus erythematosus patient receiving steroid therapy. Kidney Int 2005;68(2): 747–59.
12. Shapira Y, Weinberger A, Wysenbeek A. Lymphadenopathy in systemic lupus er-ythematosus. Prevalence and relation to disease manifestations. Clin Rheumatol 1996;15(4):335–8.

13. Kamen DL, Zollars ES. Corticosteroids in Lupus Nephritis and Central Nervous System (CNS) Lupus. Rheum Dis Clin N Am 2016, in press.
14. Blanford AT, Murphy BE. In vitro metabolism of prednisolone, dexamethasone, betamethasone, and cortisol by the human placenta. Am J Obstet Gynecol 1977;127(3):264–7.
15. Østensen M, Khamashta M, Lockshin M, et al. Anti-inflammatory and immunosuppressive drugs and reproduction. Arthritis Res Ther 2006;8(3):209.
16. Ost L, Wettrell G, Bjorkhem I, et al. Prednisolone excretion in human milk. J Pediatr 1985;106(6):1008–11.
17. Park-Wyllie L, Mazzotta P, Pastuszak A, et al. Birth defects after maternal exposure to corticosteroids: prospective cohort study and meta-analysis of epidemiological studies. Teratology 2000;62(6):385–92.
18. Bay Bjorn AM, Ehrenstein V, Hundborg HH, et al. Use of corticosteroids in early pregnancy is not associated with risk of oral clefts and other congenital malformations in offspring. Am J Ther 2014;21(2):73–80.
19. Dörner T, Giesecke C, Lipsky PE. Mechanisms of B cell autoimmunity in SLE. Arthritis Res Ther 2011;13(5):243.
20. Crispin JC, Kyttaris VC, Terhorst C, et al. T cells as therapeutic targets in SLE. Nat Rev Rheumatol 2010;6(6):317–25.
21. Knight JS, Kaplan MJ. Lupus neutrophils. Curr Opin Rheumatol 2012;24(5): 441–50.
22. Leffler J, Martin M, Gullstrand B, et al. Neutrophil extracellular traps that are not degraded in systemic lupus erythematosus activate complement exacerbating the disease. J Immunol 2012;188(7):3522–31.
23. Ruiz-Irastorza G, Danza A, Khamashta M. Glucocorticoid use and abuse in SLE. Rheumatology (Oxford) 2012;51(7):1145–53.
24. Stahn C, Buttgereit F. Genomic and nongenomic effects of glucocorticoids. Nat Clin Pract Rheumatol 2008;4(10):525–33.
25. Strand V, Buttgereit F, McCabe D, et al. A phase 2, randomized, double-blind comparison of the efficacy and safety of PF-04171327 (1, 5, 10, 15 mg QD) vs. 5 and 10 mg prednisone QD or placebo in subjects with rheumatoid arthritis (RA) over 8 weeks followed by a 4-week taper of study drug. In: American College of Rheumatology 2014 Meeting. Boston, MA, November 15-19, 2014. Late-Breaking Abstract L6.
26. Li X, Zhang FS, Zhang J-H, et al. Negative relationship between expression of glucocorticoid receptor alpha and disease activity: glucocorticoid treatment of patients with systemic lupus erythematosus. J Rheumatol 2010;37(2):316–21.
27. Spies CM, Schaumann DHS, Berki T, et al. Membrane glucocorticoid receptors are down regulated by glucocorticoids in patients with systemic lupus erythematosus and use a caveolin-1-independent expression pathway. Ann Rheum Dis 2006;65(9):1139–46.
28. Parker BJ, Bruce IN. High dose methylprednisolone therapy for the treatment of severe systemic lupus erythematosus. Lupus 2007;16:387–93.
29. Mackworth-Young CG, David J, Morgan SH, et al. A double blind, placebo controlled trial of intravenous methylprednisolone in systemic lupus erythematosus. Ann Rheum Dis 1988;47:496–502.
30. Flanc RS, Roberts MA, Strippoli GF, et al. Treatment for lupus nephritis. Cochrane Database Syst Rev 2004;(1):CD002922.
31. Trevisani V, Castro A, Neves Neto J, et al. Cyclophosphamide versus methylprednisolone for the treatment of neuropsychiatric involvement in systemic lupus erythematosus. Cochrane Database Syst Rev 2000;(3):CD002265.

32. Edwards JC, Snaith ML, Isenberg D. A double blind controlled trial of methylpred-nisolone infusions in systemic lupus erythematosus using individualised outcome assessment. Ann Rheum Dis 1987;46(10):773–6.
33. Badsha H, Kong KO, Lian TY, et al. Low-dose pulse methylprednisolone for sys-temic lupus erythematosus flares is efficacious and has a decreased risk of infec-tious complications. Lupus 2002;11(8):508–13.
34. Badsha H, Edwards CJ. Intravenous pulses of methylprednisolone for systemic lupus erythematosus. Semin Arthritis Rheum 2003;32(6):370–7.
35. Houssiau F, Vasconcelos C, D'Cruz D, et al. Immunosuppressive therapy in lupus nephritis: the Euro-Lupus Nephritis Trial, a randomized trial of low-dose versus high-dose intravenous cyclophosphamide. Arthritis Rheum 2002; 46(8):2121–31.
36. Walsh M, Jayne D, Moist L, et al. Practice pattern variation in oral glucocorticoid therapy after the induction of response in proliferative lupus nephritis. Lupus 2010;19:628–33.
37. Du J, Li M, Zhang D, et al. Flow cytometry analysis of glucocorticoid receptor expression and binding in steroid-sensitive and steroid-resistant patients with systemic lupus erythematosus. Arthritis Res Ther 2009;11(4):R108.
38. Piotrowski P, Burzynski M, Lianeri M, et al. Glucocorticoid receptor beta splice variant expression in patients with high and low activity of systemic lupus erythe-matosus. Folia Histochem Cytobiol 2007;45(4):339–42.
39. Zou Y-F, Xu J-H, Wang F, et al. Association study of glucocorticoid receptor ge-netic polymorphisms with efficacy of glucocorticoids in systemic lupus erythema-tosus: a prospective cohort study. Autoimmunity 2013;46(8):531–6.
40. Tsujimura S, Saito K, Nakayamada S, et al. Clinical relevance of the expression of P-glycoprotein on peripheral blood lymphocytes to steroid resistance in patients with systemic lupus erythematosus. Arthritis Rheum 2005;52(6):1676–83.
41. Guiducci C, Gong M, Xu Z, et al. TLR recognition of self nucleic acids hampers glucocorticoid activity in lupus. Nature 2010;465(7300):937–41.
42. Myles AB, Schiller LF, Glass D, et al. Single daily dose corticosteroid treatment. Ann Rheum Dis 1976;35(1):73–6.
43. Ballou S, Khan M, Kushner I. Intravenous pulse methylprednisolone followed by alternate day corticosteroid therapy in lupus erythematosus: a prospective eval-uation. J Rheumatol 1985;12(5):944–8.
44. Danowski A, Magder L, Petri M. Flares in Lupus: Outcome Assessment Trial (FLOAT), a comparison between oral methylprednisolone and intramuscular triamcinolone. J Rheumatol 2006;33(1):57–60.
45. Kuhn A, Ruland V, Bonsmann G. Cutaneous lupus erythematosus: update of ther-apeutic options: part I. J Am Acad Dermatol 2011;65(6):e179–93.
46. Bruce IN. "Not only…but also": factors that contribute to accelerated atheroscle-rosis and premature coronary heart disease in systemic lupus erythematosus. Rheumatology (Oxford) 2005;44(12):1492–502.
47. Gladman DD, Ginzler E, Goldsmith C, et al. The development and initial validation of the Systemic Lupus International Collaborating Clinics/American College of Rheumatology damage index for systemic lupus erythematosus. Arthritis Rheum 1996;39(3):363–9.
48. Thamer M, Hernán M, Zhang Y, et al. Prednisone, lupus activity, and permanent organ damage. J Rheumatol 2009;36(3):560–4.
49. Toloza SM, Uribe AG, McGwin G, et al. Systemic lupus erythematosus in a multi-ethnic US cohort (LUMINA): XXIII. Baseline predictors of vascular events. Arthritis Rheum 2004;50(12):3947–57.

50. Manzi S, Meilahn EN, Rairie JE, et al. Age-specific incidence rates of myocardial infarction and angina in women with systemic lupus erythematosus: comparison with the Framingham Study. Am J Epidemiol 1997;145(5):408–15.
51. Magder LS, Petri M. Incidence of and risk factors for adverse cardiovascular events among patients with systemic lupus erythematosus. Am J Epidemiol 2012;176(8):708–19.
52. Roman MJ, Shanker B-A, Davis A, et al. Prevalence and correlates of accelerated atherosclerosis in systemic lupus erythematosus. N Engl J Med 2003;349: 2399–406.
53. Ruiz-Irastorza G, Olivares N, Ruiz-Arruza I, et al. Predictors of major infections in systemic lupus erythematosus. Arthritis Res Ther 2009;11(4):R109.
54. Ramsey-Goldman R, Dunn JE, Huang CF, et al. Frequency of fractures in women with systemic lupus erythematosus: comparison with United States population data. Arthritis Rheum 1999;42(5):882–90.
55. Hromadkova L, Soukup T, Vlcek J. Important drug interactions in patients with rheumatic disorders: interactions of glucocorticoids, immunosuppressants, and antimalarial drugs. Drugs Today (Barc) 2012;48(8):545–53.
56. Hazlewood KA, Fugate SE, Harrison DL. Effect of oral corticosteroids on chronic warfarin therapy. Ann Pharmacother 2006;40:2101–6.
57. Lebrun-Vignes B, Archer VC, Diquet B, et al. Effect of itraconazole on the pharmacokinetics of prednisolone and methylprednisolone and cortisol secretion in healthy subjects. Br J Clin Pharmacol 2001;51:443–50.
58. Lam S, Partovi N, Ting LSL, et al. Corticosteroid interactions with cyclosporine, tacrolimus, mycophenolate, and sirolimus: fact or fiction? Ann Pharmacother 2008;42:1037–47.
59. Duru N, Van der Goes M, Jacobs J, et al. EULAR evidence-based and consensus-based recommendations on the management of medium to high-dose glucocorticoid therapy in rheumatic diseases. Ann Rheum Dis 2013; 72(12):1905–13.
60. Buttgereit F, Mehta D, Kirwan J, et al. Low-dose prednisone chronotherapy for rheumatoid arthritis: a randomised clinical trial (CAPRA-2). Ann Rheum Dis 2013;72(2):204–10.

Corticosteroids in Lupus Nephritis and Central Nervous System Lupus

Diane L. Kamen, MD, MSCR*, Eric S. Zollars, MD, PhD

KEYWORDS

- Systemic lupus erythematosus • Glomerulonephritis • Neuropsychiatric lupus
- Glucocorticoids • Autoimmune disease • Treatment

KEY POINTS

- The current standard of care for active proliferative lupus nephritis and severe central nervous system (CNS) lupus includes corticosteroids in high doses for immunosuppression.
- Despite the potential to be lifesaving in cases of lupus nephritis and CNS lupus, corticosteroids are also associated with long-term damage and early mortality.
- The goal of lupus therapy remains elimination of corticosteroids when possible.

INTRODUCTION

Corticosteroids, often in high doses and typically in combination with other immunosuppressive treatments, are a mainstay of therapy for severe organ-threatening systemic lupus erythematosus (SLE; lupus). The antiinflammatory effects of corticosteroids are pervasive and complex and depend on the timing, dose, and route of administration. Corticosteroids act on multiple immune cell types to inhibit the production of inflammatory mediators and stimulate the production of antiinflammatory proteins through both genomic and nongenomic pathways.

Until recently, the standard design of treatment trials for active lupus allowed, or even mandated, the use of corticosteroids for more immediate control of active disease while awaiting the anticipated benefits of the experimental intervention. It is only recently that interventional trials for active lupus have been designed with minimal use of corticosteroids. Given the known dose-related and duration-related adverse effects of corticosteroids, the potential of treating active lupus with minimal to no

Disclosure: The authors have nothing to disclose.
Division of Rheumatology and Immunology, Medical University of South Carolina, 96 Jonathan Lucas Street, Suite 816, Charleston, SC 29425, USA
* Corresponding author.
E-mail address: kamend@musc.edu

Rheum Dis Clin N Am 42 (2016) 63–73
http://dx.doi.org/10.1016/j.rdc.2015.08.008
0889-857X/16/$ – see front matter © 2016 Elsevier Inc. All rights reserved.

rheumatic.theclinics.com

corticosteroids is appealing. However, the value and lifesaving potential of high doses of corticosteroids for uncontrolled severe lupus is undeniable.

This article reviews the evidence for, and against, the efficacy of corticosteroids in the clinical setting of active lupus nephritis and/or active central nervous system (CNS) lupus. The adverse effects of corticosteroids in patients with lupus nephritis and CNS lupus are also reviewed.

EPIDEMIOLOGY OF LUPUS NEPHRITIS

Lupus nephritis remains one of the most debilitating and potentially life-threatening manifestations of lupus, occurring in 40% to 60% of adults and up to 80% of children with lupus.[1–3] The susceptibility and burden of lupus are substantially higher among black women compared with other groups, with black people having 3 times the incidence rate compared with whites and women having 9 to 10 times the prevalence compared with men.[4,5] Peak age of incidence for both lupus and lupus nephritis is also younger among black women. The disparities in lupus-related risk are most striking when examining renal involvement, with black patients and Hispanic patients having more frequent and more severe lupus nephritis compared with other groups.[2,4–6]

The prognosis of lupus nephritis is related to the degree of active renal inflammation and chronic damage, which is reflected in the renal histologic class on kidney biopsy as well as the associated clinical and laboratory features.[7] Ultimately, 10% to 20% of patients with lupus nephritis require renal-replacement therapy for end-stage renal disease, most commonly with hemodialysis, and early mortality remains unacceptably high.[8]

EVALUATION OF LUPUS NEPHRITIS

Renal biopsy histology helps not only confirm the diagnosis but also helps guide therapy for lupus nephritis. Proliferative lupus nephritis is the most common form, often presenting as proteinuria, microscopic hematuria, urinary casts, hypertension, and potentially including renal insufficiency.[9] Membranous lupus nephritis is also frequently seen histologically either alone or in conjunction with proliferative nephritis, often presenting as nephrotic syndrome with edema, wasting, and hypercoagulability.[9]

TREATMENT GOALS FOR LUPUS NEPHRITIS

Prevention of end-stage renal disease and reducing the risks of chronic kidney disease with associated comorbidities are primary goals of lupus nephritis therapy. Typical immunosuppression for lupus nephritis consists of induction with corticosteroids combined with a cytotoxic medication to achieve a rapid response, followed by a maintenance period of continued but less potent immunosuppression.

In practice, evidence supporting certain treatment regimens for specific clinical and histologic situations is considered in conjunction with other patient-specific variables. These variables influencing therapeutic decisions include patient ethnicity, age, comorbidities, pregnancy plans, fear of certain adverse effects, and any doubts about compliance,[10] which results in a shift away from one-size-fits-all protocols toward more highly individualized treatment regimens.

PROLIFERATIVE LUPUS NEPHRITIS INDUCTION THERAPY

A shift occurred in the 1970s and 1980s from using corticosteroids alone to using them in combination with cytotoxic medications to treat lupus nephritis, based on clinical trial evidence supporting combination therapy.[11] At present, the 3 most widely accepted induction regimens for proliferative lupus nephritis are corticosteroids plus either monthly high-dose intravenous (IV) cyclophosphamide (the National Institutes of Health Regimen),[12,13] low-dose IV cyclophosphamide every 2 weeks (the Euro-Lupus Regimen),[14] or daily oral mycophenolate mofetil (MMF).[15,16]

The American College of Rheumatology (ACR) published guidelines for treating lupus nephritis recommending the use of pulse-dose corticosteroids for the first 3 days of induction, followed by 0.5 to 1 mg/kg/d prednisone tapered to the lowest effective dose by the first 3 to 6 months (**Table 1**).[17] Similarly, the National Kidney Foundation's KDIGO (Kidney Disease: Improving Global Outcomes) guidelines recommend an initial prednisone dose of 1 mg/kg/d, with a slow taper over 6 to 12 months.[18]

Although a patient with lupus nephritis on induction therapy with pulse-dose corticosteroids and cyclophosphamide or MMF may start to respond clinically within the first 2 weeks, lupus nephritis biomarkers (particularly proteinuria) may take longer than 6 weeks for improvement.[19] Patient demographics influence the response to induction therapy as well, with MMF, when adequately dosed, leading to better renal responses compared with cyclophosphamide among the subgroup of black and Hispanic patients.[20]

PROLIFERATIVE LUPUS NEPHRITIS MAINTENANCE THERAPY

Following induction, the use of maintenance therapy decreases the risk of nephritis relapses and reduces cumulative corticosteroid exposure in the long term. From the results of the ALMS (Aspreva Lupus Management Study) and MAINTAIN trials in proliferative lupus nephritis, it was learned that both mycophenolate mofetil and azathioprine can be used as long-term maintenance therapy.[21,22]

Table 1
Definitions and indications for common corticosteroid regimens used in the treatment of lupus

Corticosteroid Regimen	Formulation, Dose, and Timing	Indication in Lupus Nephritis and/or CNS Lupus
Pulse-dose corticosteroids	0.5–1.0 g IV methylprednisolone per day for 1–3 d	• Life-threatening or organ-threatening complications • Active lupus refractory to high-dose corticosteroids
Very-high-dose corticosteroids	>100 mg IV or oral prednisone equivalent per day	• Life-threatening or organ-threatening complications
High-dose corticosteroids	>30 and ≤100 mg IV or oral prednisone equivalent per day	• Proliferative lupus nephritis • Severe flares of lupus
Moderate-dose corticosteroids	>7.5 and ≤30 mg IV or oral prednisone equivalent per day	• Moderate flares of lupus • Used in conjunction with pulse dose for severe lupus
Low-dose corticosteroids	≤7.5 mg oral prednisone equivalent per day	• Mild flares of lupus • Maintenance therapy
Alternate-day corticosteroids	Oral prednisone equivalent taken every other day	• Treatment of membranous lupus nephritis • Tapering from daily dosing

Doses are based on a 60-kg patient.
Adapted from Kirou KA, Boumpas DT. Systemic glucocorticoid therapy in SLE. In: Wallace DJ, Hahn BH, editors. Dubois' lupus erythematosus. 8th edition. Philadelphia: Elsevier; 2013. p. 595; with permission.

The KDIGO guidelines recommend using low-dose to moderate-dose prednisone (≤10 mg/d) for maintenance therapy (see **Table 1**).[18] For relapse of active nephritis, reinitiating the same dose of prednisone that was effective in inducing the original remission is recommended.

CHALLENGING CURRENT CORTICOSTEROID PRACTICES

The dose and duration of corticosteroids required for control of lupus nephritis have never been tested in a randomized trial design, so current recommendations are based on observation and expert opinion.[17,18]

The presumption that oral corticosteroids are a required adjunctive therapy for lupus nephritis has been called into question recently. An uncontrolled trial of 2 doses of 1000 mg of IV rituximab combined with 2 doses of 500 mg of IV methylprednisolone followed by MMF in 50 patients with lupus nephritis found that most subjects achieved complete renal remission without any oral corticosteroids.[23] Of the 50 trial participants, 72% achieved complete renal remission by a median time of 36 weeks and an additional 18% achieved persistent partial renal remission by a median time of 32 weeks.[23] These early results suggest that early initiation of a targeted biologic agent may be a safe and effective substitute for maintenance corticosteroids. A randomized controlled trial for patients with active lupus nephritis testing this hypothesis is underway.[24]

TAPERING OF CORTICOSTEROIDS

It is important to use other immunosuppressive medications as steroid-sparing agents to help allow the safe tapering of corticosteroids among patients with lupus nephritis. When tapering, the initial step is consolidation of the regimen into a once-a-day morning dose of corticosteroids. The daily dose should then be slowly decreased with the rate dependent on the patient's history of sensitivity to changes in dose, duration of corticosteroid therapy, and provider preference. There is high variability in steroid-tapering regimens between different physician practices. Standard practice in some European centers is to continue low-dose prednisone long term.[10] In our experience, tapering to less than or equal to 10 mg/d within 4 to 6 months is a reasonable goal, with subsequent tapering by 2.5 mg decrements every 2 weeks until the patient has tapered off prednisone. Patients who have been on corticosteroids longer than 6 months may require tapering less than 10 mg/d to be in decrements of 1 mg rather than 2.5 mg every 2 weeks.

EPIDEMIOLOGY OF CENTRAL NERVOUS SYSTEM LUPUS

CNS lupus, also called neuropsychiatric lupus (NPSLE), is a confusing and complex manifestation of an already confusing and complex disease. The prevalence of CNS lupus is at least as common in children with lupus as in adults, with prevalence rates overall of 30% to 40%. CNS manifestations common in patients with lupus, such as headache, anxiety, depression, and cognitive dysfunction, are also common in the general population and therefore difficult to attribute to lupus.[25] Great care must be taken with these common maladies before attributing them to increased lupus disease activity.

In a large international inception cohort of patients with lupus, 40% of patients had at least 1 neuropsychiatric event and 17% had multiple events over an average of 2 years of follow-up.[26] Less than one-third of the events could be attributed to lupus, leaving most as having nonlupus causes.[26] CNS involvement accounts for 93% of the neuropsychiatric events, with the remaining 7% involving the peripheral nervous system.[26]

Although it has a lower incidence among patients with lupus compared with nephritis, CNS lupus remains a leading cause of morbidity and accounts for approximately 13% to 17% of deaths among patients with lupus (**Fig. 1**).[27] Major events such as cerebrovascular disease, severe cognitive dysfunction, myelopathy, and optic neuritis often result in poor functional outcomes, underscoring the need for improved diagnostic tests and more effective therapeutic options.[28]

EVALUATION OF CENTRAL NERVOUS SYSTEM LUPUS

What is considered under the umbrella of CNS lupus has evolved over time based on findings from studies of its pathogenesis and from lupus population studies. An ACR Ad Hoc Neuropsychiatric Workshop Group published inclusion and exclusion criteria as well as case studies for 19 neuropsychiatric syndromes attributable to SLE.[29,30]

Distinguishing between a neuropsychiatric manifestation of lupus and a non–lupus-related cause can be difficult because the findings are generally not specific to lupus. Thus any appearance of neuropsychiatric symptoms in a patient with lupus requires a thorough investigation of other causes, most importantly to rule out metabolic disturbances, infections, or drug adverse effects.

COMMON CENTRAL NERVOUS SYSTEM FEATURES IN PATIENTS WITH LUPUS

Neurocognitive impairment is the most frequent of the 19 NPSLE syndromes defined by the ACR.[31] Up to 100% of patients with lupus have measureable abnormalities on standardized neuropsychiatric tests,[32] although one study found that 70% of detectable cognitive dysfunction is mild.[33] Complicating matters is the fact that even the low doses of corticosteroids commonly taken by patients are associated with

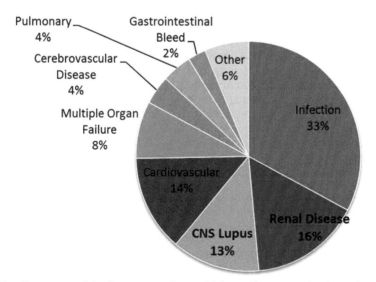

Fig. 1. Leading causes of death among patients with lupus (from 2179 deaths analyzed from 36 published studies). (*Data from* Wang Z, Wang Y, Zhu R, et al. Long-term survival and death causes of systemic lupus erythematosus in China: a systemic review of observational studies. Medicine (Baltimore) 2015;94:e794.)

neurocognitive impairment. Impairment from corticosteroid use is most commonly manifest in declarative (verbal) memory, reflecting a hippocampus-dependent process, but severe cognitive disorders induced by corticosteroids have also been reported.[31]

Headache is reported by up to 57% of patients with lupus,[34] but an isolated lupus headache that is attributable to CNS lupus is rare.[35] A headache may be a component of another NPSLE event (stroke, seizure, meningitis) but, in isolation, headache is not associated with increased disease activity. Evaluation and treatment of headache in a patient with lupus should proceed as it would in a patient without lupus. Consideration should be given to increased thrombotic risk in the presence of antiphospholipid antibodies, as well as to the possibility of lupus-related aseptic meningitis, but otherwise standard therapies for headaches apply.

Other common CNS manifestations include anxiety and mood disorder in up to 37% of patients with lupus,[36] which can also be adverse effects of corticosteroid therapy and other medications.[37] Not only can depressive symptoms increase in patients taking corticosteroids but corticosteroid withdrawal can cause symptoms of fatigue, anorexia, and depression as well.[37] Corticosteroids therefore do not play as significant a treatment role as anxiolytics and antidepressants for anxiety and mood disorders when these are the features of CNS lupus.

FEATURES OF LESS FREQUENT CENTRAL NERVOUS SYSTEM LUPUS EVENTS

Over the course of having lupus, seizures occur in 7% to 20% of patients, usually in the context of increased lupus disease activity.[38,39] Cerebrovascular disease is another common major CNS event, occurring in 5% to 18% of patients with lupus and comprising ischemic strokes in 80% of the cases.[40] Psychosis occurs in 2% to 3% of patients with lupus, characterized by delusions and/or both auditory and visual hallucinations, usually in the setting of active lupus.[36,41]

Acute confusional state (previously called acute organic brain syndrome) occurs in approximately 3% of patients with lupus and can present with disorganized thinking, loss of orientation, agitation, and delusions.[36] A poor prognosis is associated with progression to a reduced level of consciousness, such as stupor or coma, although symptoms may fluctuate.[40] Potential lupus-related causes include vasculitis, leukothrombosis, and autoantibodies, although nonlupus causes such as infection, medication effects, and metabolic disturbances are also common.

Lupus myelopathy occurs in approximately 1% of patients, can present with rapid onset, and involve either gray matter (lower motor neuron) or white matter (upper motor neuron) patterns. The lesions on MRI can involve any level of the spinal cord, typically appearing as cord edema and abnormalities of T2-weighted images. The cause is often multifactorial, with vasculitis documented in some cases, as well as thromboses related to antiphospholipid antibody syndrome in other cases.

TREATMENT STRATEGIES FOR CENTRAL NERVOUS SYSTEM LUPUS

Treatment of CNS lupus differs depending on the severity and suspected pathogenesis. As noted earlier, patients with nonspecific manifestations such as headache, anxiety, mood disorders, and mild cognitive dysfunction may not require immunosuppression to be added. Initial symptomatic treatments are wide-ranging, including analgesics, psychotropic medications (antidepressants, anxiolytics, and atypical antipsychotics), and psychological support. Anticonvulsants are used in the treatment of recurrent seizures, and antiplatelet/anticoagulation therapies are used when manifestations are related to antiphospholipid antibodies, particularly thrombotic cerebrovascular disease.[28] Hydroxychloroquine should be used as maintenance therapy to help prevent disease flare and reduce the risk of thromboembolic events.

The use of corticosteroids in patients with lupus and neurocognitive impairment is complicated. Nishimura and colleagues[31] compared cognitive functioning between corticosteroid-naive patients with lupus and healthy controls and found that reduced psychomotor speed is a lupus-specific pattern of neurocognitive impairment and is associated with increased general lupus disease activity. These findings suggest that at least a portion of the neurocognitive impairment prevalent among patients with lupus may be attributable to corticosteroids use rather than lupus disease activity. When treatment decisions hinge on knowing the attribution, formal neurocognitive testing to determine the patterns of impairment may be helpful.

Psychosis is another presentation of CNS lupus for which it can be difficult to determine attribution if the patient is already on corticosteroids when symptoms start, raising the question of steroid psychosis. Steroid psychosis is suspected especially if the prednisone dose has been increased to greater than 30 mg/d in the previous 2 weeks,[40] and rarely occurs in children. An approach suggested by West[40] includes doubling the dose of corticosteroids for 3 days while diagnostic testing is ongoing. Psychosis caused by CNS lupus should improve because of increased corticosteroids, whereas failure to improve makes CNS lupus less likely (at which point the corticosteroids can be tapered).

Corticosteroids are the first-line immunosuppressants indicated for severe or progressive CNS lupus manifestations such as acute confusional state, myelitis, psychosis, and refractory seizures. Ideally, nonlupus causes of the CNS presentations should be excluded before initiating or increasing immunosuppression; however, that is not always feasible. For example, lupus myelitis requires rapid initiation of pulse-dose corticosteroids, often in combination with IV cyclophosphamide, to avoid permanent and disabling neurologic deficits.

IMMUNOSUPPRESSION FOR CENTRAL NERVOUS SYSTEM LUPUS REFRACTORY TO CORTICOSTEROIDS

In 2010, the European League Against Rheumatism taskforce published recommendations for the treatment of neuropsychiatric manifestations of lupus. Their recommendations included the levels of evidence supporting corticosteroid use and potential use of additional or alternative immunosuppressive agents for each of the NPSLE manifestations.[28] However, with so few controlled trials conducted that have included patients with CNS lupus, the use of immunosuppression other than corticosteroids is largely empiric.

If CNS lupus remains unresponsive to high-dose corticosteroids, then the use of pulse-dose corticosteroids or additional immunosuppressive agents, or both, is warranted. Uncontrolled trials report success with B-cell depletion therapy with rituximab,[42] IV immunoglobulin, plasma exchange, hematopoietic stem cell transplantation, and high-dose cyclophosphamide therapy.[43]

ADVERSE EFFECTS OF CORTICOSTEROIDS

Despite their potential to be lifesaving in cases of lupus nephritis and CNS lupus, there is no question that corticosteroids are also associated with long-term damage and early mortality. Sergent and colleagues[44] showed increased infection-related mortality in patients with CNS lupus when treated with prednisone doses of more than 100 mg/d for an average of 37 days (range, 8–68 days). Corticosteroid use also contributes to cardiovascular risk factors in patients with lupus, including dyslipidemia, diabetes, and hypertension. Prednisone at doses greater than 10 mg/d has been shown to independently predict hypercholesterolemia in patients with lupus.[45]

When treating severe lupus manifestations such as lupus nephritis and CNS lupus, the impact of corticosteroids on bone health is often overlooked until fractures occur. Up to 24% of patients with lupus have osteoporosis, including premenopausal patients, and there is a 1.2-fold increased fracture risk compared with age-matched and sex-matched controls.[46] In addition to the known corticosteroid risk, renal disease and neuropsychiatric organ damage are also associated with an increased risk of fractures, emphasizing the added importance of adequate screening and prophylactic therapy in patients with lupus nephritis or CNS disease.[46]

As discussed earlier, corticosteroid therapy can also cause neuropsychiatric disorders, with depression, hypomania, and overt psychosis being the most common.[37] Low-dose corticosteroid therapy, albeit better tolerated overall, is still not free of risks. Common complications of even low-dose corticosteroids include growth suppression in children, osteoporosis, infections, and cataract formation.

SUMMARY

Lupus is a complex disease with the potential to involve nearly every organ system. Despite advances in therapy for lupus, the current standard of care for active proliferative lupus nephritis and severe CNS lupus still includes rapid initiation of corticosteroids in high doses for immunosuppression. Improving the prognosis for patients with lupus nephritis and CNS lupus requires a shift from the conventional liberal use of high-dose corticosteroids to a more targeted individualized therapeutic approach.

The ultimate goal of lupus therapy remains elimination of corticosteroids, when possible. Current practice often falls short of this goal with many patients, particularly those with renal and CNS involvement, developing morbidity and premature mortality from chronic corticosteroid exposure. Most completed trials for patients with lupus have excluded active lupus nephritis and CNS lupus, making it difficult to draw conclusions about safety and efficacy of novel therapies in those patients. As understanding of these manifestations of lupus grows, so will the ability to tailor treatment to their needs.

REFERENCES

1. Tucker LB, Menon S, Schaller JG, et al. Adult- and childhood-onset systemic lupus erythematosus: a comparison of onset, clinical features, serology, and outcome. Br J Rheumatol 1995;34:866–72.
2. Bastian HM, Roseman JM, McGwin G Jr, et al. Systemic lupus erythematosus in three ethnic groups. XII. Risk factors for lupus nephritis after diagnosis. Lupus 2002;11:152–60.
3. Brunner HI, Gladman DD, Ibanez D, et al. Difference in disease features between childhood-onset and adult-onset systemic lupus erythematosus. Arthritis Rheum 2008;58:556–62.
4. Lim SS, Bayakly AR, Helmick CG, et al. The incidence and prevalence of systemic lupus erythematosus, 2002-2004: the Georgia Lupus Registry. Arthritis Rheumatol 2014;66:357–68.
5. Somers EC, Marder W, Cagnoli P, et al. Population-based incidence and prevalence of systemic lupus erythematosus: the Michigan lupus epidemiology and surveillance program. Arthritis Rheumatol 2014;66:369–78.

6. Korbet SM, Schwartz MM, Evans J, et al. Severe lupus nephritis: racial differences in presentation and outcome. J Am Soc Nephrol 2007;18:244–54.
7. Faurschou M, Dreyer L, Kamper AL, et al. Long-term mortality and renal outcome in a cohort of 100 patients with lupus nephritis. Arthritis Care Res (Hoboken) 2010;62:873–80.
8. Costenbader KH, Desai A, Alarcon GS, et al. Trends in the incidence, demographics, and outcomes of end-stage renal disease due to lupus nephritis in the US from 1995 to 2006. Arthritis Rheum 2011;63:1681–8.
9. Ward MM. Recent clinical trials in lupus nephritis. Rheum Dis Clin North Am 2014; 40:519–35, ix.
10. Houssiau FA. Therapy of lupus nephritis: lessons learned from clinical research and daily care of patients. Arthritis Res Ther 2012;14:202.
11. Felson DT, Anderson J. Evidence for the superiority of immunosuppressive drugs and prednisone over prednisone alone in lupus nephritis. Results of a pooled analysis. N Engl J Med 1984;311:1528–33.
12. Boumpas DT, Austin HA 3rd, Vaughn EM, et al. Controlled trial of pulse methylprednisolone versus two regimens of pulse cyclophosphamide in severe lupus nephritis. Lancet 1992;340:741–5.
13. Illei GG, Austin HA, Crane M, et al. Combination therapy with pulse cyclophosphamide plus pulse methylprednisolone improves long-term renal outcome without adding toxicity in patients with lupus nephritis. Ann Intern Med 2001; 135:248–57.
14. Houssiau FA, Vasconcelos C, D'Cruz D, et al. Immunosuppressive therapy in lupus nephritis: the Euro-Lupus Nephritis Trial, a randomized trial of low-dose versus high-dose intravenous cyclophosphamide. Arthritis Rheum 2002;46: 2121–31.
15. Ginzler EM, Dooley MA, Aranow C, et al. Mycophenolate mofetil or intravenous cyclophosphamide for lupus nephritis. N Engl J Med 2005;353:2219–28.
16. Appel GB, Contreras G, Dooley MA, et al. Mycophenolate mofetil versus cyclophosphamide for induction treatment of lupus nephritis. J Am Soc Nephrol 2009;20:1103–12.
17. Hahn BH, McMahon MA, Wilkinson A, et al. American College of Rheumatology guidelines for screening, treatment, and management of lupus nephritis. Arthritis Care Res (Hoboken) 2012;64:797–808.
18. Kidney Disease: Improving Global Outcomes (KDIGO) Glomerulonephritis Work Group. Chapter 12: Lupus Nephritis. Kidney Int Suppl 2012;2:221–32.
19. Kirou KA, Boumpas DT. Systemic glucocorticoid therapy in SLE. In: Wallace DJ, Hahn BH, editors. Dubois' lupus erythematosus. 8th edition. Philadelphia: Lippincott Williams & Wilkins; 2013. p. 591–600.
20. Isenberg D, Appel GB, Contreras G, et al. Influence of race/ethnicity on response to lupus nephritis treatment: the ALMS study. Rheumatology (Oxford) 2010;49: 128–40.
21. Dooley MA, Jayne D, Ginzler EM, et al. Mycophenolate versus azathioprine as maintenance therapy for lupus nephritis. N Engl J Med 2011;365:1886–95.
22. Houssiau FA, D'Cruz D, Sangle S, et al. Azathioprine versus mycophenolate mofetil for long-term immunosuppression in lupus nephritis: results from the MAINTAIN Nephritis Trial. Ann Rheum Dis 2010;69:2083–9.
23. Condon MB, Ashby D, Pepper RJ, et al. Prospective observational single-centre cohort study to evaluate the effectiveness of treating lupus nephritis with rituximab and mycophenolate mofetil but no oral steroids. Ann Rheum Dis 2013;72: 1280–6.

24. Lightstone L. Minimising steroids in lupus nephritis–will B cell depletion pave the way? Lupus 2013;22:390–9.
25. Fanouriakis A, Boumpas DT, Bertsias GK. Pathogenesis and treatment of CNS lupus. Curr Opin Rheumatol 2013;25:577–83.
26. Hanly JG, Urowitz MB, Su L, et al. Prospective analysis of neuropsychiatric events in an international disease inception cohort of patients with systemic lupus erythematosus. Ann Rheum Dis 2010;69:529–35.
27. Wang Z, Wang Y, Zhu R, et al. Long-term survival and death causes of systemic lupus erythematosus in China: a systemic review of observational studies. Medicine (Baltimore) 2015;94:e794.
28. Bertsias GK, Ioannidis JP, Aringer M, et al. EULAR recommendations for the management of systemic lupus erythematosus with neuropsychiatric manifestations: report of a task force of the EULAR standing committee for clinical affairs. Ann Rheum Dis 2010;69:2074–82.
29. Singer J, Denburg JA. Diagnostic criteria for neuropsychiatric systemic lupus erythematosus: the results of a consensus meeting. The Ad Hoc Neuropsychiatric Lupus Workshop Group. J Rheumatol 1990;17:1397–402.
30. The American College of Rheumatology nomenclature and case definitions for neuropsychiatric lupus syndromes. Arthritis Rheum 1999;42:599–608.
31. Nishimura K, Omori M, Katsumata Y, et al. Neurocognitive impairment in corticosteroid-naive patients with active systemic lupus erythematosus: a prospective study. J Rheumatol 2015;42:441–8.
32. Kremer JM, Rynes RI, Bartholomew LE, et al. Non-organic non-psychotic psychopathology (NONPP) in patients with systemic lupus erythematosus. Semin Arthritis Rheum 1981;11:182–9.
33. Ainiala H, Loukkola J, Peltola J, et al. The prevalence of neuropsychiatric syndromes in systemic lupus erythematosus. Neurology 2001;57:496–500.
34. Mitsikostas DD, Sfikakis PP, Goadsby PJ. A meta-analysis for headache in systemic lupus erythematosus: the evidence and the myth. Brain 2004;127:1200–9.
35. Hanly JG, Urowitz MB, O'Keeffe AG, et al. Headache in systemic lupus erythematosus: results from a prospective, international inception cohort study. Arthritis Rheum 2013;65:2887–97.
36. Unterman A, Nolte JE, Boaz M, et al. Neuropsychiatric syndromes in systemic lupus erythematosus: a meta-analysis. Semin Arthritis Rheum 2011;41:1–11.
37. Bhangle SD, Kramer N, Rosenstein ED. Corticosteroid-induced neuropsychiatric disorders: review and contrast with neuropsychiatric lupus. Rheumatol Int 2013; 33:1923–32.
38. Andrade RM, Alarcon GS, Gonzalez LA, et al. Seizures in patients with systemic lupus erythematosus: data from LUMINA, a multiethnic cohort (LUMINA LIV). Ann Rheum Dis 2008;67:829–34.
39. Hanly JG, Urowitz MB, Su L, et al. Seizure disorders in systemic lupus erythematosus results from an international, prospective, inception cohort study. Ann Rheum Dis 2012;71:1502–9.
40. West SG. Clinical aspects of the nervous system. In: Wallace DJ, Hahn BH, editors. Systemic glucocorticoid therapy in SLE. 8th edition. Philadelphia: Lippincott Williams & Wilkins; 2013. p. 368–81.
41. Pego-Reigosa JM, Isenberg DA. Psychosis due to systemic lupus erythematosus: characteristics and long-term outcome of this rare manifestation of the disease. Rheumatology (Oxford) 2008;47:1498–502.
42. Ramos-Casals M, Soto MJ, Cuadrado MJ, et al. Rituximab in systemic lupus erythematosus: a systematic review of off-label use in 188 cases. Lupus 2009;18:767–76.

43. Sanna G, Bertolaccini ML, Khamashta MA. Neuropsychiatric involvement in systemic lupus erythematosus: current therapeutic approach. Curr Pharm Des 2008; 14:1261–9.

44. Sergent JS, Lockshin MD, Klempner MS, et al. Central nervous system disease in systemic lupus erythematosus. Therapy and prognosis. Am J Med 1975;58: 644–54.

45. Petri M, Spence D, Bone LR, et al. Coronary artery disease risk factors in the Johns Hopkins Lupus Cohort: prevalence, recognition by patients, and preventive practices. Medicine (Baltimore) 1992;71:291–302.

46. Bultink IE, Harvey NC, Lalmohamed A, et al. Elevated risk of clinical fractures and associated risk factors in patients with systemic lupus erythematosus versus matched controls: a population-based study in the United Kingdom. Osteoporos Int 2014;25:1275–83.

Glucocorticoids for Management of Polymyalgia Rheumatica and Giant Cell Arteritis

Eric L. Matteson, MD, MPH[a,b],*, Frank Buttgereit, MD[c],
Christian Dejaco, MD, PhD, MBA[d,e], Bhaskar Dasgupta, MD[f]

KEYWORDS

- Glucocorticoids • Polymyalgia rheumatica • Giant cell arteritis • Treatment

KEY POINTS

- Polymyalgia rheumatica (PMR) and giant cell arteritis (GCA) are diseases of older persons most common in persons of Northern European ancestry. There is considerable clinical overlap between the diseases, and there are many disease mimics.
- Advanced imaging can be useful in support of the diagnosis of the diseases.
- In PMR, typical ultrasonographic findings include subdeltoid bursitis and bicipital tendonitis, which resolve on successful treatment.
- Prompt initiation of treatment is important to avoid complications of visual loss in GCA and severe functional impairment in PMR.
- The course of the diseases is variable. They generally require treatment with glucocorticoids for 1 to 3 years and often longer.

Conflict of Interest: Dr E.L. Matteson: investigator, clinical trials, Bristol-Meyers-Squibb; Hoffman LA Roche, Janssen/Centocor; Dr F. Buttgereit: investigator, Mundipharma; Dr C. Dejaco: none; Dr B. Dasgupta: clinical trials design advisory board consultancies: Roche, Servier, GSK, Mundipharma, Pfizer, Merck, Sobi; unrestricted grants: Napp, Roche; speaker's honoraria: UCB, Merck.
[a] Division of Rheumatology, Department of Internal Medicine, Mayo Clinic College of Medicine, 200 1st Street Southwest, Rochester, MN 55902, USA; [b] Division of Epidemiology, Department of Health Sciences Research, Mayo Clinic College of Medicine, 200 1st Street Southwest, Rochester, MN 55902, USA; [c] Department of Rheumatology and Clinical Immunology, Charité University Medicine, Charitéplatz 1, Berlin 10117, Germany; [d] Department of Rheumatology, Medical University Graz, Auenbruggerplatz 15, Graz 8036, Austria; [e] Department of Immunology, Medical University Graz, Auenbruggerplatz 15, Graz 8036, Austria; [f] Department of Rheumatology, Southend University Hospital, Prittlewell Chase, Westcliff, Essex SS0-0RY, UK
* Corresponding author. Division of Rheumatology, Department of Internal Medicine, Mayo Clinic College of Medicine, 200 1st Street Southwest, Rochester, MN 55902.
E-mail address: Matteson.eric@mayo.edu

INTRODUCTION

Polymyalgia rheumatica (PMR) and giant cell arteritis (GCA) are both inflammatory disorders of older people, generally older than 50 years, with a peak incidence about the age of 73 years.[1,2] PMR is the second most common inflammatory rheumatic disease in the elderly after rheumatoid arthritis (RA), and GCA is the most frequent form of idiopathic vasculitis of older persons.[3] PMR and GCA affect similar patient populations, predominately but not exclusively persons of Northern European ancestry. Women are affected 2 to 3 times more frequently than men.[2,4]

Features of PMR occur in 40% to 60% of patients with GCA, and 16% to 21% of patients with PMR may also have GCA.[1,5]

PMR is a disabling condition because of the severe musculoskeletal pain, stiffness, and limitations of joint mobility, especially in the shoulder and hip. GCA may lead to sudden visual loss, including blindness in 1 or both eyes, and it is associated with morbidity caused by large-vessel disease, including acute or chronic large-vessel stenosis as well as aortic aneurysms.[2,5,6] Regular evaluation and monitoring of patients with GCA for vascular complications is essential.[7] Besides, optimal management of risk factors for atherosclerosis is necessary given that both patients with PMR and GCA are at an increased risk for peripheral arterial disease.[8,9]

Although life expectancy of patients with PMR and GCA is generally not different from the general population, patients who develop aneurysms have a markedly reduced life expectancy.[10,11]

CLINICAL FEATURES

The cardinal symptoms of PMR include bilateral pain and stiffness of the shoulders and hips.[1,5] Symptoms often begin acutely, over a matter of a few days to a few weeks. Bilateral shoulder and hip pain and stiffness can quickly lead to functional impairment. Even rising out of a chair or bed may become impossible because of pain and stiffness, not muscle weakness. Other symptoms may include peripheral arthritis, constitutional features such as weight loss, flulike symptoms, fatigue, and depression.[1] Inflammatory markers including the erythrocyte sedimentation rate (ESR) and C-reactive protein (CRP) levels are elevated at diagnosis in more than 90% of patients with PMR.

All these features have been captured by the provisional classification criteria for PMR set forth by the American College of Rheumatology (ACR) and the European League Against Rheumatism (EULAR) developed for the study of this disease (**Table 1**).[12]

Clinical features of GCA include scalp tenderness and jaw claudication. Headache occurs in only about 50% to 70% of patients.[2,5] Occasionally, the temporal artery or other superficial cranial arteries may feel nodular and thickened to palpation. Diplopia and partial or complete loss of vision occur in up to 20% of patients; stroke and cranial nerve palsy may also be observed.[2,5] Systemic features include polymyalgia symptoms, weight loss, fatigue, and fever.

Some patients with GCA, particularly those with extracranial GCA, may present with extensive systemic inflammation suffering from constitutional symptoms (eg, fever of unknown origin) or treatment-resistant PMR (referred to 60 years ago as polymyalgia arteritica) rather than ischemic complications.[13] Another subset of patients with GCA ($\leq$25%) develops symptoms related to extracranial large-vessel vasculitis such as arm claudication, arterial bruits, and heart murmurs.[14]

Inflammatory markers including CRP and ESR are increased in about 95% of patients with GCA at disease onset. Biopsy of the temporal artery is the standard for definitive diagnosis of cranial disease, which can be aided or even replaced in

Table 1
Provisional European League Against Rheumatism/American College of Rheumatology classification criteria for the polymyalgia rheumatica scoring algorithm (required criteria: age ≥50 y, bilateral shoulder aching, and abnormal C-reactive protein or erythrocyte sedimentation rate)

Criteria	Points Without Ultrasonography (0–6)	Points with Ultrasonography[a] (0–8)
Morning stiffness duration >45 min	2	2
Hip pain or limited range of movement	1	1
Absence of RF or ACPA	2	2
Absence of other joint involvement	1	1
≥1 shoulder with subdeltoid bursitis and/or biceps tenosynovitis and/or glenohumeral synovitis (either posterior or axillary) and ≥1 hip with synovitis and/or trochanteric bursitis	n/a	1
Both shoulders with subdeltoid bursitis, biceps tenosynovitis, or glenohumeral synovitis	n/a	1

A score of ≥4 is categorized as PMR in the algorithm without ultrasound and a score of ≥5 is categorized as PMR in the algorithm with ultrasonographic identification of inflammatory changes typical of PMR in the shoulders and hips.

Abbreviations: ACPA, anticitrullinated protein antibody; n/a, not applicable; RF, rheumatoid factor.

[a] Optional ultrasonographic criteria.

Adapted from Dasgupta B, Cimmino MA, Maradit-Kremers H, et al. 2012 provisional classification criteria for polymyalgia rheumatica: a European League Against Rheumatism/American College of Rheumatology collaborative initiative. Ann Rheum Dis 2012;71(4):489; with permission.

individual cases by ultrasonographic imaging.[2,5] Sonography of affected arteries may reveal a halo (ie, a hypoechoic thickening of the arterial wall), stenosis, or occlusion in the active phase of the disease.[15,16] MRI and computed tomography-aided arteriography are especially useful for defining structural abnormalities including aneurysm and stenosis of extracranial large vessels, whereas for the assessment of disease activity, ultrasonography, MRI, and fluorodeoxyglucose (FDG) PET may be more useful as imaging tools.

Key features of GCA are included in the 1990 ACR Classification Criteria for this disease, developed to distinguish GCA from other forms of systemic vasculitis (**Box 1**).[17]

Misdiagnosis of PMR and GCA is common; up to 30% of patients initially diagnosed with PMR were found to have another condition during follow-up.[18] The most important differential diagnosis is RA, given that 65% of patients with PMR whose diagnosis was corrected during follow-up suffered from this condition.[16] Other important differential diagnostic considerations include osteoarthritis, spondyloarthritis, crystalline arthropathy, systemic lupus erythematosus and other connective tissue diseases, other forms of vasculitis, systemic infections, hematologic malignancy, thyroid and parathyroid disease, and Parkinson disease.

There is no specific laboratory test for PMR and GCA. The presence of abnormal results of electrophoresis or autoantibody testing (such as antinuclear antibodies [ANA], anticitrullinated protein antibodies [ACPA], or antineutrophil cytoplasmic antibodies [ANCA]) may suggest another diagnosis.

Basic laboratory tests in patients being evaluated for new-onset PMR and GCA include ESR, CRP, serum electrophoresis, ACPA (PMR only), ANCA (GCA only), full

> **Box 1**
> **ACR classification criteria for GCA**
>
> 1. Age at onset of disease greater than 50 years
> 2. New headache
> 3. Temporal artery abnormality (tenderness to palpation or decreased pulse)
> 4. Increased ESR greater than 50 mm/h
> 5. Abnormal findings on biopsy of the temporal artery. The histopathology of the artery shows vasculitis with predominant mononuclear cells or granulomatous inflammation usually with multinucleated giant cells
>
> *Adapted from* Hunder GG, Bloch DA, Michel BA, et al. The American College of Rheumatology 1990 criteria for the classification of giant cell arteritis. Arthritis Rheum 1990;33:1125; with permission.

blood count, liver function tests, serum glucose, urea, creatinine, electrolytes, serum lipids, creatine kinase, urine analysis, and thyroid-stimulating hormone. Depending on the clinical scenario, other tests may be requested such as ANA or tuberculosis testing. Patients should be evaluated for the presence of comorbidities such as hypertension, diabetes, or osteoporosis.

MANAGEMENT

Rapid diagnosis and initiation of treatment are essential to reduce pain and stiffness in those with PMR and to prevent blindness and other ischemic complications in patients with GCA. Fast-track pathways with initial assessment and treatment of patients with suspected GCA within 1 to a few days are gaining ground as the standard of care. In Southend, UK, this strategy has led to a significant reduction of permanent sight loss compared with a historical cohort (**Fig. 1**).[19] Accordingly, patients with suspected GCA

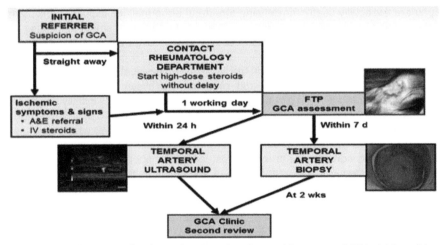

Fig. 1. Fast-track strategy for the evaluation of patients with suspected GCA. A&E, accident and emergency; FTP, Fast Track Pathway; IV, intravenous. (*From* Patil P, Maw WW, Achilleos K, et al. Outcomes of the fast-track pathway in giant cell arteritis: a sight saver. ACR 2013; [abstract: 1928]. *Courtesy of* B. Dasgupta, MD, Essex, UK.)

are immediately started on prednisone 40 to 60 mg daily and referred to the fast-track clinic, where they are seen within a working day by a rheumatologist. Patients with ischemic symptoms or jaw pain in addition receive intravenous pulse glucocorticoids (GCs) immediately. Patients then undergo full assessments, including temporal artery ultrasonography and biopsy, and are seen back within 2 weeks, during which time oral GCs are continued at 40 to 60 mg daily. In cases in which a diagnosis is confirmed, patients are followed up in the rheumatology outpatient clinic; otherwise, GCs are rapidly tapered off and patients further evaluated as dictated by symptoms and disease course.

General principles of management of PMR and GCA include (1) assurance of proper diagnosis, (2) evaluation of comorbidities, relevant medications, and risk factors for GC-related side effects, (3) assessment of risk factors for relapse/prolonged therapy, (4) an individualized disease management plan considering the patient's perspective/ preferences and shared decision making between the patient and the treating physician, (5) patient education about the disease; and (6) regular monitoring and management of disease activity, side effects, and comorbidities.

PMR is commonly treated in primary care but it is suggested to consider specialist referral, particularly in cases of atypical presentation and complex disease course and therapy. It is important to pay attention to patients' physical function, encouraging physical fitness and mobility, to maintain long-term independence and a satisfying quality of life.

Because PMR and GCA are associated with an increased risk of peripheral arterial disease and patients with GCA are prone to cardiovascular complications over the course of the disease, management should include periodic evaluation for these conditions.

GLUCOCORTICOIDS FOR TREATMENT OF POLYMYALGIA RHEUMATICA AND GIANT CELL ARTERITIS

Since the 1950s, GCs have been the mainstay of treatment of GCA and not long thereafter, PMR. Both their genomic and nongenomic effects contribute to successful treatment of these diseases.

MECHANISMS OF GLUCOCORTICOID ACTIONS

The reasons for the successful use of GCs are their strong antiinflammatory and immunosuppressive effects. To understand their established effectiveness in PMR and GCA (and many other) diseases, a short description of their mechanisms of action may be helpful. This description seems to be especially appropriate in this context because different dosages are used in the treatment of PMR and GCA, ranging from maintenance treatment in PMR with low dosages of 5 mg/d or less prednisone equivalent to pulse therapy with grams of methylprednisolone (MP) in complicated GCA (**Fig. 2**).

GCs exert their main antiinflammatory and immunosuppressive effects primarily on leucocytes and secondary immune cells, where their functions as well as their distribution are affected.[20] These antiinflammatory and immunosuppressive effects are primarily produced via so-called genomic mechanisms, that is, the classic mechanism of action mediated by the cytosolic GC receptor (cGR). This genomic mechanism of GC action can be divided into the transactivation and the transrepression processes. The so-called transrepression results in a decreased expression of proinflammatory cytokines, whereas the increased synthesis of antiinflammatory (and other) proteins is termed transactivation.[21,22] The current view is that transactivation could account

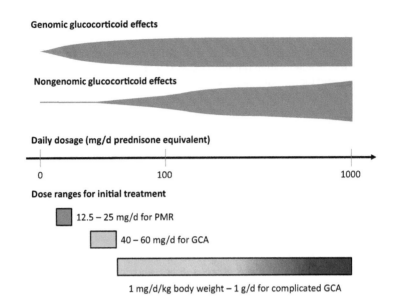

Fig. 2. Relationships between GC dosage, strengths of induced GC effects, and the use of these drugs in PMR and GCA. (*From* Tyrrell JB. Glucocorticoid therapy. In: Felig P, Baxter JD, Frohman LA, editors. Endocrinology and metabolism. 3rd edition. New York: McGraw-Hill; 1995. p. 862; with permission.)

for several adverse effects (but also mediating immunosuppressive effects), whereas transrepression is to a greater extent responsible for the main part of the therapeutic effects of GCs.

The higher the administered GC dose, the more cGR are recruited and the more intense are the genomic effects induced. It has been reported that 7.5 and 15 mg/d of prednisone would result in blood concentrations 8 hours after the dose that would bind the receptors to 42% and 63% of saturation, respectively (see **Fig. 2**).[23] According to this calculation, higher doses (ie, ≥100 mg prednisone equivalent) result in nearly complete receptor saturation (see **Fig. 2**).[23] With increasing GC doses, more cGR are recruited. This situation leads to more intense genomic effects, achieving about 100% at around 100 mg/d. Therefore, additional therapeutic benefits with dosages of 100 mg/d or greater are considered to be obtained via qualitatively different, nongenomic effects that come increasingly into play at dosages of 50 to 100 mg/d and higher. Dosages greater than 100 mg/d cannot produce stronger clinical effects via genomic effects. Therefore, additional therapeutic benefits produced by these higher doses are considered to be obtained via qualitatively different, nongenomic effects (see **Fig. 2**).

These nongenomic effects are mediated via (1) nonspecific interactions of GCs with cellular membranes, (2) nongenomic effects mediated by the cGR, and (3) specific interactions with a membrane-bound GR (mGR).[21,22] Experimental data suggest that these differential effects come increasingly into play greater than 50 to 100 mg/d.[24]

From these considerations, there are 3 major messages that are relevant for the treatment of PMR and GCA with GC:

1. GCs form the mainstay of therapy for PMR and GCA because they exert manifold and strong antiinflammatory and immunosuppressive effects.

2. Therapeutically, most important are the classic genomic mechanisms that are mediated via the cGR. These effects occur at any dosages, also at low ones, but the higher the dosage, the more receptors are activated and the stronger the GC effects reaching a maximum at a dosage of around 100 mg/d.
3. At higher GC dosages (as with pulse therapy in GCA), rapid nongenomic effects also come into play that contribute to their therapeutic efficacy.

WHY DOES CLINICAL EFFICACY OF GLUCOCORTICOID THERAPY VARY AMONG DIFFERENT PATIENTS?

The efficacy of certain (especially lower) GC dosages varies among different patients. The reasons for this situation are not entirely known, but this observation explains why GC dosing recommendations are for dose ranges rather than specific dosages for the treatment of diseases such as PMR and GCA.

There are several reasons for variation in efficacy of specific GC dosages, including (1) interindividual variability in pharmacokinetics, including differences in both number of cGC sites and binding affinities[25,26]; (2) mediation of (relative) glucocorticoid receptor (GCR) resistance, including polymorphic changes or overexpression of (co-)chaperones, overexpression of the GCR β isoform, the multidrug-resistance pump, and an altered membrane-bound GCR expression[20]; (3) variation in activation of mitogen-activated protein kinase pathways by certain cytokines; (4) excessive activation of the transcription factor activator protein 1; (5) reduced histone deacetylase-2 expression; (6) increased macrophage migration inhibitory factor; and (7) increased P-glycoprotein-mediated drug efflux.[27]

ADVERSE EFFECTS OF GLUCOCORTICOIDS

GCs also exert undesired effects, especially if higher dosages have to be given over longer periods. In this regard, GC-induced osteoporosis, metabolic and cardiovascular adverse effects, and the increased risk of infection are counted among the most important adverse effects of GC therapy, by both rheumatologists and patients (**Fig. 3**).[28] In addition, gastrointestinal, dermatologic, and ophthalmologic adverse effects, possible development of avascular necrosis, mood alteration, and development of a cushingoid phenotype need to be mentioned as important GC-related adverse effects.

However, the available data describing frequency and severity of these adverse effects are fragmentary. For example, it is difficult to distinguish specific adverse effects of GC therapy from other causations (eg, the treated disease itself, other concomitant diseases, or concomitant therapies). Nevertheless, the potential of GC to produce adverse effects may prompt both patients and prescribing physicians to take a critical view of these drugs. As with all diagnostic and therapeutic approaches in medicine, the primary aim is a positive benefit/risk ratio when using these drugs.

In the following, we consider how the goal of maximizing benefit and limiting risk of GC therapy in PMR and GCA are considered. These recommendations are mostly based on expert opinion and consensus rather than on high-quality evidence.

CLINICAL ASPECTS OF THERAPY WITH GLUCOCORTICOIDS IN POLYMYALGIA RHEUMATICA AND GIANT CELL ARTERITIS

Treatment of PMR and GCA usually exceeds 1 to 2 years. Most patients experience relapses despite effective treatment and up to 85% are affected by adverse effects of chronic GC therapy.

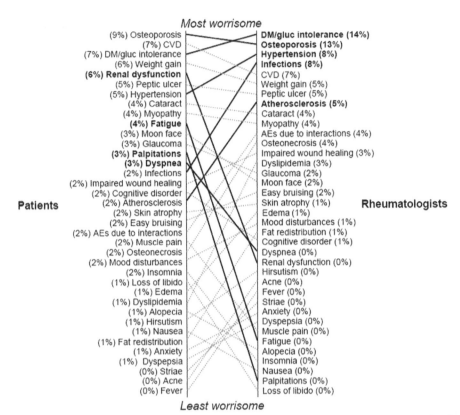

Most worrisome

Patients	Rheumatologists
(9%) Osteoporosis	DM/gluc intolerance (14%)
(7%) CVD	Osteoporosis (13%)
(7%) DM/gluc intolerance	Hypertension (8%)
(6%) Weight gain	Infections (8%)
(6%) Renal dysfunction	CVD (7%)
(5%) Peptic ulcer	Weight gain (5%)
(5%) Hypertension	Peptic ulcer (5%)
(4%) Cataract	**Atherosclerosis (5%)**
(4%) Myopathy	Cataract (4%)
(4%) Fatigue	Myopathy (4%)
(3%) Moon face	AEs due to interactions (4%)
(3%) Glaucoma	Osteonecrosis (4%)
(3%) Palpitations	Impaired wound healing (3%)
(3%) Dyspnea	Dyslipidemia (3%)
(2%) Infections	Glaucoma (2%)
(2%) Impaired wound healing	Moon face (2%)
(2%) Cognitive disorder	Easy bruising (2%)
(2%) Atherosclerosis	Skin atrophy (1%)
(2%) Skin atrophy	Edema (1%)
(2%) Easy bruising	Mood disturbances (1%)
(2%) AEs due to interactions	Fat redistribution (1%)
(2%) Muscle pain	Cognitive disorder (1%)
(2%) Osteonecrosis	Dyspnea (0%)
(2%) Mood disturbances	Renal dysfunction (0%)
(2%) Insomnia	Hirsutism (0%)
(1%) Loss of libido	Acne (0%)
(1%) Edema	Fever (0%)
(1%) Dyslipidemia	Striae (0%)
(1%) Alopecia	Anxiety (0%)
(1%) Hirsutism	Dyspepsia (0%)
(1%) Nausea	Muscle pain (0%)
(1%) Fat redistribution	Fatigue (0%)
(1%) Anxiety	Alopecia (0%)
(1%) Dyspepsia	Insomnia (0%)
(0%) Striae	Nausea (0%)
(0%) Acne	Palpitations (0%)
(0%) Fever	Loss of libido (0%)

Least worrisome

Fig. 3. GC side effects: most worrisome effects. Most worrisome adverse events (AEs) ranked by patients (*left*) and rheumatologists (*right*). Scores are corrected for the different numbers of participants per country and expressed as percentages of total score per group (the scores per country were recalculated in percentages of the total score of all countries per group, being 100%). Discordant scores, defined as a difference of at least 3%, are depicted in bold type. CVD, cardiovascular disease; DM, diabetes mellitus; gluc, glucose. (*From* van der Goes MC, Jacobs JW, Boers M, et al. Patient and rheumatologist perspectives on glucocorticoids: an exercise to improve the implementation of the EULAR recommendations on the management of systemic glucocorticoid therapy in rheumatic diseases. Ann Rheum Dis 2010;69(6):1018; with permission.)

Polymyalgia Rheumatica

As initial therapy for PMR, a minimum effective GC dose within a range of 12.5 to 25 mg/d prednisone equivalent has recently been suggested by EULAR-ACR recommendations.[29] The dose should be administered as a single morning dose, except for cases with prominent night pain, tapering GCs lower than the low dose range (ie, prednisone or equivalent <5 mg daily), where a divided dose may be acceptable.

Clinical improvement should be noted 2 weeks after initiation of GC treatment, and almost complete response can be expected after 4 weeks. In general, a prednisone dose at the upper end of the range as suggested earlier may be considered in patients with a high risk for relapse and low risk for adverse events, whereas patients with comorbidities such as diabetes, osteoporosis, and other risk factors for GC-related side effects may benefit from a lower initial dose.[18,28,29]

This recommendation has been supported by clinical trial data, experience of the authors, and national PMR guidelines.[2,18,28,29] Current ACR and EULAR guidelines on the use of GCs in rheumatic diseases suggest carefully balancing the GC dose with respect to symptom/disease control and side effects of chronic disorders.[30–33]

Although GCs are the most important drugs for PMR treatment, high-quality prospective studies comparing different initial doses and tapering regimens are not available. A single prospective study of 39 patients with PMR compared starting doses of 20 mg/d and 10 mg/d prednisone and reported a lower short-term relapse rate in the higher dose group, whereas retrospective studies suggested no difference in the long-term between doses greater than and less than 15 mg/d prednisone in this regard. There is some limited evidence for a higher risk of adverse events in patients receiving a high initial GC dose.[34,35]

Starting doses less than 7.5 mg/d and greater than 30 mg/d prednisone equivalent are explicitly discouraged for PMR by EULAR-ACR. For very small doses of GCs, there is no supporting evidence, and clinical experts believed that too small a starting dose may unnecessarily prolong patients' suffering. For high GC doses, there are data from retrospective studies[36,37] reporting no benefit of high compared with medium doses, and we know from patients with other rheumatic diseases that high doses of GCs are associated with significant treatment-related morbidity.

A fundamental principle of PMR treatment with GCs is that dose reductions should be gradual. There is no evidence from clinical trials supporting any specific tapering regimen, and we therefore suggest individualizing the treatment plan in accordance with clinical response and adverse events. EULAR-ACR recommendations suggest that a dose of 10 mg/d prednisone equivalent should be reached within 4 to 8 weeks; thereafter, the dose should be decreased by 1 mg every 4 weeks or similar. If a relapse occurs, GCs may be increased to the last effective dose.

The diagnosis should be questioned/reevaluated in case of insufficient response or frequent relapses. Up to 30% of patients with other conditions (mainly RA) may initially be misclassified as having PMR.

According to the GC regimen suggested by the EULAR-ACR recommendations, duration of PMR treatment is at least 1 year. However, data from observational studies and clinical experience indicate variable disease duration, ranging from 1 to greater than 10 years and even lifelong in some patients.

We have limited evidence that patients with a high initial inflammatory response as reflected by a high initial ESR or the presence of peripheral arthritis have a longer duration of GC therapy[30,31]; however, there are also data contradicting these observations.[31–37] New, prospective high-quality studies are thus needed to identify reliable predictors of PMR prognosis.

Intramuscular (i.m.) MP, initially administered at a dose of 120 mg given once every 3 weeks for 12 weeks, with subsequent tapering by reducing the MP dose by 20 mg every 12 weeks until off or symptom return for 48 weeks follow-up, was reported to have equal clinical efficacy in PMR to oral GCs in 1 multicenter 96-week randomized controlled trial (RCT) conducted in England.[38] i.m. MP treatment resulted in a lower cumulative GC dose and in a lower weight gain, whereas other GC-related side effects did not differ between groups. In clinical practice, i.m. MP may be used as an alternative to oral GCs in individual patients, particularly if a lower cumulative GC dose is desired; however, this substance may not be available in each country. Further trials confirming the favorable benefit/risk profile of i.m. MP compared with oral GCs are warranted.

Another unresolved issue is the possible benefit of modified oral GC preparations for treatment of PMR. In RA, treatment with modified-release prednisone resulted in a greater reduction of morning stiffness compared with standard oral prednisone, and it might be possible that this effect can be obtained in PMR as well. Further, a lower dose of modified-release prednisone might be equally effective in reducing PMR activity as a higher dose of standard GCs. Prospective studies addressing these issues are still needed.

Giant Cell Arteritis

The treatment goals in GCA include resolution of disease-related symptoms and prevention of disease-related complications, minimizing medication-related adverse effects. In patients with suspected GCA, treatment with GCs should be initiated promptly to avoid visual loss (which occurs almost exclusively in untreated patients), even as the diagnostic evaluation (including ultrasonography and temporal artery biopsy) proceeds.

Although it is known that the halo sign resolves in most patients after a few weeks of treatment, there is no clear evidence that sensitivity of ultrasonographic assessment significantly declines within a few days of GC therapy.[39] Abnormal findings on histopathologic examination of temporal artery biopsy might even be detected after weeks to months of GC therapy.[2]

Initial treatment of GCA is 1 mg/kg oral prednisone equivalent daily; however, a dose of 60 mg/d is usually not exceeded.[2] Patients with acute or fluctuating impending vision loss should receive pulse GC therapy in the form of intravenous MP, up to 1000 mg daily for 3 to 5 days, and then oral prednisone at 40 to 60 mg a day.[2] Alternative day GC dosing is not regarded as reliably effective and should be avoided.

The initial dose of prednisone should be continued for 4 weeks. As in PMR, the daily dose should then be reduced gradually. One example for a tapering schedule is the decrement of the dose by ~10% every 2 weeks to a dose of 10 mg daily, assuming disease control. Thereafter, the prednisone may be tapered more slowly, for example, by 1 mg each month. Similar regimens may work equally well, for example, in countries where 1-mg tablets are not available, the daily prednisone dose may be lowered by 2.5 mg every 2 to 3 months. The British Society of Rheumatology (BSR) guidelines suggest 40 to 60 mg prednisolone until symptoms and laboratory abnormalities resolve (at least 3–4 weeks), and then, the dose is reduced by 10 mg every 2 weeks to 20 mg a day. Thereafter, the daily dose may be reduced by 2.5 mg every 2 to 4 weeks to 10 mg a day, and then, by 1 mg every 1 to 2 months if there is no relapse.

Regarding initial GC doses in GCA, there is only a single prospective study on 35 patients with GCA comparing 40 mg/d with 20 mg/d oral prednisone. No difference regarding relapse rates at 2 months was found, although this short follow-up period may be inadequate to assess the long-term effectiveness of this smaller dose as initial therapy for GCA.[40] Other trials investigated the value of i.v. pulse MP therapy in uncomplicated GCA with contradictory results. One study[41] investigated 27 patients with GCA receiving either 15 mg/kg/d intravenous MP for 3 days or placebo + 40 mg/d oral prednisone. A lower cumulative oral GC dose as well as higher remission rates while on 5 mg or less oral prednisone at 36 to 78 weeks were found in the pulse compared with the control group. However, another study of 164 patients investigating the effect of lower pulse doses (240 mg/d MP for 3 days) found no difference between the intervention and conventional therapy with oral prednisone (1 mg/kg body weight) in the control group regarding several outcomes such as the cumulative GC dose or discontinuation of GCs.[42] No evidence is available concerning the possible value of i.m. MP or modified-release prednisone for GCA treatment.

No high-quality trials are available comparing different GC tapering schedules. The regimen proposed in this study, which closely parallels that of the BSR, is entirely based on clinical experience and expert opinion.

The average disease course of GCA is longer than in PMR, usually about 3 years; however, a disease duration of 5 to 10 years, or even lifelong treatment, are possible. As in PMR, relapse is common, with 40% to 68% of patients having at least 1 relapse. About half of patients experience disease recurrence after discontinuation of GC therapy.[2] As the GC dose is tapered, patients should be evaluated on a regular basis for signs, symptoms, and laboratory evidence of active disease. CRP seems to be a more sensitive marker of GCA-related inflammation than ESR; however, an increase of acute-phase reactants alone (ie, without clinical signs of active GCA) does not justify a change of therapy. Increases in inflammatory markers should be used in clinical context, and if isolated ESR/CRP increases persist, we suggest performing further investigations to detect large-vessel complications or mimicking conditions.

Patients with GCA and extracranial manifestation are difficult to monitor. Patients who have accelerated acute-phase reactants without specific symptoms may require further evaluation by advanced imaging techniques for the presence of active vasculitis.

NONSTEROIDAL ANTIINFLAMMATORY DRUGS AND ANALGESICS IN POLYMYALGIA RHEUMATICA AND GIANT CELL ARTERITIS

There is no evidence that nonsteroidal antiinflammatory drugs (NSAIDs) or analgesics are effective for PMR or GCA. Given the known gastrointestinal, cardiovascular, or renal side effects, NSAIDs should be avoided in these disorders except for the treatment of coexisting osteoarthritis or other causes of pain.[43,44]

GLUCOCORTICOID-SPARING AGENTS IN POLYMYALGIA RHEUMATICA AND GIANT CELL ARTERITIS
Nonbiological Agents

There is only limited evidence supporting use of GC-sparing agents for either PMR or GCA. Perhaps best studied is methotrexate (MTX), which can be considered in patients with PMR at risk for relapses/prolonged therapy or GC-related side effects in accordance with the new EULAR-ACR recommendations. The GC-sparing effect of MTX is likely best if MTX is introduced early in disease management, but MTX can also be considered in patients with GC-resistant or relapsing disease.[45–50]

According to EULAR and BSR guidelines for GCA, early introduction of MTX should be considered for each patient, although there is limited evidence supporting the efficacy of MTX for GCA therapy. A meta-analysis pooling the data of these 3 trials[51] showed a marginal reduction of the risk for the first relapse, higher rates of GC-free remission and lower cumulative GC doses.

Studies of other chemotherapies have failed to show their usefulness, for reasons of either safety or efficacy. These chemotherapies include azathioprine, cyclosporine A, and dapsone.[52–55] Two case series from Southend, UK and Kristiansand, Norway (total n = 46) reported a benefit of leflunomide for GC-resistant PMR and GCA cases. Leflunomide was generally well tolerated, with an impact on both clinical and laboratory response, and helped in steroid tapering in most cases.[56]

Biological Agents

No biological agents have shown adequate benefit in routine management of PMR and GCA. EULAR-ACR recommendations strongly discourage the routine application of tumor necrosis factor α blocking agents for PMR. Studies of adalimumab, infliximab, and etanercept have failed to show their usefulness for management of GCA as well.[57–61]

Other agents are under evaluation, including anti-interleukin (IL) 6 antibodies. Serum IL-6 levels are increased in most cases of active PMR and GCA, correlating with large-vessel involvement. Several cases of relapsing PMR and GCA were already treated with tocilizumab (an IL-6 receptor blocker) at a dose of 8 mg/kg, with satisfactory clinical and biochemical response without significant adverse events.[62,63] FDG-PET findings also showed improvement of patients with large-vessel disease, suggesting that recanalization of arteries and therefore reversal of tissue ischemia may be possible with tocilizumab therapy.[62] The GiACTA (Gi[ant cell arteritis]ACT[emr]A) trial (NCT01791153) is a an ongoing multicenter RCT investigating the efficacy of tocilizumab to maintain remission in patients with GCA.

The results of other recently completed or ongoing RCTs on other biological agents, for example, on the safety and efficacy of secukinumab (anti-IL-17A) and canakinumab (anti-IL-1β) in PMR (NCT01364389), or the value of the anti-IL-1β antibody, gevokizumab (EudraCT number 2013–002778–38) in GCA, are expected within coming months or years.

ASPIRIN USE IN GIANT CELL ARTERITIS

Aspirin is frequently added to the therapeutic regimen with the intention to reduce the likelihood of blindness. EULAR recommends giving aspirin to every patient with GCA to reduce the risk of cardiovascular and cerebrovascular events. However, evidence for the efficacy of aspirin in GCA is conflicting; prospective clinical studies of this approach have not yet been performed.[64–66]

MANAGEMENT OF GLUCOCORTICOID-RELATED COMPLICATIONS IN POLYMYALGIA RHEUMATICA AND GIANT CELL ARTERITIS

Given the high rate of GC-related adverse events (affecting ≤90% of patients) in PMR and GCA, including infections, hypertension, cardiovascular disease, osteoporosis, avascular necrosis, diabetes mellitus, and cataracts, prophylaxis and monitoring for GC-related complications should be part of the therapeutic approach to all patients with PMR/GCA, as also pointed out by the EULAR recommendations on the management of medium-dose to high-dose GC therapy in rheumatic diseases.[30] These measures include age-appropriate immunizations, including influenza and pneumococcal vaccines. Varicella zoster vaccination should be considered in patients once the GC dose is less than about 15 mg/d.

Because of concern about *Pneumocystis jirovecii* pneumonia (PJP) in patients on high-dose GC, patients with GCA who also have another cause of immunocompromise should be considered for PJP prophylaxis (eg, single-strength once daily or double-strength tablet of trimethoprim-sulfamethoxazole 3 times per week).[67,68]

SUMMARY

For more than 6 decades, GCs have been the sole or anchor therapy for treatment of PMR and GCA. Although effective, they are associated with considerable side effects and often exacerbate comorbidities from which elderly patients with these diseases suffer. The need is great for improved disease management, in terms of better tools for accurate disease diagnosis and disease activity and prognosis assessment and for better GC-sparing therapy. New therapeutic modalities with fewer side effects that can be tailored to the individual patient and that not only treat but cure these diseases are the dreams of patients and physicians alike.

REFERENCES

1. Kermani TA, Warrington KJ. Polymyalgia rheumatica. Lancet 2013;381(9860): 63–72.
2. Weyand CM, Goronzy JJ. Medium- and large-vessel vasculitis. N Engl J Med 2003;349(2):160–9.
3. Lawrence RC, Felson DT, Helmick CG, et al. Estimates of the prevalence of arthritis and other rheumatic conditions in the United States. Part II. Arthritis Rheum 2008;58(1):26–35.
4. Crowson CS, Matteson EL, Myasoedova E, et al. The lifetime risk of adult-onset rheumatoid arthritis and other inflammatory autoimmune rheumatic diseases. Arthritis Rheum 2011;63(3):633–9.
5. Salvarani C, Pipitone N, Versari A, et al. Clinical features of PMR and GCA. Nat Rev Rheumatol 2012;8(9):509–21.
6. Aiello PD, Trautmann JC, McPhee TJ, et al. Visual prognosis in GCA. Ophthalmology 1993;100(4):550–5.
7. Warrington KJ, Matteson EL. Management guidelines and outcome measures in giant cell arteritis (GCA). Clin Exp Rheumatol 2007;25(6, Suppl 47):137–41.
8. Warrington KJ, Jarpa EP, Crowson CS, et al. Increased risk of peripheral arterial disease in polymyalgia rheumatica: a population-based cohort study. Arthritis Res Ther 2009;11(2):R50.
9. Kermani TA, Warrington KJ, Crowson CS, et al. Large-vessel involvement in GCA: a population-based cohort study of the incidence-trends and prognosis. Ann Rheum Dis 2013;72(12):1989–94.
10. Matteson EL, Gold KN, Bloch DA, et al. Long-term survival of patients with GCA in the American College of Rheumatology GCA classification criteria cohort. Am J Med 1996;100(2):193–6.
11. Gran JT, Myklebust G, Wilsgaard T, et al. Survival in PMR and temporal arteritis: a study of 398 cases and matched population controls. Rheumatology 2001; 40(11):1238–42.
12. Dasgupta B, Cimmino MA, Maradit-Kremers H, et al. 2012 provisional classification criteria for polymyalgia rheumatica: a European League Against Rheumatism/ American College of Rheumatology collaborative initiative. Ann Rheum Dis 2012; 71(4):484–92.
13. Forster S, Tato F, Weiss M, et al. Patterns of extracranial involvement in newly diagnosed GCA assessed by physical examination, colour coded duplex sonography and FDG-PET. Vasa 2011;40(3):219–27.
14. Ball EL, Walsh SR, Tang TY, et al. Role of ultrasonography in the diagnosis of temporal arteritis. Br J Surg 2010;97(12):1765–71.
15. Schmidt WA. Role of ultrasound in the understanding and management of vasculitis. Ther Adv Musculoskelet Dis 2014;6(2):39–47.
16. Caporali R, Montecucco C, Epis O, et al. Presenting features of polymyalgia rheumatica (PMR) and rheumatoid arthritis with PMR-like onset: a prospective study. Ann Rheum Dis 2001;60(11):1021–4.

17. Hunder GG, Bloch DA, Michel BA, et al. The American College of Rheumatology 1990 criteria for the classification of GCA. Arthritis Rheum 1990;33(8):1122–8.

18. Dasgupta B, Borg FA, Hassan N, et al. BSR and BHPR guidelines for the management of polymyalgia rheumatica. Rheumatology 2010;49(1):186–90.

19. Patil P, Williams M, Maw W, et al. Fast track pathway reduces sight loss in giant cell arteritis: results of a longitudinal observational cohort study. Clin Exp Rheumatol 2015;33(2 Suppl 89):S103–6.

20. Buttgereit F, Saag KG, Cutolo M, et al. The molecular basis for the effectiveness, toxicity, and resistance to glucocorticoids: focus on the treatment of rheumatoid arthritis. Scand J Rheumatol 2005;34(1):14–21.

21. Stahn C, Buttgereit F. Genomic and nongenomic effects of glucocorticoids. Nat Clin Pract Rheumatol 2008;4(10):525–33.

22. Strehl C, Buttgereit F. Optimized glucocorticoid therapy: teaching old drugs new tricks. Mol Cell Endocrinol 2013;380(1–2):32–40.

23. Tyrrell JB. Glucocorticoid therapy. In: Felig P, Baxter JD, Frohman LA, editors. Endocrinology and metabolism. 3rd edition. New York: McGraw-Hill; 1995. p. 912–9.

24. Buttgereit F, da Silva JA, Boers M, et al. Standardised nomenclature for glucocorticoid dosages and glucocorticoid treatment regimens: current questions and tentative answers in rheumatology. Ann Rheum Dis 2002;61(8):718–22.

25. Sanden S, Tripmacher R, Weltrich R, et al. Glucocorticoid dose dependent downregulation of glucocorticoid receptors in patients with rheumatic diseases. J Rheumatol 2000;27(5):1265–70.

26. Andreae J, Tripmacher R, Weltrich R, et al. Effect of glucocorticoid therapy on glucocorticoid receptors in children with autoimmune diseases. Pediatr Res 2001;49(1):130–5.

27. Barnes PJ, Adcock IM. Glucocorticoid resistance in inflammatory diseases. Lancet 2009;373(9678):1905–17.

28. van der Goes MC, Jacobs JW, Boers M, et al. Patient and rheumatologist perspectives on glucocorticoids: an exercise to improve the implementation of the European League Against Rheumatism (EULAR) recommendations on the management of systemic glucocorticoid therapy in rheumatic diseases. Ann Rheum Dis 2010;69(6):1015–21.

29. Dejaco C, Singh Y, Perel P, et al. Current evidence for therapeutic interventions in polymyalgia rheumatica (PMR): a systematic literature review informing the ACR/EULAR recommendations for the management of PMR. Ann Rheum Dis 2014; 73(S2):552.

30. Duru N, van der Goes MC, Jacobs JWG, et al. EULAR evidence-based and consensus-based recommendations on the management of medium to high-dose glucocorticoid therapy in rheumatic diseases. Ann Rheum Dis 2013;72: 1905–13.

31. Grossman JM, Gordon R, Ranganath VK, et al. American College of Rheumatology 2010 recommendations for the prevention and treatment of glucocorticoid-induced osteoporosis. Arthritis Care Res 2010;62:1515–26.

32. Van der Goes MC, Jacobs JWG, Boers M, et al. Monitoring adverse events of low-dose glucocorticoid therapy: EULAR recommendations for clinical trials and daily practice. Ann Rheum Dis 2010;69:1913–9.

33. Hoes JN, Jacobs JWG, Boers M, et al. EULAR evidence-based recommendations on the management of systemic glucocorticoid therapy in rheumatic diseases. Ann Rheum Dis 2007;66:1560–7.

34. Delecoeuillerie G, Joly P, Cohen de Lara A, et al. Polymyalgia rheumatica and temporal arteritis: a retrospective analysis of prognostic features and different

corticosteroid regimens (11 year survey of 210 patients). Ann Rheum Dis 1988; 47:733–9.

35. Mackie SL, Hensor EM, Haugeberg G, et al. Can the prognosis of polymyalgia rheumatica be predicted at disease onset? Results from a 5-year prospective study. Rheumatology (Oxford) 2010;49:716–22.

36. Kanemaru K, Nagura H, Ooyama T, et al. Report of 6 cases with polymyalgia rheumatica and a review of the literature. Nihon Ronen Igakkai Zasshi 1986;23: 469–76 [in Japanese].

37. Myklebust G, Gran JT. Prednisolone maintenance dose in relation to starting dose in the treatment of polymyalgia rheumatica and temporal arteritis. A prospective two-year study in 273 patients. Scand J Rheumatol 2001;30:260–7.

38. Dasgupta B, Dolan AL, Panayi GS, et al. An initially double-blind controlled 96 week trial of depot methylprednisolone against oral prednisolone in the treatment of polymyalgia rheumatica. Br J Rheumatol 1998;37(2):189–95.

39. Hauenstein C, Reinhard M, Geiger J, et al. Effects of early corticosteroid treatment on magnetic resonance imaging and ultrasonography findings in giant cell arteritis. Rheumatology (Oxford) 2012;51:1999–2003.

40. Kyle V, Hazleman BL. Treatment of polymyalgia rheumatica and giant cell arteritis. I. Steroid regimens in the first two months. Ann Rheum Dis 1989;48(8):658–61.

41. Mazlumzadeh M, Hunder GG, Easley KA, et al. Treatment of giant cell arteritis using induction therapy with high-dose glucocorticoids: a double-blind, placebo-controlled, randomized prospective clinical trial. Arthritis Rheum 2006;54(10): 3310–8.

42. Chevalet P, Barrier JH, Pottier P, et al. A randomized, multicenter, controlled trial using intravenous pulses of methylprednisolone in the initial treatment of simple forms of giant cell arteritis: a one year followup study of 164 patients. J Rheumatol 2000;27(6):1484–91.

43. Gabriel SE, Sunku J, Salvarani C, et al. Adverse outcomes of antiinflammatory therapy among patients with polymyalgia rheumatica. Arthritis Rheum 1997;40: 1873–8.

44. Hochberg MC, Altman RD, April KT, et al. American College of Rheumatology 2012 recommendations for the use of nonpharmacologic and pharmacologic therapies in osteoarthritis of the hand, hip, and knee. Arthritis Care Res 2012; 64:465–74.

45. Caporali R, Cimmino MA, Ferraccioli G, et al. Prednisone plus methotrexate for polymyalgia rheumatica: a randomized, double-blind, placebo-controlled trial. Ann Intern Med 2004;141(7):493–500.

46. Ferraccioli G, Salaffi F, De Vita S, et al. Methotrexate in polymyalgia rheumatica: preliminary results of an open, randomized study. J Rheumatol 1996;23(4):624–8.

47. van der Veen MJ, Dinant HJ, van Booma-Frankfort C, et al. Can methotrexate be used as a steroid sparing agent in the treatment of polymyalgia rheumatica and giant cell arteritis? Ann Rheum Dis 1996;55(4):218–23.

48. Jover JA, Hernandez-Garcia C, Morado IC, et al. Combined treatment of giant-cell arteritis with methotrexate and prednisone. a randomized, double-blind, placebo-controlled trial. Ann Intern Med 2001;134(2):106–14.

49. Spiera RF, Mitnick HJ, Kupersmith M, et al. A prospective, double-blind, randomized, placebo controlled trial of methotrexate in the treatment of giant cell arteritis (GCA). Clin Exp Rheumatol 2001;19(5):495–501.

50. Hoffman GS, Cid MC, Hellmann DB, et al. A multicenter, randomized, double-blind, placebo-controlled trial of adjuvant methotrexate treatment for giant cell arteritis. Arthritis Rheum 2002;46(5):1309–18.

51. Mahr AD, Jover JA, Spiera RF, et al. Adjunctive methotrexate for treatment of giant cell arteritis: an individual patient data meta-analysis. Arthritis Rheum 2007;8:2789–97.
52. De Silva M, Hazleman BL. Azathioprine in giant cell arteritis/polymyalgia rheumatica: a double-blind study. Ann Rheum Dis 1986;45(2):136–8.
53. Schaufelberger C, Andersson R, Nordborg E. No additive effect of cyclosporin A compared with glucocorticoid treatment alone in giant cell arteritis: results of an open, controlled, randomized study. Br J Rheumatol 1998;37(4):464–5.
54. Schaufelberger C, Mollby H, Uddhammar A, et al. No additional steroid-sparing effect of cyclosporine A in giant cell arteritis. Scand J Rheumatol 2006;35(4): 327–9.
55. Lizon F, Vidal E, Barrier J. Does dapsone have a role in the treatment of giant cell arteritis with regard to efficacy and toxicity? Clin Exp Rheumatol 1993;11(8): 694–5.
56. Diamantopoulos AP, Hetland H, Myklebust G. Leflunomide as a corticosteroid-sparing agent in giant cell arteritis and polymyalgia rheumatica: a case series. Biomed Res Int 2013;2013:120638.
57. Kreiner F, Galbo H. Effect of etanercept in polymyalgia rheumatica: a randomized controlled trial. Arthritis Res Ther 2010;12(5):R176.
58. Salvarani C, Macchioni P, Manzini C, et al. Infliximab plus prednisone or placebo plus prednisone for the initial treatment of polymyalgia rheumatica: a randomized trial. Ann Intern Med 2007;146(9):631–9.
59. Seror R, Baron G, Hachulla E, et al. Adalimumab for steroid sparing in patients with giant-cell arteritis: results of a multicentre randomised controlled trial. Ann Rheum Dis 2014;73(12):2074–81.
60. Hoffman GS, Cid MC, Rendt-Zagar KE, et al. Infliximab for maintenance of glucocorticosteroid-induced remission of giant cell arteritis: a randomized trial. Ann Intern Med 2007;146(9):621–30.
61. Martinez-Taboada VM, Rodriguez-Valverde V, Carreno L, et al. A double-blind placebo controlled trial of etanercept in patients with giant cell arteritis and corticosteroid side effects. Ann Rheum Dis 2008;67(5):625–30.
62. Unizony S, Arias-Urdaneta L, Miloslavsky E, et al. Tocilizumab for the treatment of large-vessel vasculitis (giant cell arteritis, Takayasu arteritis) and polymyalgia rheumatica. Arthritis Care Res 2012;64:1720–9.
63. Prieto-González S, Depetris M, García-Martínez A, et al. Positron emission tomography assessment of large vessel inflammation in patients with newly diagnosed, biopsy-proven giant cell arteritis: a prospective, case-control study. Ann Rheum Dis 2014;73(7):1388–92.
64. Nesher G, Berkun Y, Mates M, et al. Low-dose aspirin and prevention of cranial ischemic complications in GCA. Arthritis Rheum 2004;50:1332–7.
65. Lee MS, Smith SD, Galor A, et al. Antiplatelet and anticoagulant therapy in patients with GCA. Arthritis Rheum 2006;54:3306–9.
66. Edwards MJ, Plant GT. Should we prescribe aspirin for patients with GCA? A review of the evidence. Neuroophthalmology 2009;33:1–4.
67. Yale SH, Limper AH. Pneumocystis carinii pneumonia in patients without acquired immunodeficiency syndrome: associated illness and prior corticosteroid therapy. Mayo Clin Proc 1996;71:5–13.
68. Kermani TA, Ytterberg SR, Warrington KJ. Pneumocystis jiroveci pneumonia in GCA: a case series. Arthritis Care Res 2011;63:761–5.

Corticosteroids in Antineutrophil Cytoplasmic Antibody–Associated Vasculitis

Sarah F. Keller, MD[a], Eli M. Miloslavsky, MD[b],*

KEYWORDS

- Glucocorticoids • ANCA-associated vasculitis • Granulomatosis with polyangiitis
- Microscopic polyangiitis

KEY POINTS

- Glucocorticoids (GCs) are an important component of antineutrophil cytoplasmic anti-body–associated vasculitis (AAV) treatment, in part because of their rapid onset of action.
- Intravenous GCs are important to consider in severe AAV, although the evidence base for their use is limited.
- There is considerable variation in the duration of GC therapy, ranging from less than 6 months to more than 24 months.
- Local GCs can be an important adjunctive treatment of sinonasal, ocular, and subglottic disease, but are generally not sufficient as monotherapy.
- Studies are currently underway examining the dose and duration of GC therapy in AAV as well as the effectiveness of GC-sparing therapies.

INTRODUCTION

Antineutrophil cytoplasmic antibody (ANCA)-associated vasculitides (AAV) are a group of conditions associated with inflammation of small and medium-sized blood vessels. This article focuses on the 2 major categories of AAV, granulomatosis with polyangiitis (GPA; formerly Wegener's granulomatosis) and microscopic polyangiitis.

Disclosures: Dr S.F. Keller has nothing to disclose. Dr E.M. Miloslavsky has received research support from Genentech (#224513).
[a] Department of Medicine, Massachusetts General Hospital, 55 Fruit Street, Boston, MA 02114, USA; [b] Division of Rheumatology, Department of Medicine, Yawkey Center for Outpatient Care, Massachusetts General Hospital, Harvard Medical School, Suite 2C, Boston, MA 02114, USA
* Corresponding author.
E-mail address: emiloslavsky@mgh.harvard.edu

Glucocorticoids (GCs) have been the cornerstone of AAV management therapy since the 1950s.[1–4] Long before cytotoxic agents became the mainstay of management, GCs were relied on as the primary treatment modality in AAV. Several case reports and patient series highlight the early role of GCs in AAV and their ability to reduce disease activity.[5,6] Historical studies showed that untreated systemic vasculitis is typically fatal. However 5-year survival rates increased from less than 15% to 48% when GC therapy was used.[4]

In 1971, Fauci and colleagues[7] published the first experience with the use of cyclophosphamide in GPA. Subsequent studies showed that the addition of cyclophosphamide to prednisone leads to remission in more than 90% of cases.[6,8,9] Most patients are now able to achieve clinical remission with cyclophosphamide-based, rituximab-based, or methotrexate-based regimens. However, GCs remain a mainstay of therapy, in part because of their rapid onset of action.[10] It is notable that despite major advances in the treatment of AAV, mortality still exceeds that of the general population, with most deaths having causes other than active vasculitis.[8] Therefore, in order to achieve successful outcomes, a careful balance between GC treatment efficacy and toxicity must be achieved.

Herein we discuss the current role of GCs in various phases of AAV treatment, including remission induction, maintenance therapy, treatment of relapses, and the local use of GCs. We also review current controversies relating to GC use as well as research efforts that seek to reduce GC toxicity in AAV.

REMISSION INDUCTION THERAPY

A critical goal in the treatment of AAV is achieving rapid and durable remission with minimal toxicity. According to the European League Against Rheumatism (EULAR), remission is defined as "the complete absence of disease activity attributable to active vasculitis."[11,12] When choosing the initial treatment regimen for remission induction of active disease (whether caused by new-onset vasculitis or disease relapse), clinicians must decide whether to administer GCs as an intravenous (IV) pulse (typically 500–1000 mg daily for 3 days), what starting dose of GCs to use, and how to reduce oral GCs, maintaining a balance between efficacy and toxicity. Despite extensive experience with GCs in AAV, there is no published consensus on induction dosing or tapering schedules.

Intravenous Glucocorticoids

The question of whether GCs should be initially administered as an IV or oral formulation in AAV is most relevant when treating severe disease. Definitions of severe disease have differed in the literature and may be defined as a Five-Factor Score of 1 or more,[13] a Birmingham Vasculitis Activity Score for Wegener Granulomatosis with 1 major item or greater than 3 points,[14] or as "disease that poses an immediate threat to either the patient's life or vital organ function."[15,16] Although definitions of severe AAV vary, generally pulse GCs are considered in patients who have glomerulonephritis, diffuse alveolar hemorrhage, mesenteric ischemia, and central or peripheral nervous system involvement, such as mononeuritis multiplex.[2,17] In addition, pulse GCs should be considered if there is insufficient response or progression of disease despite high-dose oral GCs.

Little is known about the comparative efficacy of IV GCs. Support for pulse GCs arose from a study by Bolton and Sturgill[18] that retrospectively analyzed 63 patients with acute crescentic rapidly progressive glomerulonephritis. Forty-six patients received pulse GCs (at a dose of 30 mg/kg, maximum daily dose of 3 g, every other day for 3 days), resulting in fewer patients on dialysis, substantial decrease in creatinine levels, and overall improved disease compared with patients receiving oral GCs. In AAV, pulse GCs have been compared with plasma exchange and oral GCs in a randomized trial that showed improved renal survival in the plasma exchange arm; however, no studies directly comparing IV and oral GCs have been conducted in AAV to date.[19]

Despite the lack of studies examining treatment with pulse GCs, many experts support the use of IV GCs in the treatment of severe AAV. An examination of treatment protocols of recent randomized controlled trials in AAV shows that many have required the use of pulse GCs during remission induction, including Rituximab versus Cyclophosphamide for ANCA-Associated Vasculitis (RAVE), Rituximab versus Cyclophosphamide in ANCA-Associated Renal Vasculitis (RITUXVAS), and Azathioprine or Methotrexate Maintenance for ANCA-Associated Vasculitis (WEGENET).[14,20–22] Other investigators have left the choice of pulse GCs up to the treating physician.[15–17,23,24] However, some studies that included patients with severe disease used only oral GCs, including the Pulse versus Daily Oral Cyclophosphamide for Induction of Remission in Antineutrophil Cytoplasmic Antibody-Associated Vasculitis (CYCLOPS) trial.[25,26] Therefore, although many clinicians advocate the use of pulse GCs, an absolute consensus on this question does not yet exist.

Several questions with respect to pulse GCs have yet to be answered. Does the use of IV GCs halt disease progression and lead to better outcomes; for example, with respect to renal recovery? Do pulse GCs lead to more durable remissions or the ability to taper oral GCs faster? Do pulse steroids cause more GC-related adverse events? A study of patients with giant cell arteritis (GCA) by Mazlumzadeh and colleagues[27] provides some insight into some of these questions. In this study, patients were randomized to receive IV pulse GCs or oral GCs. Patients in the IV pulse group were able to reduce GCs more rapidly, received a significantly reduced cumulative dose of oral prednisone compared with the group that did not receive IV GCs (5636 mg vs 7860 mg; $P = .001$), and had fewer relapses. However, when the IV dose of GCs was taken into account, the total GC dose received by patients in the two groups was similar. Although additional studies are needed to assess the role of IV GCs in GCA, similar studies are needed in AAV to clarify the utility of pulse GCs for remission induction of severe disease.

Oral Glucocorticoids

No prospective studies comparing different GC tapering regimens have been conducted in AAV. Examination of GC tapering strategies in AAV clinical trials shows that the rate and duration of tapers varies substantially. **Fig. 1** shows the GC treatment schedules used in several major randomized controlled trials that enrolled patients with severe disease. Regardless of whether or not the treatment protocol included an IV pulse, oral steroid regimens were started at 1.0 mg/kg/day, and typically tapered to 30 to 40 mg/day by month 1 and 10 to 20 mg/day by 3 months. The rate of further decreases depended largely on the duration of GC therapy. The RAVE and Wegener's Granulomatosis Etanercept (WGET) trials used the most rapid tapering regimens, tapering prednisone to 5 mg by 4 months and discontinuing GCs by 5 to 6 months, assuming that remission was reached and maintained.[14,15] However, in trials in which GCs were continued until 18 to 24 months, prednisone dosing varied from 5 mg per day to 12.5 mg per day at the 6-month time point (**Fig. 2**).[20,21,23–25]

Several other considerations with respect to the use of oral GCs in AAV deserve mention. Disease that is localized or nonsevere may respond to lower dose GCs than are shown in **Fig. 1**. For example, patients with nonsevere disease relapses in

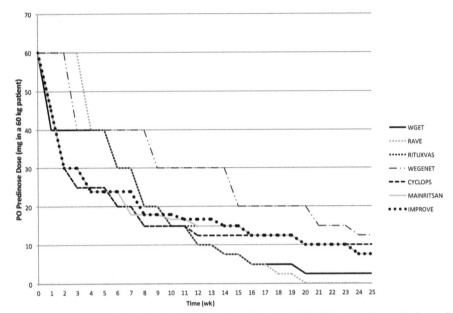

Fig. 1. GC tapering schedules during remission induction. CYCLOPS, Pulse Versus Daily Oral Cyclophosphamide for Induction of Remission in Antineutrophil Cytoplasmic Antibody-Associated Vasculitis: a randomized trial; IMPROVE, Mycophenolate Mofetil Versus Azathioprine for Remission Maintenance in Antineutrophil Cytoplasmic Antibody-Associated Vasculitis: a randomized controlled trial; MAINRITSAN, Rituximab Versus Azathioprine for Maintenance in ANCA-Associated Vasculitis; WGET, Wegener Granulomatosis Etanercept.

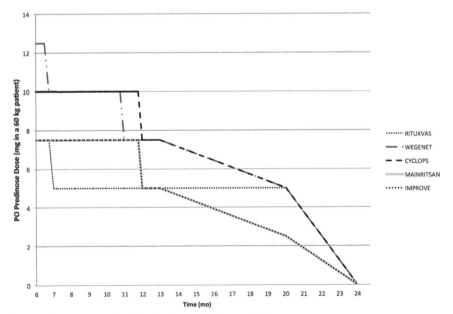

Fig. 2. GC tapering schedules during remission maintenance.

the RAVE trial were treated with a median dose of prednisone of 17.5 mg (range, 2.5–80 mg) and a shorter GC tapering schedule.[28] Prophylaxis against *Pneumocystis jiroveci* pneumonia (PJP) should be considered in all patients with AAV during remission induction, particularly those receiving high-dose GCs (0.5–1 mg/kg). The risk of PJP in AAV has been shown to be higher than in several other rheumatologic conditions.[29] The reasons for this may be several, including the need for multiple immunosuppressive agents, use of high-dose GCs with prolonged tapers, and the nature of the disease itself.[30]

MAINTENANCE THERAPY

Most patients with AAV are able to achieve remission with current treatment regimens. However, managing patients in remission, particularly with respect to GC dosing, remains a major therapeutic challenge. Considerable practice variation with regard to duration of GC treatment currently exists (see **Fig. 2**). As discussed previously, clinical trials have used GC regimens ranging in duration from less than 6 months to more than 24 months. In order to determine the optimal duration of GC use in AAV maintenance therapy it is important to balance the risks and benefits of GCs.

To understand the benefits of GCs in the maintenance of remission it is critical to determine whether or not prolonged treatment with GCs prevents disease relapse. Several studies have investigated this controversial topic. A retrospective study by McGregor and colleagues[31] compared rates of relapse, end-stage renal disease (ESRD), and mortality in patients receiving GCs beyond 6 months of treatment with those in whom GCs were discontinued by 6 months. Their single-center analysis revealed that there was no statistically significant difference in time to relapse, relapse-free survival, ESRD, or death among patients in the two groups. However, they detected an increase in infection and new-onset diabetes in patients who received GC maintenance therapy beyond 6 months. Similarly, a recently published randomized trial by Pagnoux and colleagues[32] in patients 65 years and older with AAV compared a 9-month course of GCs with 26 months, both in conjunction with reduced-dose cyclophosphamide. There was no difference in the percentage of patients achieving remission or experiencing a relapse. However, patients in the prolonged GC arm experienced more adverse events. In contrast, a meta-analysis of 13 trials by Walsh and colleagues[33] concluded that patients enrolled in trials that used longer courses of GCs had fewer relapses. Specifically, the investigators found that in studies in which the GC target dose was zero, there were 3-fold more relapses than in studies with a nonzero target dose. Furthermore, the investigators concluded that earlier withdrawal of GCs (defined as discontinuation of GC use before 12 months) was associated with increased relapses. Given the conflicting results of previous studies, a randomized controlled trial, The Assessment of Prednisone in Remission (TAPIR) trial, is currently underway and will enroll patients with GPA in remission on 5 mg/day of prednisone and randomize them to continue prednisone at 5 mg/day or to discontinue prednisone.[34] This study is designed to contribute important information to the debate about the use of low-dose GCs in remission maintenance. Although there is no consensus on duration of GC treatment, pending results of the TAPIR study, our practice is to discontinue prednisone by 6 months in patients in remission.

The possible benefits of continuing GCs must be balanced against possible toxicities, including those associated with low-dose GCs. GC toxicity has not been examined specifically in the AAV population to date, therefore what is known about this topic is extrapolated from other patient populations whose risk of GC toxicity may be different than that of patients with AAV. Nevertheless, several studies suggest that GCs at doses that are considered low may lead to morbidity. For example, del Rincón and colleagues[35] found that a dosage of prednisone of more than 8 mg/day was associated with an increase in all-cause mortality in patients with rheumatoid arthritis. Examining the risk of infection in patients treated with GCs, Dixon and colleagues[36] showed that prednisone, even at doses as low as 5 mg, was associated with an increased risk of infection and that the risk increased with longer duration of treatment. In contrast, some experts have argued that there is little evidence linking low-dose GCs and morbidity.[37] Further studies of GC toxicity, particularly in patients with AAV, are needed to better assess the risks and benefits of using low-dose prednisone for maintenance of disease remission.

TREATMENT OF RELAPSES

Although most patients with AAV are able to achieve remission, relapses remain common over long-term follow-up.[24,38,39] Most such relapses are nonsevere and do not pose immediate threats to major organs.[15,25,26] Treatment of nonsevere relapses has not been studied extensively in AAV and one treatment strategy that has been used in such instances has been to increase GCs without changing the non-GC immunosuppressive regimen. This strategy was used in the RAVE trial, in which nonsevere relapses were treated with a prednisone increase at the discretion of the investigator followed by a prespecified taper with decreases every 2 weeks until tapering off completely.[28] Using this strategy led to remission in 80% of patients; however, 70% of patients had a second relapse within a mean of 9.4 months. Although additional studies are needed to investigate the optimal treatment of nonsevere relapses, data from the RAVE trial suggest that a short-term increase in GCs without changing the background immunosuppression may lead to unacceptably high rates of subsequent relapse. Our practice is to treat nonsevere relapses with a change in the background non-GC immunosuppression or an increase in the dose (if using methotrexate or azathioprine) in combination with a short-term increase in GC dose followed by a taper.

LOCAL GLUCOCORTICOIDS

Local GCs may be a useful adjunct in the treatment of subglottic stenosis, sinus disease, and ocular manifestations of AAV. Subglottic stenosis of the trachea occurs in up to 23% of all patients diagnosed with AAV and can be refractory to immunosuppressive therapy, although some reports document improvement with immunosuppression.[40] Endoscopic dilation has been used to treat subglottic stenosis occurring in a variety of diseases, such as tracheal cancers, tracheal compression, sarcoidosis, and GPA.[41–44] Single-center series have shown that adding intralesional GCs to dilation is effective and can be repeated safely to maintain patency of the trachea.[40] Randomized studies of intralesional GCs in addition to dilation are needed to establish whether this modality leads to more effective results and prolongs time to restenosis.

Local GCs can be used as an adjunctive treatment of sinonasal disease. GC nasal rinses, such as saline with budesonide inhalation suspension, can have utility, although little literature is available on their efficacy.[45] Topical GCs can also be used as adjunctive treatment in ocular inflammatory disease, including episcleritis, scleritis, and uveitis; however, concomitant systemic therapy is usually necessary to prevent additional disease manifestations, even if the ocular disease responds to topical therapy.[46]

FUTURE CONSIDERATIONS

With expanding treatment options in AAV, several ongoing studies are investigating regimens designed to reduce GC toxicity, during both induction and maintenance of remission. Several non-GC treatment options are being investigated during remission induction for their potential role in GC sparing. The Plasma Exchange and Glucocorticoids for Treatment of AAV (PEXIVAS) trial is comparing a reduced-dose GC regimen with and without plasma exchange with a conventional GC regimen in patients with severe renal disease or pulmonary hemorrhage.[47] Treatment with plasma exchange has previously been shown to be potentially more effective than IV GC pulse[19]; however, its ability to spare oral GCs has not previously been investigated. Therefore PEXIVAS may further clarify the role of plasma exchange and its ability to spare GCs in severe AAV.

Efforts are also underway to identify an agent that has the potential to replace GCs in the treatment of active AAV. The alternative complement pathway may play an important role in AAV pathogenesis.[48] The development of an oral complement C5a receptor inhibitor (CCX 168) has led to the first study to use a GC-free treatment regimen in ANCA-associated renal vasculitis. The currently ongoing phase II CLEAR (C5aR Inhibitor on Leukocytes Exploratory ANCA-associated Renal Vasculitis) trial is using two treatment arms with CCX 168 in conjunction with IV cyclophosphamide (administered at a dosage of 15 mg/kg every 2 to 3 weeks): one arm with low-dose prednisone and the other with no GCs. The comparator arm is standard therapy with IV cyclophosphamide and high-dose prednisone.[49] A second phase II study of CCX 168 CLASSIC (Clinical ANCA Vasculitis Safety and Efficacy Study of Inhibitor C5aR) trial - is examining CCX 168 in conjunction with IV cyclophosphamide or rituximab and low-dose prednisone compared with standard therapy with high-dose GCs and cyclophosphamide or rituximab.[50] Although GCs are likely to remain a necessary treatment option in AAV, at least in the near future, efforts to replace GCs are also ongoing in other diseases that have historically relied on GC-based regimens. For example, Condon and colleagues[51] investigated a GC-free remission induction regimen in lupus nephritis with promising results. In addition, Stone and colleagues[52,53] are currently conducting a study to determine whether tocilizumab, an interleukin 6 inhibitor, is able to reduce the need for GCs in GCA.

Limiting disease relapses is important for minimizing lifetime exposure to GCs because GC use is considerably increased in patients with relapses.[54] Identifying the most effective remission maintenance agent has been a considerable focus of research in AAV over the past 2 decades. Since the US Food and Drug Administration's approval of rituximab for remission induction in AAV, several studies are investigating the efficacy of rituximab in the maintenance of remission. Building on the retrospective experience with continuous B-cell depletion,[55–57] and the positive outcome of the MAINRITSAN (Rituximab Versus Azathioprine for Maintenance in ANCA-Associated Vasculitis study), which showed superiority of fixed-dose rituximab to azathioprine,[23] MAINRITSAN II and RITAZAREM (Rituximab Vasculitis Maintenance Study) seek to further elucidate the role of rituximab in remission maintenance. RITAZAREM is investigating an alternate fixed-dose rituximab regimen compared with azathioprine,[58] whereas MAINRITSAN II is investigating several rituximab dosing strategies, including one driven by B-cell counts and ANCA titers.[59]

As new therapies with the potential to replace or limit GCs are investigated, the ability to measure their GC-sparing potential has become increasingly important. The accurate measurement of GC toxicity in patients with AAV will allow investigators to document not only the dose of GCs spared but the adverse events that were avoided as a result of using GC-sparing medications. This information is critical in assessing both the medical and the economic utility of such agents. To date, clinical trials have not systematically measured GC-related toxicity in a comprehensive fashion. EULAR has attempted to address this by identifying a set of adverse events that should be monitored during clinical trials in order to better capture GC toxicity.[60] As clinicians weigh the costs and benefits of new agents, a better understanding of GC toxicity is necessary.

SUMMARY

GCs have revolutionized the treatment of AAV and continue to be an important component of AAV management, both in remission induction and remission maintenance. However, there is considerable variation in their use, with treatment regimens ranging from less than 6 months to more than 24 months. Given considerable treatment-related morbidity and mortality, refining the role of GCs is becoming increasingly important. Studies are currently underway examining the dose and duration of GC therapy in AAV as well as the effectiveness of GC-sparing therapies.

REFERENCES

1. Jennette JC, Falk RJ. Small-vessel vasculitis. N Engl J Med 1997;337(21): 1512–23.
2. Lally L, Spiera R. Current landscape of antineutrophil cytoplasmic antibody-associated vasculitis: classification, diagnosis, and treatment. Rheum Dis Clin North Am 2015;41(1):1–19, vii.
3. Bacon PA. Therapy of vasculitis. J Rheumatol 1994;21(5):788–90.
4. Fauci AS, Katz P, Haynes BF, et al. Cyclophosphamide therapy of severe systemic necrotizing vasculitis. N Engl J Med 1979;301(5):235–8.
5. Moore P, Beard E, Thoburn T, et al. Idiopathic (lethal) granuloma of the midline facial tissues treated with cortisone: report of a case. Laryngoscope 1951; 61(4):320–31.
6. Walton E. Giant-cell granuloma of the respiratory tract (Wegener's granulomatosis). Br Med J 1958;2(5091):265–70.
7. Fauci AS, Wolff SM, Johnson JS. Effect of cyclophosphamide upon the immune response in Wegener's granulomatosis. N Engl J Med 1971;285(27):1493–6.
8. Flossmann O, Berden A, de Groot K, et al. Long-term patient survival in ANCA-associated vasculitis. Ann Rheum Dis 2011;70(3):488–94.
9. Fauci AS, Haynes BF, Katz P, et al. Wegener's granulomatosis: prospective clinical and therapeutic experience with 85 patients for 21 years. Ann Intern Med 1983;98(1):76–85.
10. Rhen T, Cidlowski JA. Antiinflammatory action of glucocorticoids—new mechanisms for old drugs. N Engl J Med 2005;353(16):1711–23.
11. Hellmich B, Flossmann O, Gross WL, et al. EULAR recommendations for conducting clinical studies and/or clinical trials in systemic vasculitis: focus on anti-neutrophil cytoplasm antibody-associated vasculitis. Ann Rheum Dis 2007; 66(5):605–17.
12. Mukhtyar C, Hellmich B, Jayne D, et al. Remission in antineutrophil cytoplasmic antibody-associated systemic vasculitis. Clin Exp Rheumatol 2006;24(6 Suppl 43). S-93-8.
13. Guillevin L, Lhote F, Gayraud M, et al. Prognostic factors in polyarteritis nodosa and Churg-Strauss syndrome. A prospective study in 342 patients. Medicine (Baltimore) 1996;75(1):17–28.

14. Stone JH, Merkel PA, Spiera R, et al. Rituximab versus cyclophosphamide for ANCA-associated vasculitis. N Engl J Med 2010;363(3):221–32.
15. Wegener's Granulomatosis Etanercept Trial (WGET) Research Group. Etanercept plus standard therapy for Wegener's granulomatosis. N Engl J Med 2005;352(4): 351–61.
16. WGET Research Group. Design of the Wegener's Granulomatosis Etanercept Trial (WGET). Control Clin Trials 2002;23(4):450–68.
17. Stone JH. Limited versus severe Wegener's granulomatosis: baseline data on patients in the Wegener's granulomatosis etanercept trial. Arthritis Rheum 2003; 48(8):2299–309.
18. Bolton WK, Sturgill BC. Methylprednisolone therapy for acute crescentic rapidly progressive glomerulonephritis. Am J Nephrol 1989;9(5):368–75.
19. Jayne DR, Gaskin G, Rasmussen N, et al. Randomized trial of plasma exchange or high-dosage methylprednisolone as adjunctive therapy for severe renal vasculitis. J Am Soc Nephrol 2007;18(7):2180–8.
20. Jones RB, Tervaert JWC, Hauser T, et al. Rituximab versus cyclophosphamide in ANCA-associated renal vasculitis. N Engl J Med 2010;363(3):211–20.
21. Pagnoux C, Mahr A, Hamidou MA, et al. Azathioprine or methotrexate maintenance for ANCA-associated vasculitis. N Engl J Med 2008;359(26):2790–803.
22. Specks U, Merkel PA, Seo P, et al. Efficacy of remission-induction regimens for ANCA-associated vasculitis. N Engl J Med 2013;369(5):417–27.
23. Guillevin L, Pagnoux C, Karras A, et al. Rituximab versus azathioprine for maintenance in ANCA-associated vasculitis. N Engl J Med 2014;371(19):1771–80.
24. Hiemstra TF, Walsh M, Mahr A, et al. Mycophenolate mofetil vs azathioprine for remission maintenance in antineutrophil cytoplasmic antibody-associated vasculitis: a randomized controlled trial. JAMA 2010;304(21):2381–8.
25. De Groot K, Harper L, Jayne DRW, et al. Pulse versus daily oral cyclophosphamide for induction of remission in antineutrophil cytoplasmic antibody-associated vasculitis: a randomized trial. Ann Intern Med 2009;150(10): 670–80.
26. Jayne D, Rasmussen N, Andrassy K, et al. A randomized trial of maintenance therapy for vasculitis associated with antineutrophil cytoplasmic autoantibodies. N Engl J Med 2003;349(1):36–44.
27. Mazlumzadeh M, Hunder GG, Easley KA, et al. Treatment of giant cell arteritis using induction therapy with high-dose glucocorticoids: a double-blind, placebo-controlled, randomized prospective clinical trial. Arthritis Rheum 2006;54(10): 3310–8.
28. Miloslavsky EM, Specks U, Merkel PA, et al. Outcomes of non-severe relapses in ANCA-associated vasculitis treated with glucocorticoids. Arthritis Rheumatol 2015;67(6):1629–36.
29. Ward MM, Donald F. *Pneumocystis carinii* pneumonia in patients with connective tissue diseases: the role of hospital experience in diagnosis and mortality. Arthritis Rheum 1999;42(4):780–9.
30. Sowden E, Carmichael AJ. Autoimmune inflammatory disorders, systemic corticosteroids and pneumocystis pneumonia: a strategy for prevention. BMC Infect Dis 2004;4:42.
31. McGregor JG, Hogan SL, Hu Y, et al. Glucocorticoids and relapse and infection rates in anti-neutrophil cytoplasmic antibody disease. Clin J Am Soc Nephrol 2012;7(2):240–7.
32. Pagnoux C, Quéméneur T, Ninet J, et al. Treatment of systemic necrotizing vasculitides in patients aged sixty-five years or older: results of a multicenter, open-label,

randomized controlled trial of corticosteroid and cyclophosphamide-based induction therapy. Arthritis Rheumatol 2015;67(4):1117–27.

33. Walsh M, Merkel PA, Mahr A, et al. Effects of duration of glucocorticoid therapy on relapse rate in antineutrophil cytoplasmic antibody-associated vasculitis: a meta-analysis. Arthritis Care Res (Hoboken) 2010;62(8):1166–73.

34. Merkel PA, University of Pennsylvania. The Assessment of Prednisone in Remission trial—center of excellence approach (TAPIR). Bethesda (MD): National Library of Medicine (US); 2000. Available at: ClinicalTrials.gov. Accessed June 1, 2015.

35. del Rincón I, Battafarano DF, Restrepo JF, et al. Glucocorticoid dose thresholds associated with all-cause and cardiovascular mortality in rheumatoid arthritis. Arthritis Rheumatol 2014;66(2):264–72.

36. Dixon WG, Abrahamowicz M, Beauchamp M-E, et al. Immediate and delayed impact of oral glucocorticoid therapy on risk of serious infection in older patients with rheumatoid arthritis: a nested case-control analysis. Ann Rheum Dis 2012; 71(7):1128–33.

37. Da Silva JAP, Jacobs JWG, Kirwan JR, et al. Safety of low dose glucocorticoid treatment in rheumatoid arthritis: published evidence and prospective trial data. Ann Rheum Dis 2006;65(3):285–93.

38. De Groot K, Rasmussen N, Bacon PA, et al. Randomized trial of cyclophosphamide versus methotrexate for induction of remission in early systemic antineutrophil cytoplasmic antibody-associated vasculitis. Arthritis Rheum 2005;52(8):2461–9.

39. Springer J, Nutter B, Langford CA, et al. Granulomatosis with polyangiitis (Wegener's): impact of maintenance therapy duration. Medicine (Baltimore) 2014;93(2): 82–90.

40. Hoffman GS, Thomas-Golbanov CK, Chan J, et al. Treatment of subglottic stenosis, due to Wegener's granulomatosis, with intralesional corticosteroids and dilation. J Rheumatol 2003;30(5):1017–21.

41. Solans-Laqué R, Bosch-Gil J, Canela M, et al. Clinical features and therapeutic management of subglottic stenosis in patients with Wegener's granulomatosis. Lupus 2008;17(9):832–6.

42. Holle JU, Voigt C, Both M, et al. Orbital masses in granulomatosis with polyangiitis are associated with a refractory course and a high burden of local damage. Rheumatology (Oxford) 2013;52(5):875–82.

43. Kopstein AB, Kristopaitis T, Gujrati TM, et al. Orbital Wegener granulomatosis without systemic findings. Ophthal Plast Reconstr Surg 1999;15(6):467–9.

44. Nouraei SAR, Sandhu GS. Outcome of a multimodality approach to the management of idiopathic subglottic stenosis. Laryngoscope 2013;123(10):2474–84.

45. Pagnoux C, Wolter NE. Vasculitis of the upper airways. Swiss Med Wkly 2012; 142:w13541.

46. Schmidt J, Pulido JS, Matteson EL. Ocular manifestations of systemic disease: antineutrophil cytoplasmic antibody-associated vasculitis. Curr Opin Ophthalmol 2011;22(6):489–95.

47. Merkel P. Plasma Exchange and Glucocorticoids for Treatment of Anti-Neutrophil Cytoplasm Antibody (ANCA) - Associated Vasculitis (PEXIVAS).

48. Flint SM, McKinney EF, Smith KGC. Emerging concepts in the pathogenesis of antineutrophil cytoplasmic antibody-associated vasculitis. Curr Opin Rheumatol 2015;27(2):197–203.

49. ChemoCentryx. Clinical trial to evaluate safety and efficacy of CCX168 in ANCA-associated vasculitis. Bethesda (MD): National Library of Medicine (US); 2000. Available at: ClinicalTrials.gov. Accessed June 1, 2015.

50. ChemoCentryx. A study to evaluate the safety and efficacy of CCX168 in subjects with ANCA-associated vasculitis. Bethesda (MD): National Library of Medicine (US); 2000. Available at: ClinicalTrials.gov. Accessed June 1, 2015.
51. Condon MB, Ashby D, Pepper RJ, et al. Prospective observational single-centre cohort study to evaluate the effectiveness of treating lupus nephritis with rituximab and mycophenolate mofetil but no oral steroids. Ann Rheum Dis 2013; 72(8):1280–6.
52. Unizony SH, Dasgupta B, Fisheleva E, et al. Design of the tocilizumab in giant cell arteritis trial. Int J Rheumatol 2013;2013:912562.
53. Collinson N, Tuckwell K, Habeck F, et al. Development and implementation of a double-blind corticosteroid-tapering regimen for a clinical trial. Int J Rheumatol 2015;2015:589841.
54. Miloslavsky EM, Specks U, Merkel PA, et al. Rituximab for the treatment of relapses in antineutrophil cytoplasmic antibody-associated vasculitis. Arthritis Rheumatol 2014;66(11):3151–9.
55. Pendergraft WF, Cortazar FB, Wenger J, et al. Long-term maintenance therapy using rituximab-induced continuous B-cell depletion in patients with ANCA vasculitis. Clin J Am Soc Nephrol 2014;9(4):736–44.
56. Cartin-Ceba R, Golbin JM, Keogh KA, et al. Rituximab for remission induction and maintenance in refractory granulomatosis with polyangiitis (Wegener's): ten-year experience at a single center. Arthritis Rheum 2012;64(11):3770–8.
57. Smith RM, Jones RB, Guerry M-J, et al. Rituximab for remission maintenance in relapsing antineutrophil cytoplasmic antibody-associated vasculitis. Arthritis Rheum 2012;64(11):3760–9.
58. Jayne D, Cambridge University Hospitals NHS Foundation Trust. Rituximab Vasculitis Maintenance Study (RITAZAREM). Bethesda (MD): National Library of Medicine (US); 2000. Available at: ClinicalTrials.gov. Accessed June 1, 2015.
59. Assistance Publique – Hôpitaux de Paris. Comparison study of two rituximab regimens in the remission of ANCA associated vasculitis (MAINRITSAN 2). Bethesda (MD): National Library of Medicine (US); 2000. Available at: ClinicalTrials.gov. Accessed June 1, 2015.
60. Van der Goes MC, Jacobs JWG, Boers M, et al. Monitoring adverse events of low-dose glucocorticoid therapy: EULAR recommendations for clinical trials and daily practice. Ann Rheum Dis 2010;69(11):1913–9.

Corticosteroids in Myositis and Scleroderma

Anna Postolova, MD, MPH[a], Jennifer K. Chen, MD[b], Lorinda Chung, MD, MS[a,c],*

KEYWORDS

- Idiopathic inflammatory myopathies • Myositis • Systemic sclerosis • Scleroderma
- Morphea • Corticosteroids • Glucocorticoids

KEY POINTS

- Treatment with corticosteroids is the standard of care for idiopathic inflammatory myopathies with muscle and organ involvement.
- Extracutaneous features of scleroderma occasionally warrant treatment with corticosteroids; however, high doses have been associated with the development of scleroderma renal crisis in high-risk patients.
- Corticosteroid monotherapy is not recommended for cutaneous manifestations of dermatomyositis and scleroderma.
- The significant side effect profile of corticosteroids encourages concomitant treatment with other immunosuppressive medications to enable timely tapering.

IDIOPATHIC INFLAMMATORY MYOPATHIES
Background and Clinical Manifestations

Idiopathic inflammatory myopathies (IIMs) are rare systemic diseases that involve muscle inflammation and manifest clinically as an insidious onset of weakness over weeks to months. IIMs are classified based on the patterns of presentation and immunohistopathologic features on skin and muscle biopsy into 4 major categories: dermatomyositis (DM), polymyositis (PM), inclusion body myositis (IBM), and immune-mediated necrotizing myopathy (IMNM).[1]

Disclosures: The authors have no relationships to disclose.
[a] Division of Rheumatology and Immunology, Stanford University School of Medicine, 300 Pasteur Drive, Stanford, CA 94305, USA; [b] Department of Dermatology, Stanford Hospital and Clinics, 450 Broadway Street, Pavilion C, Suite 242, Redwood City, CA 94063, USA; [c] Division of Rheumatology, VA Palo Alto Health Care System, 3801 Miranda Avenue, Palo Alto, CA 94304, USA
* Corresponding author. Division of Rheumatology, VA Palo Alto Health Care System, 3801 Miranda Avenue, Palo Alto, CA 94304.
E-mail address: Shauwei@stanford.edu

Rheum Dis Clin N Am 42 (2016) 103–118
http://dx.doi.org/10.1016/j.rdc.2015.08.011
0889-857X/16/$ – see front matter Published by Elsevier Inc.

rheumatic.theclinics.com

Diagnostic Evaluation

Increased serum levels of muscle enzymes (aspartate aminotransferase, alanine aminotransferase, creatine kinase [CK], aldolase, and lactate dehydrogenase) are present in at least 90% of patients with an IIM.[2] Although CK is the most sensitive and specific marker of muscle damage, patients can have increased levels of aldolase or other muscle enzymes without accompanying increases in CK levels.[2]

Further evaluation with electromyography (EMG), magnetic resonance imaging (MRI), and muscle biopsy may be necessary to identify evidence of muscle inflammation.[1,2] EMG activity depends on the degree of inflammation.[2] MRI can detect muscle necrosis, degeneration, and inflammation through increased signal intensity on short tau inversion recovery (STIR) imaging.[2,3] T1-weighted images identify atrophy and chronic muscle damage, whereas T2-weighted images can identify active inflammation.[3] Muscle biopsies show inflammatory infiltrates, vascular involvement, and necrosis, depending on the subtype of IIM. Additional evaluation for extramuscular involvement and cancer screening may be warranted depending on the subtype of IIM.[1]

Classification Criteria for Idiopathic Inflammatory Myopathy

The most commonly used classification criteria for PM and DM was proposed by Bohan and Peter[4] in 1975 and includes (1) symmetric proximal muscle weakness; (2) increased muscle enzyme levels; (3) a myopathic pattern on EMG; (4) muscle biopsy showing myofiber necrosis, regeneration, variation in fiber diameter, and an inflammatory exudate; and (5) characteristic skin findings (DM). The American College of Rheumatology (ACR) and European League Against Rheumatism (EULAR) are currently validating updated classification criteria, which include weakness involving particular muscle groups, hallmark cutaneous manifestations, and specific muscle biopsy findings.[5]

Treatment Options

Systemic corticosteroids (CS) are the most commonly used medications for IIM with muscle involvement, either as monotherapy or in combination with other immunomodulatory agents.[6–8] The significant side effect profile of CS, including myopathy, avascular necrosis of the bone, osteoporosis, hyperglycemia, infection, and cataract formation, motivates a multitherapy treatment plan with the goal of minimizing CS dose.[7]

POLYMYOSITIS
Background and Clinical Manifestations

PM presents with bilateral, symmetric proximal muscle weakness that progresses over weeks to months.[1,2] Neck flexor weakness, dysphagia, and dysphonia can occur from pharyngeal and laryngeal muscle involvement. Interstitial lung disease (ILD) can affect 5% to 46% of patients with PM and up to 70% to 100% of those with antisynthetase syndrome.[9] This syndrome consists of fever, mechanic's hands, Raynaud phenomenon (RP), myositis, ILD, and arthritis, and is frequently associated with the anti–Jo-1 antibody.[1] In addition, patients with PM have a 2-fold increase in the incidence of malignancy compared with the general population within the first 5 years of disease onset.[2]

Diagnostic Evaluation

Up to a 50-fold increase in CK levels can be observed in active PM.[3] More than half of patients with PM present with myositis-associated (MAA) or myositis-specific antibodies (MSA) (**Table 1**).[10,11] EMG of affected muscles shows short-duration, low-amplitude, polyphasic motor unit potentials.[2] Muscles with active inflammation show irritable myopathy with spontaneous activity (positive sharp waves and fibrillation potentials) and/or complex repetitive discharges.[2] MRI may show edema and increased signal in the muscles on T2-weighted imaging. In addition, characteristic muscle biopsy findings of PM include scattered necrotic and regenerating myofibers of variable size, perivascular and endomysial inflammatory infiltrates of major histocompatibility complex (MHC-I)/CD8+ T-cell complexes, and macrophages without microvascular involvement.[3,6]

Treatment

Corticosteroids

Although no randomized controlled trials using CS have been conducted, studies have shown decreased muscle inflammation with CS use,[12,13] and 60% to 80% of patients show improvement in muscle strength.[1,6,7] Initial treatment usually consists of oral prednisone (0.5–1.5 mg/kg/d), with intravenous (IV) methyprednisolone treatment (500–1000 mg/d for 3–5 days) reserved for severe cutaneous disease or muscle weakness, dysphagia, respiratory muscle involvement, and ILD.[1,8,9] One randomized controlled trial comparing monthly oral pulse dexamethasone (6 cycles of 40 mg/d for 4 consecutive days at 28-day intervals) with daily prednisolone (70–90 mg/d) for 28 days followed by a slow taper, did not show improved efficacy with pulse dosing, but did show fewer adverse effects.[14] High-dose (60–80 mg/d) oral prednisone treatment is usually continued for 2 to 4 weeks with slow tapers extending for 3 to 6 months.[1,6] In patients with severe disease and ILD, or in patients with comorbidities such as osteoporosis and diabetes, combination therapy with another immunosuppressant is initiated immediately.[9]

Corticosteroid-sparing options

Another immunosuppressive drug is typically started concurrently with CS to enable timely tapering of the CS (**Table 2**).[1] Azathioprine (AZA) in combination with prednisone has been shown to result in less functional disability and lower CS dosing at 3 years compared with prednisone monotherapy.[1] When AZA/CS combination therapy was compared with methotrexate (MTX)/CS, both had similar efficacy, but MTX was better tolerated.[8] In addition, cyclosporine has been shown to be as effective as MTX for myositis, with favorable outcomes for treatment of ILD.[1,9] Mycophenolate mofetil (MMF) has also shown efficacy and tolerability, and is generally considered the CS-sparing drug of choice when PM is complicated by ILD.[1,9] A growing body of evidence supports the use of IV immunoglobulin (IVIG) for more severe disease presentations, including dysphagia, respiratory muscle involvement, and refractory cases.[1] Cyclophosphamide (CYC) may be required for recalcitrant cases and patients with significant cardiac or pulmonary disease.[1,9] In addition, data from the Rituximab in Myositis Trial, the largest randomized placebo-controlled myositis trial to date, showed that 83% of patients treated with rituximab experienced disease improvement and required less CS.[15]

DERMATOMYOSITIS
Background and Clinical Manifestations

DM has pathognomonic cutaneous features including heliotrope rash, periorbital edema, Gottron papules, Gottron sign, shawl sign, holster sign, mechanic's hands, malar erythema, and nail-fold capillary changes (**Fig. 1**).[1] Euwer and Sontheimer[16] described the variable presentations of DM as symptomatic myositis with evidence

Table 1
Myositis-associated and myositis-specific autoantibodies

Antibody	Antigen	Frequency (%)	Disease Associations	Clinical Associations
Myositis-associated Autoantibodies				
Anti-56 kDa	Ribonucleoprotein component	Up to 90	Overlap syndromes	—
Anti-U1-RNP	U1 small nuclear ribonucleoprotein	12	Myositis-SLE Myositis-SSc	Erosive arthritis, alopecia, ILD, oral ulcer, rarely renal disease
Anti-Ro/SSA	RNA-protein particle	10–30	Overlap syndromes	Sicca symptoms
Anti-La/SSB	RNA-protein particle	10	Overlap syndromes	Sicca symptoms
Anti-PM-Scl	Nucleolar protein complex	8	50%–60% have myositis-SSc overlap	RP, myositis, calcinosis
Anti-U3-RNP	U3 small nuclear ribonucleoprotein	5	Myositis-SLE Myositis-SSc	—
Anti-Ku	DNA-binding proteins	<1	Myositis-SSc Myositis-SLE	Severe ILD, mild myopathy
Myositis-specific Autoantibodies				
Antisynthetases	—	25–30	PM/DM	Antisynthetase syndrome (myositis, ILD, arthritis, RP, mechanic's hands, fever), acute onset in spring, poor prognosis
Anti-Jo-1	His-tRNA synthetase	25		
Anti-PL-7	Thr-tRNA synthetase	3		
Anti-PL-12	Ala-tRNA synthetase	3		
Anti-OJ	Ile-tRNA synthetase	1		
Anti-EJ	Gly tRNA synthetase	1		
Anti-KS	Asp-tRNA synthetase	1		
Anti-Ha	Tyrl-tRNA synthetase	1		
Anti-Zo	Phe-tRNA synthetase	1		
Anti-Mup44/cN1A	Cytosolic 5′-nucleotidase 1A	30	IBM>PM/DM/IMNM	—
Anti-HMGCR/ Anti-200/100	3-Hydroxy-3-methylguaryl-CoA reductase	3–8	NM IMNM	Acute/subacute presentation, associated with statin use, necrotizing myopathy
Anti-SRP	Signal recognition particle proteins	3–6	PM>DM NM IMNM	Acute onset in fall, cardiac involvement, poor prognosis, necrotizing myopathy
Anti-KJ	Translation factor	<1	PM ILD	—
Anti-Fer	Elongation factor 1-alpha	<1	PM/DM	—
Anti-Mas	Small RNA	<1	PM/DM	—

Abbreviations: HMGCR, 3-Hydroxy-3-methyguaryl-CoA reductase; kDa, kilodalton; RNP, ribonucleoprotein; SLE, systemic lupus erythematosus; SRP, signal recog-

Table 2
CS-sparing immunosuppressant treatment options for myositis

Therapy	Route	Dose
Azathioprine	PO	2–3 mg/kg/d divided twice daily
Methotrexate	PO	15–25 mg/wk; single or divided dosing; 1 d/wk dosing
	SQ/IM	20–40 mg/wk; 1 d/wk dosing
Cyclosporine	PO	4–6 mg/kg/d divided twice daily
Tacrolimus	PO	0.1–0.2 mg/kg/d divided twice daily
Mycophenolate Mofetil	PO	2–3 g/d divided twice daily
Cyclophosphamide	PO	1–2 mg/kg/d
	IV	0.5–1 g/m² every 4 wk
Rituximab	IV	750 mg/m² (up to 1 g), repeat in 2 wk; course repeated every 6–9 mo
IVIG	IV	2 g/kg divided over 2–5 d every 4 wk

Abbreviations: IM, intramuscular; IVIG, IV immunoglobulin; PO, orally; SQ, subcutaneously.

of muscle inflammation on laboratory, EMG, and biopsy evaluation; a hypomyopathic presentation with asymptomatic muscle inflammation; and an amyopathic variant without muscle symptoms or muscle inflammation for at least 6 months after cutaneous symptoms arise. Similar to PM, extramuscular involvement can occur in DM, with ILD affecting 21% to 78% of patients.[9] Patients with DM (in particular those with amyopathic DM and certain autoantibodies (**Table 3**)) have a 3-fold to 6-fold increased risk for malignancy compared with the general population.[2]

Diagnostic Evaluation

Muscle enzyme levels can be normal or increased up to 50-fold in DM.[6] EMG and MRI findings in active myositis are similar to those seen in PM. Features differentiating DM from PM on muscle biopsy include CD4+ T-cell and B-cell infiltrates in perimysial, perifascicular, and vascular areas causing microangiopathic ischemia.[1] Skin biopsies

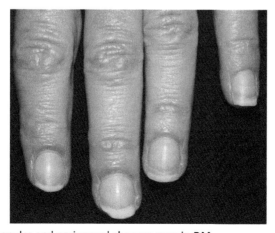

Fig. 1. Gottron papules and periungual changes seen in DM.

Table 3
DM-predominant myosis-specific autoantibodies

Antibody	Antigen	Frequency (%)	Clinical Associations
Anti-MDA5/ CADM140/IFIh1	Melanoma differentiation– associated protein 5	15–30 (in Asian populations)	Mild or no muscle disease, rapidly progressive ILD in Asian populations, poor prognosis, cutaneous ulcers, alopecia, arthritis
Anti-p155/140/ TRIM33/TIF1-γ	Transcriptional intermediary factor 1-γ	20–40	Cancer in adults (60%–80%), widespread/severe skin disease, less ILD
Anti-Mi-2	Nuclear helicase	10–30	Classic skin and muscle disease, good prognosis, low ILD/cancer
Anti-SAE-1/2	SUMO-1 activating enzyme	8	Disease progresses from skin to muscle, dysphagia, good prognosis
Anti-NXP-2/MJ	Nuclear matrix protein 2	10–25	Calcinosis, cancer in men

Abbreviations: CADM, clinically amyopathic DM; IFIH1, interferon-induced helicase C domain-containing protein 1; MDA5, melanoma differentiation-associated protein 5; SAE, small ubiquitin like modifier/SUMO-1 activating enzyme; TIF1-γ, transcriptional intermediary factor 1-gamma; TRIM33, tripartite motif containing 33.

in patients with DM show an interface dermatitis, perivascular lymphocytic infiltrate, epidermal atrophy, basement membrane thickening, increased dermal mucin, and vascular ectasia, which may be indistinguishable from findings in cutaneous lupus.[8] The discovery and phenotypic characterization of novel DM-specific autoantibodies has improved diagnostic and prognostic capabilities, because more than 80% of patients are positive for one of these antibodies, which tend to be mutually exclusive (see **Table 3**).[10,17]

Treatment

Corticosteroids
In cases of DM with muscle and organ involvement, CS are the first line of treatment, with an algorithm similar to PM. However, cutaneous manifestations are often not as responsive to CS as is muscle disease, and skin lesions can flare after discontinuation of CS.[7,8] Steroid-induced myopathy may be confusing as patients develop, rather than present with, symmetric muscle weakness; however, there is no evidence of muscle inflammation, and termination of CS results in improvement in strength.[18] The American Academy of Dermatology[19] recommends topical CS (tCS) under occlusion for patients with limited skin involvement. Lower potency tCS (hydrocortisone 2.5%, desonide 0.05%) are advised for the face, axillae, and groin to decrease the risk for skin atrophy.[7]

Corticosteroid-sparing options
Photoprotective clothing, sunscreen with sun protection factor (SPF) greater than 50, and sun avoidance are vital because cutaneous DM may be worsened by ultraviolet A (UVA)/ultraviolet B (UVB) radiation.[7] Topical calcineurin inhibitors can be used on areas with thinner skin.[7,8] Hydroxychloroquine (HCQ) can be effective for cutaneous DM[7]; however, up to 31% of patients with DM develop a rash to HCQ.[20] In a randomized controlled trial, Dalakas and colleagues[21] showed efficacy of IVIG for both skin

and muscle inflammation in patients with DM. Case series have shown some benefit from MTX, MMF, and AZA for skin and muscle disease.[1,7–9] MMF, CYC, cyclosporine, and rituximab have been used for DM-associated ILD.[1,7,9]

INCLUSION BODY MYOSITIS
Background and Clinical Manifestations

IBM is characterized by the insidious onset of weakness in an asymmetric distribution, involving both proximal and distal extremities.[22] The Griggs diagnostic criteria for IBM include (1) age greater than 45 years, (2) symptom duration greater than or equal to 12 months, (3) CK level less than 15-fold the upper limit of normal, (4) pronounced weakness of the long finger flexors and/or knee extensors, and (5) histology with vacuolization and/or protein accumulation.[23] IBM presents in association with other connective tissues diseases (CTD) in 15% of patients; however, unlike PM and DM, it is not associated with an increased risk of ILD or malignancy.[24]

Diagnostic Evaluation

Myositis-specific and myositis-associated antibodies are not typically observed in IBM; however, antibodies to cytosolic 5'-nucleotidase 1A (anti-Mup44/cN1A antibodies) have been identified in up to 30% of patients.[22] EMG findings are similar to those in PM/DM, but some patients show a mixed neurogenic and myopathic pattern.[25] MRI shows atrophy and signal abnormalities in affected muscle groups.[24] Classic findings on muscle biopsy include CD8+ T-cell infiltration of non-necrotic myofibers, accumulation of abnormal protein aggregates, and the presence of rimmed vacuoles.[22]

Treatment

Corticosteroids
An effective treatment of IBM has yet to be identified. CS can decrease muscle enzyme levels, but do not affect symptoms or disease progression.[22] One study showed decreased inflammatory infiltrates, but increased amyloid deposition on muscle biopsy after CS treatment, which was concerning for disease acceleration.[25] Treatment with CS may be more effective for patients with IBM with an associated CTD.

Corticosteroid-sparing options
Case series with AZA, MTX, and MMF have not shown durable improvement in strength in patients with IBM.[24,25] IVIG can decrease CK levels, but without symptomatic improvement.[25]

NECROTIZING MYOPATHIES
Background and Clinical Presentation

Necrotizing myopathies (NM) present as acute or subacute symmetric, proximal muscle weakness, and are associated with necrosis without significant inflammation on muscle biopsy.[26] NM can be classified as non–immune-mediated NM (NIMNM), triggered by medications or toxins, and immune-mediated NM (IMNM), triggered by CTDs, viruses, cancers, and statin medications in the setting of positive serology.[1,26] In NIMNM, patients experience symptom resolution in several weeks to months after discontinuation of the offending agent.[1] If symptoms persist despite discontinuation of the offending agent, IMNM should be considered.[26] To be classified as having IMNM, patients must fulfill clinical criteria of adult DM or PM, have MSA, have no clinical features of IBM, and have characteristic histologic findings on muscle biopsy.[27]

Diagnostic Evaluation

In statin-induced cases, variable CK level increases can be seen.[1] Sixty percent of patients with antibodies against 3-hydroxy-3-methylglutaryl-coenzyme A reductase (anti-HMGCR) have had prior exposure to statins, suggesting the medication is an immunologic trigger.[28] Patients who were never exposed had an indistinguishable clinical myopathy, evoking a pathomechanistic role of these antibodies in IMNM. Note that 25% to 37% of patients with other IIMs have anti-HMGCR antibodies.[28] Anti–signal recognition particle (anti-SRP) antibodies are also found in up to 15% of cases of IMNM and are associated with more severe disease.[26] Typical histopathologic findings of IMNM include myofiber necrosis, membrane attack complex deposition in small vessels, variable MHC-1 expression, and regeneration of muscle fibers without significant inflammation.[26] NIMNM appears similarly on biopsy, but the immunohistochemical abnormalities are often absent.[26] EMG can show irritable myopathy similar to other IIMs and MRI shows muscle edema, atrophy, or fatty replacement.[26]

Treatment

Corticosteroids

If discontinuation of potentially offending agents does not lead to symptomatic improvement over several weeks and biopsy suggests IMNM, high-dose oral prednisone (40–100 mg/d) or pulse IV methylprednisolone (1 g/d for 3–5 days) is initiated.[26] Grable-Esposito and colleagues[29] reported that 60% of patients with statin–induced anti-HMGCR+ IMNM required long-term immunosuppression for symptom control.

Corticosteroid-sparing options

Similar to other IIMs, small studies suggest that other immunosuppressants, in conjunction with or in lieu of CS, have shown benefit in refractory IMNM cases.[26]

SCLERODERMA: LOCALIZED SCLERODERMA (MORPHEA) AND SYSTEMIC SCLEROSIS

The term scleroderma refers to fibrosis of the skin. Localized scleroderma (morphea) is skin limited, whereas systemic sclerosis (SSc) is associated with vascular and internal organ involvement.[30] Unlike SSc, morphea is not typically associated with RP, nailfold capillary changes, or the presence of SSc-specific autoantibodies (**Table 4**).[31,32]

LOCALIZED SCLERODERMA (MORPHEA)
Background and Clinical Manifestations

In contrast with SSc, morphea is less symmetric, better demarcated, and typically spares the hands.[33] Linear, pansclerotic, and generalized variants are most frequently associated with extracutaneous complications (**Table 5**).[34,35] Morphea lesions have an initial inflammatory stage characterized by erythematous patches or plaques. Over time, the center becomes less erythematous, and the borders develop a violaceous appearance. Most lesions become inactive over 3 to 5 years, gradually softening and leaving behind patches or plaques with postinflammatory hyperpigmentation.[34] Linear morphea tends to have a more chronic course. Reactivation may occur in all subtypes, with one study showing reactivation at the same site in 3.7% of patients after greater than 6 months off medication.[36]

Diagnostic Evaluation

Clinical evaluation is the gold standard for morphea diagnosis and assessment. Although antinuclear antibody (ANA) is the most commonly reported positive autoantibody, this is typically low titer and not considered part of the diagnostic work-up.[31]

Table 4
SSc-associated autoantibodies

Antibody	Frequency (%)	Typical Disease Subtype	Clinical Associations
Anti-centromere	20–38	lcSSc	PAH, digital ulcers, calcinosis
Anti-topoisomerase I	15–42	dcSSc	ILD, cardiac involvement, digital ulcers
Anti-RNA polymerase III	5–31	dcSSc	SRC, tendon friction rubs, synovitis, myositis, joint contractures, malignancy, GAVE
Anti-U1-RNP	2–14	Overlap	RP, puffy fingers, arthritis, myositis, PAH
Anti-Th/To	1–13	lcSSc	ILD, pulmonary hypertension
Anti-PM-Scl	4–11	Myositis-lcSSc	RP, arthritis, myositis, calcinosis
Anti-U3-RNP (fibrillarin)	4–10	dcSSc	African Americans, cardiac involvement, ILD, PAH
Anti-hUBF (NOR 90)	<5	lcSSc	Mild organ involvement
Anti-U11/U12- RNP	3	lcSSc	RP, GI involvement, severe ILD
Anti-Ku	2–4	Myositis-lcSSc	Myositis, arthritis, joint contractures, ILD, dysphagia

Abbreviations: dSSc, diffuse cutaneous SSc; GAVE, gastric antral vascular ectasia; GI, gastrointestinal; lcSSc, limited cutaneous SSc; PAH, pulmonary arterial hypertension; SRC, scleroderma renal crisis.

Other autoantibodies that have been associated with morphea include anti–single-stranded DNA antibodies, antihistone antibodies, and anti–topoisomerase II-a antibodies.[35] In early stage disease, skin biopsies show perivascular lymphocytes in the reticular dermis.[34] In late stages, inflammation disappears and collagen bundles of the reticular dermis become thickened in association with atrophic eccrine glands and a dearth of blood vessels.[34]

Treatment

Corticosteroids
It is important to differentiate active from inactive morphea lesions, because the latter are unlikely to respond to treatment with immunosuppression.[35] Active disease may be indicated by growth or spread of lesions; appearance of new lesions; or clinical signs of inflammation, such as a violaceous or lilac border.

Morphea lesions that are not associated with systemic complications are best treated with topical therapy. Class 1 to 2 high-potency tCS applied twice daily are commonly used[35–37]; however, there have been no studies evaluating their efficacy other than 1 case series showing improvement with topical calcipotriol and betamethasone.[38] Intralesional triamcinolone (5 mg/mL monthly for 3 months) can be used, especially for the treatment of linear morphea of the en coup de sabre variant.[36]

CS may be indicated in cases of morphea associated with risk for functional impairment or systemic complications (see **Table 5**).[39] Methylprednisolone 1 g/d for adults and 30 mg/kg/d (for a maximum of 500 mg/d) for children may be administered intravenously over 3 consecutive days per month for at least 3 months.[40] Oral CS dosing is more variable and may be dosed in the form of prednisone 0.5 to 2 mg/kg/d, with a

Table 5
Subtypes and clinical associations of morphea

Classification	Included Subtypes	Definition	Clinical Pearls	Potential Complications
Plaque	Superficial (morphea en plaque, guttate, keloidal)	Areas of induration limited to epidermis and dermis	Often develop plaques in areas of pressure, such as the waistline, bra line	—
	Deep (morphea profunda, subcutaneous morphea)	Areas of induration including the subcutaneous tissue (may include fascia and muscle); overlying skin may not be involved	Bound-down or pseudocellulite appearance	
Generalized	—	4 or more plaques >3 cm in size, involving 2 or more anatomic areas (head-neck, each extremity, anterior trunk, posterior trunk)	Spares the face and hands	Myalgia, arthralgia, fatigue
Linear	Linear morphea of the extremities	Linear induration involving the dermis and subcutaneous tissue (may involve underlying muscle and bone)	—	Joint contractures, limb length discrepancy, muscle atrophy, muscle cramps, ulcers
	En coup de sabre	Linear induration involving the dermis of the face and scalp (may involve underlying muscle, bone, and central nervous system)	—	Facial disfigurement, central nervous system/ocular involvement, seizure
	Progressive facial hemiatrophy (Parry-Romberg syndrome)	Loss of dermis, subcutaneous tissue, muscle, and bone of the unilateral face	—	Facial disfigurement, central nervous system/ocular involvement, seizure

(continued on next page)

Table 5
(continued)

Classification	Included Subtypes	Definition	Clinical Pearls	Potential Complications
Pansclerotic	—	Circumferential involvement of limbs involving epidermis, dermis, subcutaneous tissue, muscle, and bone; may affect other areas of the body with full-depth sclerosis	—	Joint contractures, muscle atrophy, nonhealing ulcers, squamous cell carcinoma
Mixed	—	Combination of 2 or more subtypes of morphea	—	Arthralgia, decreased range of motion, limb contracture, myalgia

maximum of 50 to 60 mg daily, tapered to 0.25 to 0.5 mg/kg/d maintenance over at least 2 months.[36,41,42] Prednisone monotherapy may be associated with increased rates of relapse[43]; thus, combination treatment with other modalities, usually MTX, is recommended.[40]

Corticosteroid-sparing options
For patients without severe disfigurement or systemic complications, non-CS treatments include topical tacrolimus or calcipotriene (±tCS) under occlusion (**Table 6**).[40,44] Topical imiquimod may be helpful.[40,44] Phototherapy, including psoralen UVA and narrow-band UVB, may be useful for widespread active lesions both as monotherapy and as adjunctive treatment.[40,44]

For patients at risk for significant cosmetic or functional impairment, combination therapy with IV or oral CS and MTX is recommended,[36,40,42,44] with MMF as second-line CS-sparing therapy.[40,44] Variable success has been reported with cyclosporine, abatacept, penicillin, D-penicillamine, photopheresis, bosentan, infliximab, HCQ, and imatinib.[40,44,45]

Table 6
Evidence-based treatment algorithm for morphea

	First Line	Second Line
Uncomplicated morphea	Tacrolimus Calcipotriene ± betamethasone dipropionate Phototherapy (if large body surface area)	Topical imiquimod MTX and systemic CS (if progressing and treatment refractory)
If involving face, crossing joints, or risk of functional impairment	MTX and systemic CS	MMF

SYSTEMIC SCLEROSIS
Background and Clinical Presentation

In 2013 ACR/EULAR revised the classification criteria for SSc to include skin thickening of the fingers or hands, puffy fingers, digital pits and ulcers, telangiectasias, abnormal nail-fold capillaries, pulmonary arterial hypertension (PAH), ILD, RP, and SSc-related autoantibodies.[46] Most patients with SSc experience RP and have nail-fold capillary changes, but the extent of cutaneous fibrosis and the pattern of internal organ involvement is highly variable, correlating to some degree with autoantibody profile.[35] Patients with limited cutaneous SSc (lcSSc) characteristically have skin thickening distal to the elbows and knees with or without facial involvement; however, up to 9% of patients remain sine sclerosis (SSc sine scleroderma).[35,47] Patients with diffuse cutaneous SSc (dcSSc) develop skin thickening proximal to the elbows and knees, which may also involve the trunk.[35]

Organ manifestations in SSc vary depending on cutaneous and autoantibody subtypes (see **Table 4**).[32] Myositis and synovitis are twice as common in patients with dcSSc versus lcSSc. Clinically significant ILD with pulmonary fibrosis is reported in up to 53% of patients with dcSSc and 35% of patients with lcSSc.[48] PAH has a similar occurrence rate between the two subsets and affects 7% to 12% of patients with SSc overall.[48] Gastrointestinal manifestations, including dysphagia and gastroesophageal reflux, occur in 70% to 80% of patients with SSc, and gastric antral vascular ectasia (GAVE) occurs in up to 22% of patients.[48] Cardiac involvement occurs in 10% to 30% of patients.[48] Scleroderma renal crisis (SRC) presenting with progressive renal failure and microangiopathy occurs in 7% to 17% of patients with dcSSc and 2% to 9% of patients with lcSSc.[49]

Diagnostic Evaluation

Basic laboratory evaluation and muscle enzyme levels should be performed on all patients with SSc. Evaluation for SSc-specific antibodies is warranted for diagnostic and prognostic information regarding internal organ involvement (see **Table 4**).[32] Pulmonary function testing and transthoracic echocardiography should be performed at baseline and annually to screen for pulmonary involvement. High-resolution computed tomography (HRCT) is useful for assessing extent and progression of ILD. Right heart catheterization is necessary to confirm the presence of PAH.

Treatment

Treatment of SSc is guided by cutaneous and organ-specific involvement, and as such, this article reviews treatment by organ system, with particular attention to those that may benefit from CS. CS are not used in the treatment of gastrointestinal and vascular manifestations of SSc, including RP, digital ulcers, and PAH, and therefore management of these symptoms is not be discussed here.

Skin

Mild skin disease, limited to the face and fingers, does not warrant systemic therapy.[50] For more severe skin disease, treatment with CS-sparing agents has shown improvement.[50] About a quarter of patients with SSc develop calcinosis.[51]

Corticosteroids Because of lack of efficacy and risk for inducing SRC, particularly in patients with early dcSSc or with RNA polymerase III antibodies, CS are not recommended for cutaneous SSc.[52] Nevertheless, a recent survey reported that 31% of patients with lcSSc and 49% of patients with dcSSc received CS for treatment of various manifestations.[53] Case reports have shown some benefit from intralesional steroids for calcinosis.[51]

Corticosteroid-sparing options MTX and MMF have been shown to be effective for skin disease in small studies.[50] For diffuse, rapidly progressive disease, IVIG, CYC, and rituximab are alternative options.[50] Hematopoietic stem cell transplantation can be considered in patients with rapidly progressive skin disease.[50]

Musculoskeletal

Musculoskeletal involvement in SSc includes painful tendon friction rubs, development of contractures related to tight skin over the joints, or overlap features with inflammatory myopathies and/or arthritis.[50]

Corticosteroids CS are most commonly used as treatment of the inflammatory components of SSc, such as arthritis and myositis. Low doses (10–15 mg daily) of oral prednisone may improve pain control and quality of life.[50] High-dose CS may be necessary to control active myositis, but should be avoided if possible in patients at high risk for SRC.

Corticosteroid-sparing options Treatment of myositis in patients with SSc is similar to that for patients with IIMs. HCQ, MTX, or leflunomide may be helpful for inflammatory arthritis.[30,50] Small studies have shown benefit with tumor necrosis factor inhibitors, IVIG, abatacept, and tocilizumab for SSc-associated arthritis.[30]

Interstitial lung disease

ILD is confirmed by ground-glass opacities or fibrotic changes on HRCT and is associated with depressed forced vital capacity on pulmonary function tests.[30,50] The most prevalent pattern of SSc-ILD is nonspecific interstitial pneumonia (NSIP), seen in up to 78% of cases, followed by usual interstitial pneumonia (UIP) in 25% to 40% of cases.[54,55]

Corticosteroids SSc-ILD is treated with low-dose CS (up to 15 mg oral prednisone daily), usually in conjunction with other immunosuppressants,[55] particularly in patients with NSIP and significant ground-glass opacification.

Corticosteroid-sparing options The use of CYC has evidence-based support for the treatment of SSc-ILD and is recommended based on a placebo-controlled trial that showed improvement in pulmonary function, dyspnea, and quality of life.[56] Given the toxicity associated with CYC, most experts, on completion of the course of CYC, continue maintenance immunosuppression with MMF, and a multicenter trial is underway comparing CYC with MMF as first-line therapy in SSc-ILD.

Scleroderma renal crisis

SRC is defined as rapidly progressive renal failure with or without arterial hypertension.[50] It is associated with dcSSc and anti–RNA polymerase III antibodies. CS treatment (oral prednisone 15 mg daily or higher) during the first 4 years of disease can trigger SRC, often without accompanying hypertension.[52] Although first-line treatment of SRC is angiotensin-converting enzyme (ACE) inhibitor therapy, studies have shown worse outcomes when ACE inhibitors are used prophylactically.[52] There is no role for CS in the treatment of SRC.

SUMMARY

Immunosuppressive therapies remain the mainstay of treatment of IIMs and some manifestations of scleroderma, although randomized controlled trials are limited and most recommendations are guided by clinical practice. Despite an increasing number of available immunosuppressive agents, CS continue to be a first-line treatment of IIMs and some manifestations of scleroderma, especially synovitis, myositis, and ILD. Nonetheless, given the sequelae of long-term CS use, prompt tapering and use of other immunosuppressants for maintenance therapy is recommended.

REFERENCES

1. Ernste FC, Reed AM. Idiopathic inflammatory myopathies: current trends in pathogenesis, clinical features, and up-to-date treatment recommendations. Mayo Clin Proc 2013;88:83–105.
2. Mammen AL. Autoimmune myopathies: autoantibodies, phenotypes and pathogenesis. Nat Rev Neurol 2011;7:343–54.
3. Findlay AR, Goyal NA, Mozaffar T. An overview of polymyositis and dermatomyositis. Muscle Nerve 2015;51(5):638–56.
4. Bohan A, Peter JB, Bowman RL, et al. A computer-assisted analysis of 153 patients with polymyositis and dermatomyositis. Medicine 1977;86:255–86.
5. Tjarnlund A, Bottai M, Rider LG, et al. Progress report on development of classification criteria for adult and juvenile idiopathic inflammatory myopathies. Washington, DC: ACR Annual Meeting. 2012. Abstract.
6. Dimachkie MM, Barohn RJ, Amato AA. Idiopathic inflammatory myopathies. Neurol Clin 2014;32:595–628.
7. Femia AN, Vleugels RA, Callen JP. Cutaneous dermatomyositis: an updated review of treatment options and internal associations. Am J Clin Dermatol 2013; 14:291–313.
8. Strowd LC, Jorizzo JL. Review of dermatomyositis: establishing the diagnosis and treatment algorithm. J Dermatolog Treat 2013;24:418–21.
9. Miller SA, Glassberg MK, Ascherman DP. Pulmonary complications of inflammatory myopathy. Rheum Dis Clin North Am 2015;41:249–62.
10. Tansley SL, Betteridge ZE, McHugh NJ. The diagnostic utility of autoantibodies in adult and juvenile myositis. Curr Opin Rheumatol 2013;25:772–7.
11. Sarkar K, Miller F. Autoantibodies as predictive and diagnostic markers of idiopathic inflammatory myopathies. Autoimmunity 2004;37:291–4.
12. Winkelmann RK, Mulder DW, Lambert EH, et al. Course of dermatomyositis-polymyositis: comparison of untreated and cortisone-treated patients. Mayo Clin Proc 1968;43:545–56.
13. Lundberg I, Kratz AK, Alexanderson H, et al. Decreased expression of interleukin-1alpha, interleukin-1beta, and cell adhesion molecules in muscle tissue following corticosteroid treatment in patients with polymyositis and dermatomyositis. Arthritis Rheum 2000;43:336–48.
14. van de Vlekkert J, Hoogendijk JE, de Haan RJ, et al. Oral dexamethasone pulse therapy versus daily prednisolone in sub-acute onset myositis, a randomised clinical trial. Neuromuscul Disord 2010;20:382–9.
15. Oddis CV, Reed AM, Aggarwal R, et al. Rituximab in the treatment of refractory adult and juvenile dermatomyositis and adult polymyositis: a randomized, placebo-phase trial. Arthritis Rheum 2013;65:314–24.
16. Euwer RL, Sontheimer RD. Amyopathic dermatomyositis (dermatomyositis sine myositis) presentation of six new cases and review of the literature. J Am Acad Dermatol 1991;24:959–66.
17. Ghirardello A, Borella E, Beggio M, et al. Myositis autoantibodies and clinical phenotype. Auto Immun Highlights 2014;5:69–75.

18. Gil B, Merav L, Pnina L, et al. Diagnosis and treatment of clinically amyopathic dermatomyositis (CADM): a case series and literature review. Clin Rheumatol 2015. [Epub ahead of print].
19. Drake LA, Dinehart SM, Farmer ER, et al. Guidelines of care for dermatomyositis. American Academy Dermatology. J Am Acad Dermatol 1996;34: 824–9.
20. Pelle MT, Callen JP. Adverse cutaneous reactions to hydroxychloroquine are more common in patients with dermatomyositis than in patients with lupus erythematosus. Arch Dermatol 2002;138:1231–3.
21. Dalakas MC, Illa I, Dambrosia JM, et al. A controlled trial of high-dose intravenous immune globulin infusions as treatment for dermatomyositis. N Engl J Med 1993; 329:1993–2000.
22. Schmidt J, Dalakas MC. Inclusion body myositis: from immunopathology and degenerative mechanisms to treatment perspectives. Expert Rev Clin Immunol 2013;9:1125–33.
23. Griggs RC, Askanas V, DiMauro S, et al. Inclusion body myositis and myopathies. Ann Neurol 1995;38:705–13.
24. Amato AA, Barohn RJ. Inclusion body myositis: old and new concepts. J Neurol Neurosurg Psychiatry 2009;80:1186–93.
25. Breithaupt M, Schmidt J. Update on treatment of inclusion body myositis. Curr Rheumatol Rep 2013;15:329.
26. Quinn C, Salameh JS, Smith T, et al. Necrotizing myopathies: an update. J Clin Neuromuscul Dis 2015;16:131–40.
27. Hoogendijk JE, Amato AA, Lecky BR, et al. 119th ENMC international workshop: trial design in adult idiopathic inflammatory myopathies, with the exception of inclusion body myositis. Neuromuscul Disord 2004;14:337–45.
28. Christopher-Stine L, Casciola-Rosen LA, Hong G, et al. A novel autoantibody recognizing 200-kd and 100-kd proteins is associated with an immune-mediated necrotizing myopathy. Arthritis Rheum 2010;62:2757–66.
29. Grable-Esposito P, Katzberg HD, Greenberg SA, et al. Immune-mediated necrotizing myopathy associated with statins. Muscle Nerve 2010;41:185–90.
30. Barsotti S, Bellando Randone S, Guiducci S, et al. Systemic sclerosis: a critical digest of the recent literature. Clin Exp Rheumatol 2014;32:S194–205.
31. Nashel J, Steen V. Scleroderma mimics. Curr Rheumatol Rep 2012;14:39–46.
32. Kayser C, Fritzler MJ. Autoantibodies in systemic sclerosis: unanswered questions. Front Immunol 2015;15:167.
33. Laxer RM, Zulian F. Localized scleroderma. Curr Opin Rheumatol 2006;18: 606–13.
34. Fett N, Werth VP. Update on morphea: part I. Epidemiology, clinical presentation, and pathogenesis. J Am Acad Dermatol 2011;64:217–28.
35. Fett N. Scleroderma: nomenclature, etiology, pathogenesis, prognosis, and treatments: facts and controversies. Clin Dermatol 2013;31:432–7.
36. Christen-Zaech S, Hakim MD, Afsar FS, et al. Pediatric morphea (localized scleroderma): review of 136 patients. J Am Acad Dermatol 2008;59:385–96.
37. Nagai Y, Hattori T, Ishikawa O. Unilateral generalized morphea in childhood. J Dermatol 2002;29:435–8.
38. Dytoc MT, Kossintseva I, Ting PT. First case series on the use of calcipotriol-betamethasone dipropionate for morphoea. Br J Dermatol 2007;157:615–8.
39. Unterberger I, Trinka E, Engelhardt K, et al. Linear scleroderma "en coup de sabre" coexisting with plaque-morphea: neuroradiological manifestation

and response to corticosteroids. J Neurol Neurosurg Psychiatry 2003;74: 661–4.

40. Zwischenberger BA, Jacobe HT. A systematic review of morphea treatments and therapeutic algorithm. J Am Acad Dermatol 2011;65:925–41.

41. Zulian F, Martini G, Vallongo C, et al. Methotrexate treatment in juvenile localized scleroderma: a randomized, double-blind, placebo-controlled trial. Arthritis Rheum 2011;63:1998–2006.

42. Torok KS, Arkachaisri T. Methotrexate and corticosteroids in the treatment of localized scleroderma: a standardized prospective longitudinal single-center study. J Rheumatol 2012;39:286–94.

43. Joly P, Bamberger N, Crickx B, et al. Treatment of severe forms of localized scleroderma with oral corticosteroids: follow-up study on 17 patients. Arch Dermatol 1994;130:663–4.

44. Fett N, Werth VP. Update on morphea: part II. Outcome measures and treatment. J Am Acad Dermatol 2011;64:231–42.

45. Stausbol-Gron B, Olesen AB, Deleuran B, et al. Abatacept is a promising treatment for patients with disseminated morphea profunda: presentation of two cases. Acta Derm Venereol 2011;91:686–8.

46. van den Hoogen F, Khanna D, Fransen J, et al. 2013 classification criteria for systemic sclerosis: an American College of Rheumatology/European League against Rheumatism collaborative initiative. Arthritis Rheum 2013;65:2737–47.

47. Poormoghim H, Lucas M, Fertig N, et al. Systemic sclerosis sine scleroderma: demographic, clinical, and serologic features and survival in forty-eight patients. Arthritis Rheum 2000;43:444–51.

48. Walker UA, Tyndall A, Czirjak L, et al. Clinical risk assessment of organ manifestations in systemic sclerosis: a report from the EULAR Scleroderma Trials And Research Group database. Ann Rheum Dis 2007;66:754–63.

49. Gabrielli A, Avvedimento EV, Krieg T. Scleroderma. N Engl J Med 2009;360: 1989–2003.

50. Shah AA, Wigley FM. My approach to the treatment of scleroderma. Mayo Clin Proc 2013;88:377–93.

51. McMahan ZH, Hunners LK. Systemic sclerosis—challenges for clinical practice. Nat Rev Rheumatol 2013;9:90–100.

52. Steen VD. Kidney involvement in systemic sclerosis. Presse Med 2014;43: e305–14.

53. Hunzelmann N, Moinzadeh P, Genth E, et al. High frequency of corticosteroid and immunosuppressive therapy in patients with systemic sclerosis despite limited evidence for efficacy. Arthritis Res Ther 2009;11:R30.

54. Wells AU, Margaritopoulos GA, Antoniou KM, et al. Interstitial lung disease in systemic sclerosis. Semin Respir Crit Care Med 2014;35:213–21.

55. Schoenfeld SR, Castelino FV. Interstitial lung disease in scleroderma. Rheum Dis Clin North Am 2015;41:237–48.

56. Tashkin DP, Elashoff R, Clements PJ, et al. Cyclophosphamide versus placebo in scleroderma lung disease. N Engl J Med 2006;354:2655–66.

Corticosteroids in Sarcoidosis

Marc A. Judson, MD

KEYWORDS

- Sarcoidosis • Corticosteroids • Treatment • Toxicity

KEY POINTS

- Corticosteroids are almost universally effective for the treatment of sarcoidosis. The treatment of sarcoidosis is indicated if the disease causes a dangerous health situation or significantly impairs the patient's quality of life.
- Treatment should not be based on biomarkers of active granulomatous inflammation.
- Pulmonary sarcoidosis can usually be adequately treated with modest doses of corticosteroids.
- It is unusual for patients to be refractory to corticosteroid therapy. Alternative medications are almost exclusively used because of the frequent development of corticosteroid toxicity.

INTRODUCTION

Corticosteroids are considered the drug of choice for the treatment of almost all forms of sarcoidosis. Nonetheless, there is considerable controversy and confusion concerning the use of corticosteroids in the management of sarcoidosis for several reasons. First, sarcoidosis may be a self-limiting disease that may spontaneously remit and/or never cause significant clinical problems. In such patients, toxicity from corticosteroid treatment may cause more harm than that caused by the natural course of the disease. Second, the optimal dose of corticosteroids has not been established for sarcoidosis. Third, the duration of therapy depends on the natural course of the disease, which is highly variable and often unpredictable. Fourth, the indications for adding a corticosteroid-sparing agent have not been standardized. This article discusses an approach to corticosteroid therapy in sarcoidosis based on the available clinical data plus our understanding of the disease.

Division of Pulmonary and Critical Care Medicine, Albany Medical College, MC-91, Albany, NY 12208, USA
E-mail address: judsonm@mail.amc.edu

Rheum Dis Clin N Am 42 (2016) 119–135
http://dx.doi.org/10.1016/j.rdc.2015.08.012   **rheumatic.theclinics.com**
0889-857X/16/$ – see front matter © 2016 Elsevier Inc. All rights reserved.

INDICATIONS TO TREAT SARCOIDOSIS

There are 2 indications for the treatment of sarcoidosis: (1) the development of a dangerous health situation; and (2) significant worsening of quality of life. **Table 1** lists several situations of danger resulting from sarcoidosis. Note that many of these relate to the development of fibrosis, which, unlike active granulomatous inflammation, is not corticosteroid responsive. Furthermore, most of the entities listed in **Table 1** are rare manifestations of sarcoidosis. Therefore, the overwhelmingly most common reason to treat sarcoidosis is for significant worsening of quality of life. **Fig. 1** shows the processes leading to significant quality-of-life impairment in sarcoidosis.[1] First, granulomatous inflammation occurs. This inflammation may not lead to any physiologic disturbance or the development of significant symptoms. For example, patients with pulmonary sarcoidosis who have bilateral hilar adenopathy and a normal lung parenchyma (stage I radiograph) often have no pulmonary symptoms, normal pulmonary function, and a benign clinical course.[2,3] Even if sarcoidosis causes a physiologic disturbance, it may have no significant clinical consequences and cause minimal to no symptoms.[4,5] Therefore, markers of active granulomatous inflammation, such as increased angiotensin-converting enzyme levels, pulmonary opacities on lung imaging, and positive PET scans, are not indications for treatment. Neither are the asymptomatic minor pulmonary function abnormalities that are very typically observed.[4,5] Note that the presence of quality-of-life impairment is a necessary but insufficient requirement for the treatment of sarcoidosis because (1) pulmonary symptoms may be caused by an alternative process, or (2) the quality-of-life impairment may be the result of previous granulomatous inflammation resulting in fibrosis that does not respond to antigranulomatous therapy.[6] Identifying biomarkers of granulomatous inflammation and physiologic abnormalities may provide useful evidence to support

Table 1 Dangerous health situations from sarcoidosis		
Conditions	**Estimated Frequency (%)**	**Corticosteroid Responsive**
Sudden death, severe arrhythmia, severe left ventricular dysfunction from cardiac sarcoidosis	1	Yes
End-stage fibrocystic sarcoidosis (FVC<50% of predicted)	<5	No or minimally
Sarcoidosis-associated pulmonary hypertension	5	No
Optic neuritis	<5	Yes
Severe neurosarcoidosis	1	Yes
Hemoptysis from pulmonary mycetoma	<1	No
Vitamin D dysregulation causing renal failure, severe nephrolithiasis	<1	Yes
Upper airway obstruction	<1	Usually surgical resection is required if airway obstruction is critical
Endobronchial airway obstruction	<1	Usually not (significant fibrosis present)

Abbreviation: FVC, forced vital capacity.

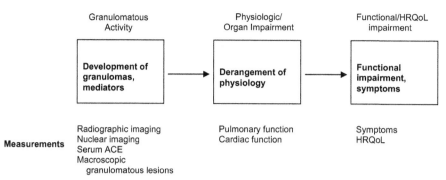

Fig. 1. The processes leading to significant quality-of-life impairment in sarcoidosis. Granulomatous inflammation may lead to physiologic/organ impairment that may lead to functional impairment/worse quality of life. Evidence of granulomatous inflammation and physiologic/organ impairment are insufficient grounds for the treatment of sarcoidosis. ACE, angiotensin-converting enzyme; HRQoL, health-related quality of life. (*Adapted from* Judson MA. The treatment of pulmonary sarcoidosis. Respir Med 2012;106(10):1353; with permission.)

or refute that sarcoidosis is the cause of the quality-of-life impairment. **Fig. 2** outlines a general algorithm for the decision to treat sarcoidosis.

Not only may corticosteroid treatment of asymptomatic or minimally symptomatic sarcoidosis create a risk of corticosteroid toxicity with minimal potential for clinical benefit, it may increase the likelihood of relapse. It is thought that granulomatous inflammation is an attempt by the host to clear a nondegradable antigen.[7] Therefore, the granulomatous inflammation of sarcoidosis may be a beneficial process. Antigranulomatous therapy may prevent a putative sarcoidosis antigen from being cleared, resulting in relapse when the antigranulomatous therapy is withdrawn. As evidence that this theoretic schema may be clinically relevant, studies have shown that patients with sarcoidosis receiving corticosteroid therapy have a higher rate of relapse than

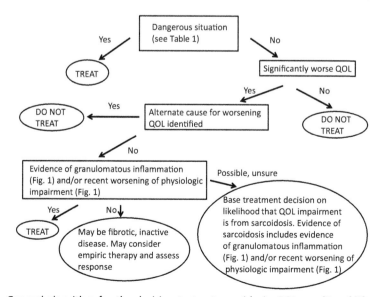

Fig. 2. General algorithm for the decision to treat sarcoidosis. QOL, quality of life.

those who are observed without antisarcoidosis therapy.[8] In addition, in a study of patients with sarcoidosis who were all treated with corticosteroids, those who relapsed received a higher mean dose (17.0 vs 10.6 mg of prednisolone; $P<.05$; N = 82).[9] These data add further support to withholding therapy in patients with active sarcoidosis who are not experiencing a potentially dangerous clinical condition, significant symptoms, or a significant quality-of-life impairment. Such patients should be closely monitored to ensure that these situations do not develop.

GENERAL APPROACH TO THE TREATMENT OF SARCOIDOSIS WITH CORTICOSTEROIDS

Corticosteroids are the initial drug of choice for the treatment of most forms of sarcoidosis because they are almost universally effective and a significant response is quickly observed, usually in a matter of a few weeks or less.[10] Alternative antisarcoidosis therapies, including methotrexate[11] antimalarials,[12] and others,[13] usually require several months to achieve a meaningful response. In addition, most alternative antisarcoidosis medications when used as monotherapy are effective as sole agents less than half of the time,[11,14,15] and, therefore, are most commonly used as corticosteroid-sparing agents.

Issues of Dose

Many of the toxicities of corticosteroids are cumulative, including weight gain and cataract formation. Other side effects may develop rapidly but continue to progress over time, such as bone loss and fluid retention. Therefore, although the corticosteroid dose-response curve for the treatment of sarcoidosis may be maximized at a dose near to or more than 20 mg of prednisone equivalent per day, a lower dose may be optimal to balance the benefits of corticosteroids versus their risks (**Fig. 3**). The optimal dose of corticosteroids depends in part on the form of sarcoidosis that is being treated, and this is discussed in detail later.

Issues of Duration

In addition to the corticosteroid dose, the duration of corticosteroid therapy is an important issue in terms of the treatment of sarcoidosis. It is important to recognize that the treatment of sarcoidosis with corticosteroids or other therapies may not affect the natural course of the disease.[16,17] As previously mentioned, sarcoidosis granulomas probably develop as a response to clear a foreign antigen, as is true for most other granulomatous diseases. Antigranulomatous therapy may impair

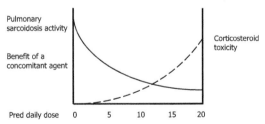

Fig. 3. The effect of corticosteroid dose (milligrams) on sarcoidosis activity (*solid line*) versus the risks of corticosteroid toxicity (*dashed line*). The need for an additional agent is related to the level of sarcoidosis activity (*solid line*). The optimal dose of corticosteroids that suppresses granulomatous activity while leading to minimal corticosteroid side effects may be near the intersection of these two lines, or at approximately 10 mg of daily prednisone in this example. Pred, prednisone.

that clearance process and thus could potentially prolong the disease. To that end, adequate therapy for sarcoidosis may be more a matter of the duration of therapy than the use of specific medications or specific doses. As long as the duration of an antisarcoidosis regimen exceeds the length of time necessary to clear the antigen, the therapy will be effective.[6] In contrast, if the regimen is discontinued while the antigen is still present, the patient will relapse (**Fig. 4**). Because the duration of sarcoidosis is highly variable and unpredictable, it is problematic to determine how long corticosteroid therapy should be continued. All biomarkers of granulomatous activity (eg, angiotensin-converting enzyme levels, lung nodules on chest imaging) are suppressed by resolution of granulomatous inflammation.[18–20] However, these biomarkers do not reliably predict relapse when therapy is withdrawn.[20] Therefore, presently, the most reliable method to determine whether the duration of therapy for sarcoidosis is adequate is to taper and discontinue therapy and monitor the patient to determine whether the patient relapses (**Fig. 5**). There is some indirect evidence that serum interleukin-2 receptor and PET scanning may be biomarkers of sarcoidosis activity that are impervious to effective therapy,[21] but this conjecture remains unproved.

Issues of When to Add Additional Agents to Corticosteroids

A corollary of the above discussion concerning the duration of antisarcoidosis therapy is that, because corticosteroid toxicity is cumulative, a longer duration of corticosteroid therapy is associated with increasing risks to the patient. Therefore, the indications for corticosteroid-sparing medications for sarcoidosis are most dependent on the required duration of corticosteroid therapy (see **Fig. 5**). It is much less common for alternative agents to be needed for sarcoidosis because the disease is truly refractory to corticosteroids.[11,22]

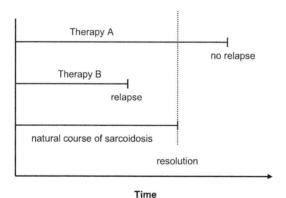

Time

Fig. 4. Evidence suggests that antisarcoidosis therapy does not affect the natural course of sarcoidosis. Two antisarcoidosis therapies are shown that are effective in controlling the granulomatous inflammation of sarcoidosis. The duration of one of these therapies (therapy A) exceeds the natural course of the disease, whereas the other (therapy B) does not. Although both therapies are effective, therapy A does not lead to relapse and therapy B leads to relapse, not because of superior efficacy of therapy A compared with therapy B but because the duration of therapy A exceeded the duration of the disease, whereas the duration of therapy B failed to exceed the duration of disease. (*Adapted from* Judson MA. The treatment of pulmonary sarcoidosis. Respir Med 2012;106(10):1355; with permission.)

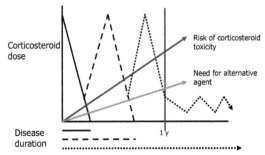

Fig. 5. Three natural courses of sarcoidosis: (1) disease of short duration (*solid line* below the X-Y axis); (2) moderate duration of less than 1 year (*dashed line* below the X-Y axis); and (3) long duration of greater than 1 year (*dotted line* below the X-Y axis). The longer the disease duration, the more failed attempts at successful corticosteroid taper trials (*solid, dashed, and dotted graphs*). The risk of corticosteroid toxicity (*blue arrow*), and hence the need for a corticosteroid-sparing agent (*green arrow*), increases over time.

CORTICOSTEROID THERAPY FOR SPECIFIC FORMS OF SARCOIDOSIS
Pulmonary Sarcoidosis

A Delphi study of sarcoidosis experts reached a consensus that corticosteroids are the drug of choice for the treatment of pulmonary sarcoidosis.[23] The American Thoracic Society/European Respiratory Society/World Association of Sarcoidosis and Other Granulomatous Diseases consensus statement recommends a daily prednisone equivalent of 20 to 40 mg for the initial treatment of pulmonary sarcoidosis.[24] It is recommended that this dose be continued for at least 1 to 3 months and then tapered to a dose of 5 to 10 mg/d for a total of 1 year before discontinuing.[24] The rationale for a total of 1 year of therapy is based on the unproven assumption that relapses are common with regimens with shorter courses. The rationale for reducing the maintenance prednisone dose to a low level relates to the observation that, after the initial burst of corticosteroid therapy, most patients with pulmonary sarcoidosis can be maintained on a small dose. Other similar dosing regimens for pulmonary sarcoidosis have also been proposed (**Fig. 6**).[25] Because there is a significant risk of relapse and

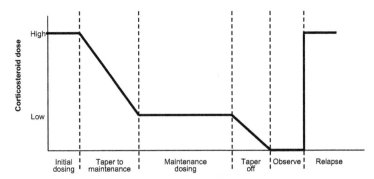

Fig. 6. The 6 phases of sarcoidosis treatment with corticosteroids: (1) initial therapy that is often moderate to high dose; (2) taper to a maintenance dose; (3) maintenance dose; (4) attempt to taper off; (5) observe off therapy (if corticosteroids can be discontinued); (6) increase corticosteroids if there is relapse. The need for corticosteroid-sparing agents depends on the duration of corticosteroid therapy (see **Fig. 5**) as well as the risks of corticosteroid toxicity.

the natural course of the disease is unpredictable, any algorithm to taper corticosteroids for pulmonary sarcoidosis must be individualized based on the specific response of the patient.[25,26]

It is our opinion that the lower range of the recommended prednisone dose is very effective for the initial treatment of pulmonary sarcoidosis, and may avoid or lessen corticosteroid toxicity. A retrospective analysis of treatment of 36 patients with acute pulmonary exacerbations of sarcoidosis who received 20 mg of prednisone per day was universally successful in returning pulmonary symptoms and spirometry to baseline levels.[10] A double-blind randomized placebo-controlled trial performed more than 4 decades ago showed a significant improvement in pulmonary sarcoidosis after 3 months of 15 mg of prednisone daily.[27] These data suggest that an initial dose of corticosteroids for the treatment of pulmonary sarcoidosis may be 20 mg of prednisone per day or even less. This dose seems quite effective and lessens the likelihood and severity of corticosteroid side effects. Although alternate-day corticosteroid therapy has been advocated as minimizing corticosteroid side effects,[24,28–30] this has never formally been studied in sarcoidosis.

The use of inhaled corticosteroids for the treatment of pulmonary sarcoidosis is controversial. A meta-analysis concerning the use of inhaled corticosteroids for pulmonary sarcoidosis did not clearly show a benefit.[16] A Delphi study of sarcoidosis experts reached a consensus that inhaled corticosteroids should not be used routinely to treat acute pulmonary sarcoidosis.[23] Inhaled corticosteroids have been advocated for sarcoidosis-associated cough, although conclusive evidence for improvement of this symptom has not been shown.[26] One well-designed study suggesting that inhaled corticosteroids may have some long-term benefit for the treatment of sarcoidosis was a double-blind randomized placebo-controlled trial of 189 recently diagnosed patients with pulmonary sarcoidosis who received either 3 months of systemic corticosteroids alone (prednisolone 20 mg/d tapered to 10 mg/d) followed by 15 months of high-dose budesonide (800 μg twice daily) or 3 months of oral placebo followed by 15 months of inhaled placebos. The active treatment group had modest improvements in spirometry and diffusing capacity at 18 months in only the patients with stage II chest radiographs (hilar adenopathy plus parenchymal lung opacities).[31] Although the clinical significance of these physiologic improvements could be argued, follow-up at 5 years showed that the stage II patients who received active therapy had significantly fewer exacerbations requiring corticosteroid treatment.[32] In assessing the available evidence, we do not recommend the routine use of inhaled corticosteroids for the treatment of pulmonary sarcoidosis. We believe that inhaled corticosteroids may have a role in selected situations, such as in patients with significant cough without significant pulmonary dysfunction, or possibly as a corticosteroid-sparing agent.

Cardiac Sarcoidosis

The criteria for the treatment of cardiac sarcoidosis remain unresolved. Symptomatic patients, those with significant arrhythmias and heart blocks, should be treated. It remains to be determined whether patients with asymptomatic cardiac sarcoidosis, such as those detected serendipitously on imaging studies, require treatment. As previously mentioned, it is a general principle that patients with sarcoidosis should not be treated for asymptomatic granulomatous inflammation. However, because cardiac sarcoidosis is a potentially life-threatening condition, some clinicians advocate an aggressive treatment approach for such patients. A recent study of asymptomatic cardiac sarcoidosis detected on nuclear magnetic imaging found that such patients had a very low risk of significant cardiac events.[33] Some electrophysiology experts have suggested performing programmed electrical stimulation studies in patients with sarcoidosis, even if asymptomatic, for risk stratification for serious cardiac events.[34] However, this approach has not yet been validated. A Delphi study of cardiac sarcoidosis experts did not reach a consensus concerning the treatment of asymptomatic cardiac sarcoidosis or using programmed electrical stimulation studies in such patients.[35]

Corticosteroids are the first-line agents for the treatment of cardiac sarcoidosis because they have high efficacy, and there is usually a short delay in obtaining a significant response.[36] Corticosteroids have been shown to improve all manifestations of cardiac sarcoidosis, including left ventricular dysfunction, ventricular tachycardia, and atrioventricular block.[36–38] Corticosteroids probably improve survival from cardiac sarcoidosis.[37,39]

Although the evidence supporting corticosteroids as the cornerstone of treatment of cardiac sarcoidosis is irrefutable, the optimal dosing regimen remains undetermined. Although many clinicians advocate higher doses, such as 1 mg/kg/d, of prednisone as initial therapy,[36] others recommend 30 mg/d of prednisone based on a longitudinal study showing no difference in the prognosis of cardiac sarcoidosis between those treated with at least 40 mg/d of prednisone and those receiving 30 mg/d or less.[39] Although there is no supporting evidence, it is rational to consider higher doses of corticosteroids in high-risk situations, such as symptomatic ventricular tachycardia and a severe acute decline in left ventricular function, to ensure that the dose is maximized. A Delphi study of cardiac sarcoidosis experts reached a consensus that 30 to 40 mg of daily prednisone should be the initial treatment dose for cardiac sarcoidosis.[35]

Skin Sarcoidosis

Skin sarcoidosis causes no significant morbidity or mortality. It rarely causes pain or pruritus.[40] Therefore, the main indication for the treatment of skin sarcoidosis is cosmetic importance of the lesions to the patient.[40] Skin sarcoidosis lesions are classified as specific when the histologic examination shows typical granulomatous inflammation of sarcoidosis.[41] Nonspecific sarcoidosis skin lesions show a nondiagnostic (nongranulomatous) inflammatory reaction pattern on histologic evaluation. Nonspecific skin lesions are often associated with acute presentations of sarcoidosis and, in general, portend a good prognosis.[41] The prototypical nonspecific sarcoidosis skin lesion is erythema nodosum, which is often associated with Lofgren syndrome.[42] The treatment of specific sarcoidosis skin lesions is discussed later.

Topical corticosteroids may be considered for a single or a few sarcoidosis skin lesions of concern. Although potent topical corticosteroids such as clobetasol propionate cream and halobetasol propionate ointment have shown benefit for skin sarcoidosis,[43,44] they are often not completely effective,[44] probably because the corticosteroid cannot penetrate deep into the dermis, which may contain the bulk of the skin lesion. Intralesional injections of corticosteroids such as triamcinolone may be more effective than topical preparations.[45,46] Even ultrasound delivery (phonophoresis) of corticosteroid has been reported to be effective.[47] However, all these topical therapies are impractical for widespread disease,[45] and there is a concern for the development of skin atrophy with chronic use.

Systemic corticosteroids are the treatment of choice for generalized or highly disfiguring skin sarcoidosis.[45,48,49] An initial dose of 20 to 60 mg/d of daily prednisone equivalent has been recommended,[45] although we recommend initiating therapy at the lower end of that dose range because this is not a life-threatening form of the disease and the dose can always be increased if the response is inadequate. Antimalarials such as chloroquine and hydroxychloroquine,[50,51] methotrexate,[11,52] and the tetracyclines[13] have been shown to be beneficial for skin sarcoidosis in case series. However, these drugs often work slowly over a range of several months to more than 1 year. Therefore, in severe cases in which there is a high likelihood of requiring chronic therapy, concomitant initial therapy with corticosteroids plus 1 or more of these alternative agents may be considered so that the alternative agent may reach a therapeutic level in the skin as quickly as possible, minimizing the time until corticosteroids can be tapered.

Lupus pernio (**Fig. 7**), or disfiguring facial sarcoidosis, is especially problematic to treat. It may be relatively refractory to corticosteroid therapy.[53] In a large retrospective review of treatment regimens for lupus pernio, corticosteroid regimens often resulted in improvement, but infrequently resulted in resolution or near resolution of the lesions.[54] Regimens that included infliximab, a monoclonal antibody against tumor necrosis factor alpha, resulted in resolution of lupus pernio lesions in more than three-quarters of the cases.[54] Noncorticosteroid, non–infliximab-containing regimens were rarely effective for this particular form of skin sarcoidosis. Because of these findings, we recommend early consideration of infliximab for patients with lupus pernio sarcoidosis skin lesions that fail to adequately respond to corticosteroids.

Eye Sarcoidosis

Eye sarcoidosis is one of the few forms of the disease that is almost always treated, even if it causes no symptoms, because active granulomatous inflammation can result in permanent vision impairment.[55,56] Therefore, every patient diagnosed with sarcoidosis requires a detailed eye examination, including a slit lamp and funduscopic examination.[24]

Corticosteroids are recommended as the initial treatment of eye sarcoidosis.[57,58] For acute anterior uveitis from sarcoidosis, topical corticosteroids are usually effective because they penetrate well into the anterior chamber.[57,58] When iritis or uveitis is

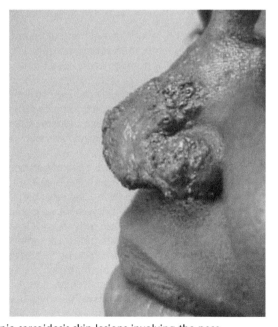

Fig. 7. Lupus pernio sarcoidosis skin lesions involving the nose.

severe, extends beyond the anterior chamber, or fails to respond to topical eye drops, then subconjunctival, periocular, and intravitreal injections of corticosteroids may be considered.[57,58] Mydriatics are almost always instilled to suppress the inflammation and to avoid adhesion of the iris to the lens (posterior synechia). Intraocular pressure must be monitored after corticosteroids are administered orally or injected because any prolonged course of corticosteroids may induce glaucoma.

Systemic corticosteroids are recommended for severe anterior uveitis, uveitis deeper to the anterior chamber, and uveitis that fails to respond to topical or injection therapy. An initial dose of 40 mg of prednisone per day has been recommended.[58] Although systemic corticosteroids are usually effective in rapidly controlling ocular inflammation, long-term corticosteroid side effects, especially cataracts and glaucoma, mandate earlier consideration of corticosteroid-sparing drugs than other forms of sarcoidosis.[57] Drugs that have shown efficacy for the treatment of sarcoid uveitis include methotrexate,[59–61] azathioprine,[61,62] leflunomide,[63] infliximab,[64,65] and adalimumab.[66,67]

Optic neuritis is a feared complication of eye sarcoidosis that can rapidly cause permanent vision loss.[68,69] Acute optic neuritis should be considered in patients with sarcoidosis with sudden loss of vision or disturbance in color perception.[68] Although the treatment of acute optic neuritis from sarcoidosis has not been subjected to a clinical trial, an aggressive initial approach seems reasonable with high-dose intravenous corticosteroids.

Neurologic

Symptomatic neurologic manifestations of sarcoidosis almost always mandate treatment. A seventh cranial nerve (Bell) palsy is the most common manifestation of neurosarcoidosis[70,71] and may spontaneously remit. However, even these patients should be considered for corticosteroid therapy in an effort to resolve this manifestation.[72,73] Asymptomatic neurosarcoidosis poses a treatment dilemma.[71] The decision to treat such patients must be individualized and based on the location of the lesions, changes in the lesions over time, and risks of therapy.[71]

Corticosteroids are the drug of choice for the treatment of neurosarcoidosis.[74] The initial corticosteroid treatment dose is 40 to 80 mg or more of daily prednisone,[75,76] which is higher than the suggested initial corticosteroid dose for almost all other forms of sarcoidosis. The dose of corticosteroids is tapered depending on the clinical response. A sarcoidosis-related Bell palsy may only require 2 to 4 weeks of corticosteroid therapy, whereas more serious forms of neurosarcoidosis may require a duration of therapy exceeding 1 year.[71] Severe acute neurosarcoidosis causing major manifestations such as visual loss, altered sensorium, or weakness may require initial high-dose intravenous corticosteroids.[75]

Neurosarcoidosis not only requires a higher initial dose of corticosteroids to control but patients are often corticosteroid dependent, and it is problematic to successfully wean the corticosteroid dose to a nontoxic level. In 2 series of patients with neurosarcoidosis, less than half achieved significant improvement on corticosteroid therapy, and most relapsed when corticosteroids were reduced to less than the 20 to 25 mg/d range.[70,77] For these reasons, corticosteroid-sparing medications are often considered, including hydroxychloroquine,[78] chloroquine,[78] methotrexate,[77] mycophenolate mofetil,[79,80] azathioprine,[81] cyclophosphamide,[77,82] infliximab,[83,84] and adalimumab.[85] Although based on limited data, infliximab seems to be particularly effective.[84,86,87] Although adalimumab and infliximab have not been compared in a controlled fashion, a Delphi study of sarcoidosis experts revealed that infliximab was more potent for the treatment of sarcoidosis than was adalimumab.[88] Most experts administered 3 to 5 mg/kg of infliximab every 4 to 6 weeks after a loading regimen. For adalimumab, the experts recommended dosages that were greater than those used for rheumatoid arthritis, with a consensus of experts using at least 40 mg subcutaneously weekly.[88]

Musculoskeletal Involvement

Acute sarcoid arthritis is the most common form of sarcoidosis joint disease. In the ankle, ultrasonography imaging suggests there may be little true arthritis, as opposed to periarticular edema.[89] Often, this form of arthritis is associated with Lofgren syndrome.[90] This arthritis is usually self-limited with remission rates as high as 90%.[91,92] Despite several investigators recommending conservative treatment of this condition, including cold packs, a training program, and nonsteroidal antiinflammatory agents,[93,94] our personal experience is that most patients are not satisfied with such therapy and immediately respond to corticosteroids. We are unaware of any formal analysis of specific treatment of acute sarcoidosis arthritis. Our experience is that an effective initial dose of prednisone is 20 to 30 mg daily, with tapering individualized, and most patients are completely tapered off corticosteroids within 4 to 8 weeks.

Chronic sarcoid arthritis is much rarer than the acute forms.[95] On occasion, the arthritis is destructive.[96] The optimum treatment regimen is unknown. Corticosteroids are the most common form of treatment, either by intra-articular or systemic administration, and, in the latter case, often with corticosteroid-sparing drugs such as methotrexate, antimalarials, azathioprine, or infliximab.[91,93,97–99] Nonsteroidal antiinflammatory agents may be used as possible corticosteroid-sparing agents.

A tenosynovitis from sarcoidosis may occur. It almost exclusively affects the upper extremities, most commonly the wrist, hand, or fingers.[100] These lesions may present as painful, palpable masses and histology reveals granulomatous inflammation on biopsy.[100] Corticosteroids are usually effective and the dose is not standardized.[100] There are reports of effective monotherapy with chloroquine[101] and methotrexate.[100]

Bone sarcoidosis usually involves the small bones of the hands and feet, although any portion of the axial or appendicular skeleton may be involved. The high frequency of hand and foot involvement reported previously may be inaccurate and relate to data collected before the advent of sophisticated scanning techniques (eg, PET and MRI scans).[94] Osseous lesions tend to be osteolytic and/or cystic. On plain radiographs, they appear as osteopenic lesions with a lacy trabecular pattern.[102] Cysts may accompany these lesions, and when they are large may show a punched-out appearance. Although these lesions are described as lytic, they do not result in bone destruction. It has been postulated that these lytic lesions represent a tunneling process rather than a destructive phenomenon.[94,103] Many of these lesions, especially in large bones, are asymptomatic and are fortuitously found on body imaging studies performed for other reasons. Treatment is not recommended for asymptomatic lesions, because it is extremely rare for them to result in pain syndromes or fractures. Corticosteroids are recommended as the drug of choice when therapy is required, although there is little evidence to support a specific regimen.[94]

Muscle involvement may occur in sarcoidosis and it often causes no symptoms.[75] Sarcoidosis muscle involvement may manifest as a nodular myopathy, acute myopathy, or chronic myopathy. Sarcoid muscle nodules are usually palpable and painless.[75] They are not usually associated with muscle weakness and serum muscle enzyme levels tend to be normal. An acute sarcoid myopathy is usually painful and associated with increased serum muscle enzyme levels. It is our experience that the serum creatine kinase is often normal, whereas the serum aldolase level is increased.

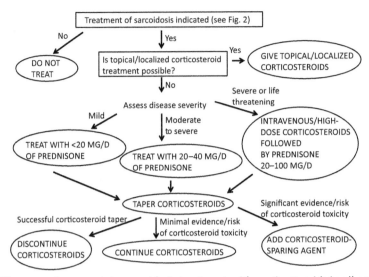

Fig. 8. The general approach to sarcoidosis treatment with corticosteroids in all organs.

Chronic sarcoid myopathy usually presents with progressive weakness and atrophy in the proximal muscles. Serum muscle enzyme levels are usually normal in chronic sarcoid myopathies. There is limited information concerning the treatment of sarcoid myositis. Our experience is that it usually responds to daily doses of 20 to 30 mg of prednisone within a matter of weeks.

Other Organs

Although there are specific nuances in treatment of sarcoidosis in each organ, **Fig. 8** outlines the general approach to sarcoidosis treatment with corticosteroids. Corticosteroids are the cornerstone of treatment in almost all cases. The addition of corticosteroid-sparing agents is usually based on the patient's response to corticosteroid therapy as well as the risks of corticosteroid therapy, the latter depending on the required dose and duration of therapy as well as patient-related comorbidities.

SUMMARY

Corticosteroids are the drug of choice for the treatment of sarcoidosis. Because of the toxicity of corticosteroids and other antisarcoidosis medications, therapy should only be considered when sarcoidosis causes a dangerous/potentially dangerous health situation or significantly affects the patient's quality of life. Topical/local therapy should be considered whenever possible to minimize the risk of corticosteroid toxicity. When systemic therapy is required, patients should be aggressively tapered to the lowest effective corticosteroid dose once the disease has been stabilized. Corticosteroid-sparing agents should be considered in patients who are at significant risk of corticosteroid toxicity, which includes the risks associated with prolonged corticosteroid therapy. Corticosteroid dosing regimens vary depending on the organ involved.

REFERENCES

1. Baughman RP, Drent M, Culver DA, et al. Endpoints for clinical trials of sarcoidosis. Sarcoidosis Vasc Diffuse Lung Dis 2012;29(2):90–8.

2. Romer FK. Presentation of sarcoidosis and outcome of pulmonary changes. Dan Med Bull 1982;29(1):27–32.
3. Judson MA, Baughman RP, Thompson BW, et al. Two year prognosis of sarcoidosis: the ACCESS experience. Sarcoidosis Vasc Diffuse Lung Dis 2003;20(3): 204–11.
4. Baydur A, Alsalek M, Louie SG, et al. Respiratory muscle strength, lung function, and dyspnea in patients with sarcoidosis. Chest 2001;120(1):102–8.
5. Judson MA, Boan AD, Lackland DT. The clinical course of sarcoidosis: presentation, diagnosis, and treatment in a large white and black cohort in the United States. Sarcoidosis Vasc Diffuse Lung Dis 2012;29(2):119–27.
6. Judson MA. The treatment of pulmonary sarcoidosis. Respir Med 2012;106(10): 1351–61.
7. Judson MA. Determining the cause of pulmonary granulomas: a multidimensional process. Respirology 2015;20(1):5–6.
8. Gottlieb JE, Israel HL, Steiner RM, et al. Outcome in sarcoidosis. The relationship of relapse to corticosteroid therapy. Chest 1997;111(3):623–31.
9. Rizzato G, Montemurro L, Colombo P. The late follow-up of chronic sarcoid patients previously treated with corticosteroids. Sarcoidosis Vasc Diffuse Lung Dis 1998;15(1):52–8.
10. McKinzie BP, Bullington WM, Mazur JE, et al. Efficacy of short-course, low-dose corticosteroid therapy for acute pulmonary sarcoidosis exacerbations. Am J Med Sci 2010;339(1):1–4.
11. Lower EE, Baughman RP. Prolonged use of methotrexate for sarcoidosis. Arch Intern Med 1995;155(8):846–51.
12. Baltzan M, Mehta S, Kirkham TH, et al. Randomized trial of prolonged chloroquine therapy in advanced pulmonary sarcoidosis. Am J Respir Crit Care Med 1999;160(1):192–7.
13. Bachelez H, Senet P, Cadranel J, et al. The use of tetracyclines for the treatment of sarcoidosis. Arch Dermatol 2001;137(1):69–73.
14. Baughman RP, Lower EE. Steroid-sparing alternative treatments for sarcoidosis. Clin Chest Med 1997;18(4):853–64.
15. Droitcourt C, Rybojad M, Porcher R, et al. A randomized, investigator-masked, double-blind, placebo-controlled trial on thalidomide in severe cutaneous sarcoidosis. Chest 2014;146(4):1046–54.
16. Paramothayan NS, Lasserson TJ, Jones PW. Corticosteroids for pulmonary sarcoidosis. Cochrane Database Syst Rev 2005;(2):CD001114.
17. Baughman RP, Culver DA, Judson MA. A concise review of pulmonary sarcoidosis. Am J Respir Crit Care Med 2011;183(5):573–81.
18. Baughman RP, Ploysongsang Y, Roberts RD, et al. Effects of sarcoid and steroids on angiotensin-converting enzyme. Am Rev Respir Dis 1983;128(4):631–3.
19. Kohn H, Klech H, Mostbeck A, et al. 67Ga scanning for assessment of disease activity and therapy decisions in pulmonary sarcoidosis in comparison to chest radiography, serum ACE and blood T-lymphocytes. Eur J Nucl Med 1982;7(9): 413–6.
20. Keir G, Wells AU. Assessing pulmonary disease and response to therapy: which test? Semin Respir Crit Care Med 2010;31(4):409–18.
21. Vorselaars AD, Verwoerd A, van Moorsel CH, et al. Prediction of relapse after discontinuation of infliximab therapy in severe sarcoidosis. Eur Respir J 2014; 43(2):602–9.
22. Judson MA, Baughman RP, Costabel U, et al. The potential additional benefit of infliximab in patients with chronic pulmonary sarcoidosis already receiving

corticosteroids: a retrospective analysis from a randomized clinical trial. Respir Med 2014;108(1):189–94.

23. Schutt AC, Bullington WM, Judson MA. Pharmacotherapy for pulmonary sarcoidosis: a Delphi consensus study. Respir Med 2010;104(5):717–23.

24. Hunninghake GW, Costabel U, Ando M, et al. ATS/ERS/WASOG statement on sarcoidosis. American Thoracic Society/European Respiratory Society/World Association of Sarcoidosis and other Granulomatous Disorders. Sarcoidosis Vasc Diffuse Lung Dis 1999;16(2):149–73.

25. Judson MA. An approach to the treatment of pulmonary sarcoidosis with corticosteroids: the six phases of treatment. Chest 1999;115(4):1158–65.

26. Baughman RP, Iannuzzi MC, Lower EE, et al. Use of fluticasone in acute symptomatic pulmonary sarcoidosis. Sarcoidosis Vasc Diffuse Lung Dis 2002;19(3): 198–204.

27. Israel HL, Fouts DW, Beggs RA. A controlled trial of prednisone treatment of sarcoidosis. Am Rev Respir Dis 1973;107(4):609–14.

28. Kiper N, Anadol D, Ozcelik U, et al. Inhaled corticosteroids for maintenance treatment in childhood pulmonary sarcoidosis. Acta Paediatr 2001;90(8):953–6.

29. DeRemee RA. Sarcoidosis. Mayo Clin Proc 1995;70(2):177–81.

30. Selroos O. Treatment of sarcoidosis. Sarcoidosis 1994;11(1):80–3.

31. Pietinalho A, Tukiainen P, Haahtela T, et al. Oral prednisolone followed by inhaled budesonide in newly diagnosed pulmonary sarcoidosis: a double-blind, placebo-controlled multicenter study. Finnish Pulmonary Sarcoidosis Study Group. Chest 1999;116(2):424–31.

32. Pietinalho A, Tukiainen P, Haahtela T, et al. Early treatment of stage II sarcoidosis improves 5-year pulmonary function. Chest 2002;121(1):24–31.

33. Nagai T, Kohsaka S, Okuda S, et al. Incidence and prognostic significance of myocardial late gadolinium enhancement in patients with sarcoidosis without cardiac manifestation. Chest 2014;146(4):1064–72.

34. Birnie DH, Sauer WH, Bogun F, et al. HRS expert consensus statement on the diagnosis and management of arrhythmias associated with cardiac sarcoidosis. Heart Rhythm 2014;11(7):1305–23.

35. Hamzeh NY, Wamboldt FS, Weinberger HD. Management of cardiac sarcoidosis in the United States: a Delphi study. Chest 2012;141(1):154–62.

36. Nunes H, Freynet O, Naggara N, et al. Cardiac sarcoidosis. Semin Respir Crit Care Med 2010;31(4):428–41.

37. Chapelon-Abric C, de Zuttere D, Duhaut P, et al. Cardiac sarcoidosis: a retrospective study of 41 cases. Medicine 2004;83(6):315–34.

38. Valantine HA, Tazelaar HD, Macoviak J, et al. Cardiac sarcoidosis: response to steroids and transplantation. J Heart Transplant 1987;6(4):244–50.

39. Yazaki Y, Isobe M, Hiroe M, et al. Prognostic determinants of long-term survival in Japanese patients with cardiac sarcoidosis treated with prednisone. Am J Cardiol 2001;88(9):1006–10.

40. Marchell RM, Judson MA. Chronic cutaneous lesions of sarcoidosis. Clin Dermatol 2007;25(3):295–302.

41. Mana J, Marcoval J, Graells J, et al. Cutaneous involvement in sarcoidosis. Relationship to systemic disease. Arch Dermatol 1997;133(7):882–8.

42. Eklund A, Rizzato G. Skin manifestations in sarcoidosis. Eur Respir J Monogr 2005;10:150–63.

43. Volden G. Successful treatment of chronic skin diseases with clobetasol propionate and a hydrocolloid occlusive dressing. Acta Derm Venereol 1992;72(1): 69–71.

44. Khatri KA, Chotzen VA, Burrall BA. Lupus pernio: successful treatment with a potent topical corticosteroid. Arch Dermatol 1995;131(5):617–8.
45. Badgwell C, Rosen T. Cutaneous sarcoidosis therapy updated. J Am Acad Dermatol 2007;56(1):69–83.
46. Callen JP. Intralesional corticosteroids. J Am Acad Dermatol 1981;4(2):149–51.
47. Gogstetter DS, Goldsmith LA. Treatment of cutaneous sarcoidosis using phonophoresis. J Am Acad Dermatol 1999;40(5 Pt 1):767–9.
48. Veien NK. Cutaneous sarcoidosis: prognosis and treatment. Clin Dermatol 1986;4(4):75–87.
49. Haimovic A, Sanchez M, Judson MA, et al. Sarcoidosis: a comprehensive review and update for the dermatologist: part I. Cutaneous disease. J Am Acad Dermatol 2012;66(5):699.e1–18 [quiz: 717–8].
50. Hawk A, English J. Cutaneous manifestations of sarcoidosis. London: BMJ Books; 2003.
51. Jones E, Callen JP. Hydroxychloroquine is effective therapy for control of cutaneous sarcoidal granulomas. J Am Acad Dermatol 1990;23(3 Pt 1):487–9.
52. Baughman RP, Lower EE. Evidence-based therapy for cutaneous sarcoidosis. Clin Dermatol 2007;25(3):334–40.
53. James DG. Lupus pernio. Lupus 1992;1(3):129–31.
54. Stagaki E, Mountford WK, Lackland DT, et al. The treatment of lupus pernio: results of 116 treatment courses in 54 patients. Chest 2009;135(2):468–76.
55. Dana MR, Merayo-Lloves J, Schaumberg DA, et al. Prognosticators for visual outcome in sarcoid uveitis. Ophthalmology 1996;103(11):1846–53.
56. Ohara K, Okubo A, Sasaki H, et al. Intraocular manifestations of systemic sarcoidosis. Jpn J Ophthalmol 1992;36(4):452–7.
57. Baughman RP, Lower EE, Kaufman AH. Ocular sarcoidosis. Semin Respir Crit Care Med 2010;31(4):452–62.
58. Ohara K, Judson MA, Baughman RP. Clinical aspects of ocular sarcoidosis. Eur Respir J Monogr 2005;10:188–209.
59. Samson CM, Waheed N, Baltatzis S, et al. Methotrexate therapy for chronic noninfectious uveitis: analysis of a case series of 160 patients. Ophthalmology 2001;108(6):1134–9.
60. Dev S, McCallum RM, Jaffe GJ. Methotrexate treatment for sarcoid-associated panuveitis. Ophthalmology 1999;106(1):111–8.
61. Baughman RP, Lower EE, Bradley DA, et al. Use of cytotoxic therapy for chronic ophthalmic sarcoidosis. Sarcoidosis Vasc Diffuse Lung Dis 1999;16(Suppl 1 (abstract issue)):17.
62. Pasadhika S, Kempen JH, Newcomb CW, et al. Azathioprine for ocular inflammatory diseases. Am J Ophthalmol 2009;148(4):500–9.e5.
63. Baughman RP, Lower EE. Leflunomide for chronic sarcoidosis. Sarcoidosis Vasc Diffuse Lung Dis 2004;21(1):43–8.
64. Baughman RP, Bradley DA, Lower EE. Infliximab in chronic ocular inflammation. Int J Clin Pharmacol Ther 2005;43(1):7–11.
65. Galor A, Perez VL, Hammel JP, et al. Differential effectiveness of etanercept and infliximab in the treatment of ocular inflammation. Ophthalmology 2006;113(12):2317–23.
66. Erckens RJ, Mostard RL, Wijnen PA, et al. Adalimumab successful in sarcoidosis patients with refractory chronic non-infectious uveitis. Graefes Arch Clin Exp Ophthalmol 2012;250(5):713–20.

67. Dragnev D, Barr D, Kulshrestha M, et al. Sarcoid panuveitis associated with etanercept treatment, resolving with adalimumab. BMJ Case Rep 2013;2013 [pii: bcr2013200552].

68. Bradley DA, Baughman RP, Raymond L, et al. Ocular manifestations of sarcoidosis. Semin Respir Crit Care Med 2002;23:543–8.

69. Mayers M. Ocular sarcoidosis. Int Ophthalmol Clin 1990;30(4):257–63.

70. Zajicek JP, Scolding NJ, Foster O, et al. Central nervous system sarcoidosis-diagnosis and management. QJM 1999;92(2):103–17.

71. Terushkin V, Stern BJ, Judson MA, et al. Neurosarcoidosis: presentations and management. Neurologist 2010;16(1):2–15.

72. Jain V, Deshmukh A, Gollomp S. Bilateral facial paralysis: case presentation and discussion of differential diagnosis. J Gen Intern Med 2006;21(7):C7–10.

73. Glocker FX, Seifert C, Lucking CH. Facial palsy in Heerfordt's syndrome: electrophysiological localization of the lesion. Muscle Nerve 1999;22(9):1279–82.

74. Patel AV, Stickler DE, Tyor WR. Neurosarcoidosis. Curr Treat Options Neurol 2007;9(3):161–8.

75. Nozaki K, Judson MA. Neurosarcoidosis: clinical manifestations, diagnosis and treatment. Presse Med 2012;41(6 Pt 2):e331–48.

76. Sharma OP. Neurosarcoidosis: a personal perspective based on the study of 37 patients. Chest 1997;112(1):220–8.

77. Lower EE, Broderick JP, Brott TG, et al. Diagnosis and management of neurological sarcoidosis. Arch Intern Med 1997;157(16):1864–8.

78. Sharma OP. Effectiveness of chloroquine and hydroxychloroquine in treating selected patients with sarcoidosis with neurological involvement. Arch Neurol 1998;55(9):1248–54.

79. Chaussenot A, Bourg V, Chanalet S, et al. Neurosarcoidosis treated with mycophenolate mofetil: two cases. Rev Neurol (Paris) 2007;163(4):471–5 [in French].

80. Androdias G, Maillet D, Marignier R, et al. Mycophenolate mofetil may be effective in CNS sarcoidosis but not in sarcoid myopathy. Neurology 2011;76(13): 1168–72.

81. Pawate S, Moses H, Sriram S. Presentations and outcomes of neurosarcoidosis: a study of 54 cases. QJM 2009;102(7):449–60.

82. Doty JD, Mazur JE, Judson MA. Treatment of corticosteroid-resistant neurosarcoidosis with a short-course cyclophosphamide regimen. Chest 2003;124(5): 2023–6.

83. Pereira J, Anderson NE, McAuley D, et al. Medically refractory neurosarcoidosis treated with infliximab. Intern Med J 2011;41(4):354–7.

84. Sodhi M, Pearson K, White ES, et al. Infliximab therapy rescues cyclophosphamide failure in severe central nervous system sarcoidosis. Respir Med 2009; 103(2):268–73.

85. Marnane M, Lynch T, Scott J, et al. Steroid-unresponsive neurosarcoidosis successfully treated with adalimumab. J Neurol 2009;256(1):139–40.

86. Chintamaneni S, Patel AM, Pegram SB, et al. Dramatic response to infliximab in refractory neurosarcoidosis. Ann Indian Acad Neurol 2010;13(3):207–10.

87. Metyas S, Tawadrous M, Yeter KC, et al. Neurosarcoidosis mimicking multiple sclerosis successfully treated with methotrexate and adalimumab. Int J Rheum Dis 2014;17(2):214–6.

88. Drent M, Cremers JP, Jansen TL, et al. Practical eminence and experience-based recommendations for use of TNF-alpha inhibitors in sarcoidosis. Sarcoidosis Vasc Diffuse Lung Dis 2014;31(2):91–107.

89. Kellner H, Spathling S, Herzer P. Ultrasound findings in Lofgren's syndrome: is ankle swelling caused by arthritis, tenosynovitis or periarthritis? J Rheumatol 1992;19(1):38–41.

90. Glennas A, Kvien TK, Melby K, et al. Acute sarcoid arthritis: occurrence, seasonal onset, clinical features and outcome. Br J Rheumatol 1995;34(1):45–50.

91. Barnard J, Newman LS. Sarcoidosis: immunology, rheumatic involvement, and therapeutics. Curr Opin Rheumatol 2001;13(1):84–91.

92. Mana J, Gomez-Vaquero C, Montero A, et al. Lofgren's syndrome revisited: a study of 186 patients. Am J Med 1999;107(3):240–5.

93. Awada H, Abi-Karam G, Fayad F. Musculoskeletal and other extrapulmonary disorders in sarcoidosis. Best Pract Res Clin Rheumatol 2003;17(6):971–87.

94. Shorr AF, Stack AL. Osseous sarcoidosis. In: Baughman RP, editor. Sarcoidosis, vol. 210. New York: Taylor and Francis; 2006. p. 605–33.

95. Torralba KD, Quismorio FP Jr. Sarcoid arthritis: a review of clinical features, pathology and therapy. Sarcoidosis Vasc Diffuse Lung Dis 2003;20(2):95–103.

96. Sokoloff L, Bunim JJ. Clinical and pathological studies of joint involvement in sarcoidosis. N Engl J Med 1959;260(17):841–7.

97. Sanchez-Cano D, Callejas-Rubio JL, Ruiz-Villaverde R, et al. Off-label uses of anti-TNF therapy in three frequent disorders: Behcet's disease, sarcoidosis, and noninfectious uveitis. Mediators Inflamm 2013;2013:286857.

98. Pettersson T. Rheumatic features of sarcoidosis. Curr Opin Rheumatol 1998; 10(1):73–8.

99. Loupasakis K, Berman J, Jaber N, et al. Refractory sarcoid arthritis in World Trade Center-exposed New York City firefighters: a case series. J Clin Rheumatol 2015;21(1):19–23.

100. Lambert L, Riemer EC, Judson MA. Rapid development of sarcoid tenosynovitis. J Clin Rheumatol 2011;17(4):201–3.

101. Mayock RL, Bertrand P, Morrison CE, et al. Manifestations of sarcoidosis. Analysis of 145 patients, with a review of nine series selected from the literature. Am J Med 1963;35:67–89.

102. Sartoris DJ, Resnick D, Resnik C, et al. Musculoskeletal manifestations of sarcoidosis. Semin Roentgenol 1985;20(4):376–86.

103. Wilcox A, Bharadwaj P, Sharma OP. Bone sarcoidosis. Curr Opin Rheumatol 2000;12(4):321–30.

Corticosteroids for Pain of Spinal Origin

Epidural and Intraarticular Administration

Louisa S. Schilling, BSc[a,b], John D. Markman, MD[c,*]

KEYWORDS

- Corticosteroid • Glucocorticoid • Epidural steroid injection • Low back pain
- Lumbar stenosis • Transforaminal • Facet joint • Sacroiliac joint

KEY POINTS

- Epidural steroid injection (ESI) is the most commonly performed outpatient procedure for the treatment of spinal pain worldwide.
- The epidural approach is most often used to optimize the local, anti-inflammatory effects of corticosteroid at the nerve root level in lumbar radiculitis and neurogenic claudication.
- Facet and sacroiliac joint injection of corticosteroid is widely practiced in pain management to target putative peripheral sources of referred, nociceptive chronic low back pain.
- There are a range of widely used corticosteroid formulations with distinct physicochemical properties that may affect outcomes and side effects profiles.
- ESIs offer the advantage of a more localized corticosteroid delivery to the putative anatomic correlate of pain such as the nerve root, thereby decreasing the likelihood of systemic side effects.

INTRODUCTION

Spinal pain syndromes are the leading cause of disability in the United States. The 2010 Global Burden of Disease Study found that the years lived with disability attributed to low back pain (3.1 million) exceeds even that of osteoarthritis (1.9 million).[1] The lifetime prevalence of a single episode of low back pain is estimated at 85%.[2] Corticosteroids are commonly used for a wide range of spinal pain syndromes, such as

Disclosure: None.
[a] Department of Neuroscience, University of Toronto, 27 Kings College Circle, Toronto, ON M5S, Canada; [b] Translational Pain Research Program, University of Rochester School of Medicine and Dentistry, 601 Elmwood Avenue, Rochester, NY 14642, USA; [c] Department of Neurosurgery, Translational Pain Research Program, University of Rochester School of Medicine and Dentistry, 601 Elmwood Avenue, Rochester, NY 14642, USA
* Corresponding author. Translational Pain Research Program, Neuromedicine Pain Management Center, 2180 South Clinton Avenue, Rochester, NY 14618.
E-mail address: john_markman@urmc.rochester.edu

Rheum Dis Clin N Am 42 (2016) 137–155
http://dx.doi.org/10.1016/j.rdc.2015.08.003   rheumatic.theclinics.com

lumbar radiculitis and neurogenic claudication associated with spinal stenosis. In the United States alone, 9 million injections of corticosteroids are administered annually and this rate is increasing steadily.[3] Sustained increase in utilization is likely owing to (1) recent studies demonstrating lack of analgesic efficacy with oral steroid treatment for acute radicular pain, and (2) growing concerns about the therapeutic index of orally administered pain relievers such as nonsteroidal antiinflammatory drugs (NSAIDs) and opioids.[4] Corticosteroids are most often delivered via the epidural route owing to this compartment's proximity to the putative source of pain. Epidural steroid injection (ESI) is the most common outpatient procedure for pain relief worldwide,[3] despite considerable controversy about the clinical indications for and effectiveness and risks of this approach.

BACKGROUND

Synthetic glucocorticoids mimic the mechanisms of endogenous glucocorticoid (cortisol) but have different levels of efficacy, potency, and affinity for glucocorticoid receptors (GRs). These hormones, whether elaborated endogenously or delivered exogenously, are characterized based on their actions in the body as either glucocorticoids (carbohydrate regulating) or mineralocorticoids (electrolyte regulating). When used clinically, the term "corticosteroids" usually designates glucocorticoids, which are administered in ESIs. Corticosteroids are anti-inflammatory agents, and it this mechanism of action that is most often thought to account for the analgesic benefit of this therapy in patients with spinal disorders; however, there is strong experimental evidence for the direct, neural antinociceptive effects of corticosteroids.[5] Corticosteroids have a broad scope of action beyond their analgesic effects. The wide-ranging effects of steroid hormones on fluid and electrolyte balance and function of the immune, cardiovascular, renal, endocrine, musculoskeletal, and nervous systems account for many of the unintended adverse effects of these agents when used as analgesics.[6] Four of the most commonly administered preparations of synthetic glucocorticoids for intraspinal injections include methylprednisolone, triamcinolone, betamethasone, and dexamethasone[7] (**Table 1**). The considerable variation among different glucocorticoid formulations with respect to potency, particle size, tendency to aggregate, pharmacokinetics, and half-life are summarized in **Table 1**.

Owing to the adverse effects associated with the use of high-dose glucocorticoids, highly potent formulations that achieve the same effect at lower doses are in demand. Efficacy of a glucocorticoid refers to the maximal activity (GR transactivation and transrepression as measured in a cell-based reporter assay) that it can achieve (usually at maximal concentration), whereas the potency of a glucocorticoid pertains to the concentration needed to reach one-half of its maximal activity. For 2 glucocorticoids of the same efficacy, a highly potent one will require a lower dose to achieve the same treatment effect.[8] Potency varies widely across corticosteroid formulations. Although there is no consensus on the ideal dose of steroid to be administered in an ESI,[9] the North American Spine Society (NASS) recommends limiting each ESI session to 80 mg of triamcinolone, 80 mg of methylprednisolone, 12 mg of betamethasone, or 15 mg of dexamethasone.[10] Approximately one-fifth the dose of dexamethasone and betamethasone is required to achieve an equivalent effect to that of methylprednisolone or triamcinolone. Notably, a glucocorticoid may have different potencies for transactivation and transrepression. In the case of dexamethasone, gene activation requires a 5-fold higher concentration than for gene repression. This variance allows for the development of highly potent glucocorticoids that can be administered in low doses to achieve repression of inflammation signaling while minimizing other side effects.[9]

Table 1
Four of the most commonly injected corticosteroids

Corticosteroid	Commercial Name	Equivalent Potency Dose (mg)	Suspension or Solution	Solubility	Particulate Aggregation	Maximum Particle Size (μm)	Benzyl Alcohol
Betamethasone acetate/ sodium phosphate	Celestone Soluspan	0.75	Suspension	Acetate form: insoluble, sodium phosphate form: freely soluble	Some	500	No
Dexamethasone sodium phosphate	Hexadrol	0.75	Solution	Freely soluble	None	0.5	Yes
Methylprednisolone acetate	Depo-Medrol	4	Suspension	Insoluble	Few	>500	Yes
Triamcinolone acetonide	Kenalog-10 Kenalog-40	4	Suspension	Insoluble	Extensive	>500	Yes

Adapted from MacMahon PJ, Eustace SJ, Kavanagh EC. Injectable corticosteroid and local anesthetic preparations: a review for radiologists 1. Radiology 2009;252(3):649.

The solubility of corticosteroid preparations has important clinical implications in the context of epidural delivery. Many preparations contain corticosteroid esters, which are insoluble in water and consequently form microcrystalline suspensions. Other preparations, such as dexamethasone, are not esters and are freely soluble in water and therefore considered "nonparticulate." The possible benefit of ester preparations is that they require hydrolysis by cellular esterases to release the active moiety and consequently should have a longer duration of action in the epidural space or injected area. In contrast, freely water-soluble preparations such as dexamethasone sodium phosphate and betamethasone sodium phosphate are taken up quickly by cells and thus have a quicker onset of effect but a shorter duration of action. Corticosteroid ester preparations vary in crystal size and in the crystals' tendency to aggregate into larger particles that are bigger than a red blood cell (RBC).[11] Some expert reviews have associated vascular adverse events (ie, infarct) with large crystal aggregations.

Corticosteroids are generally highly lipophilic, which has important implications for intraspinal injections.[12] The epidural space contains abundant fat that serves as a repository for the storage and delayed release of lipid-soluble medication. The amount of drug stored in the epidural fat is largely a function of lipid solubility. When released from this "drug depot," the lipophilic steroids migrate to nearby structures such as the dural sac, nerve roots, and nerve root dural sleeves. Corticosteroid formulations that are more lipid soluble are released more slowly into the epidural space, possibly elongating the duration of their pharmacologic effects.[13] In addition to the steroid, there are also several other chemical ingredients in any corticosteroid formulation, including preservatives.[11] The clinical importance of the variations of corticosteroid formulations in **Table 1** are discussed in more detail elsewhere in this article. The focus of this article is the treatment of pain syndromes of spinal origin because these constellations of pain syndromes constitute the most common clinical indication for glucocorticoids.

THERAPEUTIC RATIONALE

The epidural route of delivery enables localized administration of a glucocorticoid and hence a more direct effect on the nerve roots, dorsal root ganglia, cauda equina, and central nervous system. The epidural space is the compartment bound by the dura mater, spinal ligaments, and boney confines of the vertebral bodies. The content of this space includes fat cells, lymphatic tissue, arteries, areolar connective tissue, spinal nerve roots, and the epidural venous plexus.[14] The epidural space is composed of enclosed discontinuous compartments, which allows for injection into a confined space with close proximity to a specific nerve root.[15] Fat is the main component of the epidural space and therefore plays an important role in the absorption of injected corticosteroids. Lumbar epidural fat has a discontinuous and metameric distribution. The amount of fat varies along the spinal canal, which may influence the strategy used for injections.[16]

Most glucocorticoids ultimately diffuse through the blood-nerve barrier to enter the central nervous system. For a steroid to pass the blood–brain and blood–nerve barriers with ease, it must be highly lipophilic.[17] Receptors for glucocorticoids, GRs, are present in the brain and are especially abundant in the hippocampus. Endogenous glucocorticoids are involved in mood, satiety, the sleep–wake cycle, and the processes of learning and memory through interactions with specific GRs located in the prefrontal cortex, hippocampus, and basolateral amygdala.[18] Penetration of drug into these structures likely accounts for the protean effects and side effects observed following ESI. The rich expression of GRs in the hippocampus and amygdala are linked to the many behavioral and antidepressant effects of glucocorticoids.[19] In a recent study conducted by Friedly and colleagues[20] and published in the *New England Journal of Medicine* that examined the effectiveness of epidural injections of glucocorticoids, patients injected with glucocorticoids plus an anesthetic displayed decreased symptoms of depression and greater treatment satisfaction compared with patients injected with an anesthetic alone (according to scores on the Patient Health Questionnaire). The authors hypothesized that these outcomes may be explained in part by the glucocorticoid action in the brain from an epidural injection, rather than the local antiinflammatory effects in the lumbar compartment, leading to effects that reduce symptoms of depression such as fatigue.

The loci and mechanisms of action for corticosteroids' antiinflammatory effects and their relationship to analgesia are not understood fully. The antiinflammatory actions are the result of the pleiotropic effects of the GRs on multiple signaling pathways. These lipophilic hormones cross the cytoplasmic membrane and regulate gene expression by binding to specific GRs. The steroid–receptor complex can then translocate to the nucleus upregulating the transcription of antiinflammatory genes.[21] Glucocorticoids also inhibit the expression of many proinflammatory factors, including proinflammatory cytokines (eg, tumor necrosis factor-α, interleukin-1β, and interleukin-6), chemokines (eg, chemokine C-C motif ligand 2 and 19), and enzymes associated with inflammation (eg, collagenase, cyclooxygenase 2, matrix metalloproteinase 13, and phospholipase A2).[22,23] These processes occur slowly and likely account for the delayed onset of action over days to weeks of epidural steroids in contrast with the immediate onset of local anesthetic effects, which are commonly coadministered with glucocorticoids.[4]

The general assumption is that the mechanical factors (eg, compression, traction, vascular congestion owing to increased compartment pressures) that incite and exacerbate lumbar pain symptoms are associated with inflammation.[22] Well-characterized causes of inflammation in spinal pain syndromes include the release of inflammatory cytokines from an extruded intervertebral disc[24] and increased intraspinal pressure in the setting of a narrowing central, lateral, or recess or foramina as in the case of lumbar spinal stenosis associated with neurogenic claudication.[25,26] As such, corticosteroids are administered with the therapeutic rationale that they reduce inflammation and therefore pain. Putative analgesic mechanisms of action include reduction in ischemia as a consequence of diminished intraneural edema and venous congestion; however, there is an ongoing debate on the precise antinociceptive mechanism of glucocorticoids.[6]

CLINICAL INDICATIONS

Since the early 20th century, corticosteroids have been in widespread pharmacologic use for the management of pain of spinal origin owing to their powerful antiinflammatory and analgesic effects.[3] This widespread practice long predated the modern regulatory requirements for the development of an analgesic drug. As a consequence, the US Food and Drug Administration has never formally approved the use of injectable corticosteroids for various spinal pain indications.[27] More recently, as certain techniques of administration such as the cervical transforaminal approach and compounding formulation of glucocorticoids have been linked to serious adverse events such as spinal cord infarct and meningitis, the entire practice of epidural administration of steroids has come under greater scrutiny.[6] Even with this increased attention on adverse events and effectiveness, ESIs remain a mainstay of treatment recommendations based on systematic reviews and clinical practice guidelines.[28,29]

For many patient populations, this mode of therapy has the highest therapeutic index when compared with other analgesic options including chronic opioid therapy, long-term NSAID exposure, or complex spine surgery.[30-32] There is increasing concern for the complications of long-term opioid use for chronic low back pain syndromes, especially at higher doses.[33,34] Equally important, chronic NSAID therapy is linked to serious cardiovascular adverse events and commonly used therapies (eg, gabapentinoids) have not demonstrated efficacy in neurogenic claudication.[35-37] The NASS and the Agency for Healthcare of the Department of Health and Human Services have endorsed the use of ESIs as part of the nonoperative management of radicular pain from lumbar spine disorders.[38]

He structural pathology associated with acute and chronic spinal pain syndromes disclosed by axial imaging techniques and clinical evaluation (eg, straight leg raise testing) lack both sensitivity and specificity for the experience of radiating low back pain and pain-related activity limitation. The principal indications for epidural corticosteroid administration are the treatment of pain localizing to the lumbar nerve roots and the cauda equina. Inflammation of the nerve roots (so-called sciatica), with or without mechanical compression, is a leading reason to seek medical care.[39] The vast majority of cases of acute low back pain resolve spontaneously over days to weeks without the need for imaging. It is in the cases where pain is severe, persistent, and causes marked activity limitation beyond the acute window that epidural corticosteroid administration is contemplated.[40] Interestingly, oral corticosteroids have failed consistently to provide pain-relieving benefit for radicular leg pain, whereas epidural steroids reduce leg pain intensity.[41]

Advances in imaging, diagnostics, and therapy have allowed for the continued refinement of corticosteroid-based interventional techniques for managing spinal pain when surgery is deferred or not a feasible option. During the interval when definitive anatomic treatment is under consideration for intervertebral disc herniation (eg, discectomy), but there remains a likely possibility of resolution of pain associated with mechanical root compression or local inflammation, epidural steroids are a reasonable consideration for poorly controlled pain not responsive to oral medication.[42] Many patients prefer to limit the chronic use of NSAIDs and opioid medication owing to their associated risks.[30,31,43] In seniors, who are far more likely to experience the evoked pain known as neurogenic claudication associated with lumbar spinal stenosis,[20] there are no oral drugs with demonstrated analgesic benefit.[41] Many older patients are not candidates for decompressive surgery owing to comorbid conditions that increase perioperative risks, spinal deformity, or the risk of segmental instability introduced by previous spine surgeries.[44] In this growing population of patients, epidural steroids may offer improved standing and walking tolerance. Oral analgesic medications pose even higher risks of falls, vascular, and end-organ complications in the elderly. Furthermore, loss of mobility is the leading reason for transition to a nursing home.[45] Other common sites of nociceptive spine-related pain include the sacroiliac joint (SIJ) and lumbar facet joints. These articular structures are also targets for local corticosteroid delivery.

ANATOMIC TARGETS FOR CORTICOSTEROID INJECTION

The most common treatment options for the management of chronic pain of spinal origin are the use of injectable corticosteroids targeting the cauda equina, nerve root, facet joint, or SIJ.[46] Rates of injection into the facet (zygoapophyseal) joints, or blockade of the medial branches of the posterior rami of spinal nerves that innervate this articular site, increased by 231% from 1994 to 2001 among Medicare patients.

The use of injectable corticosteroid and other drugs (eg, local anesthetics) via local drug delivery optimizes the analgesic benefit relative to the oral route and limits systemic effects. Over the past 2 decades, the rate of injections of corticosteroids has increased dramatically. Between 1994 and 2001, epidural injections increased by 271% and facet joint injections increased by 231% among Medicare patients. ESIs remain the most commonly administered spinal injection of corticosteroids[28] (**Figs. 1–4**).

EPIDURAL STEROID INJECTION

ESI is the most commonly performed intervention for chronic and subacute radicular pain syndromes in the United States.[47] Lievre and colleagues[48] reported the earliest use of this technique with hydrocortisone in 1953. Over the past half century, the epidural route of drug delivery emerged as a mainstay of both obstetric anesthesia during labor and the treatment of severe radicular pain (so-called sciatica). In 2008, 61% of women who had a singleton birth in a vaginal delivery received epidural anesthesia based on data collected in 27 states in the United States.[49] In both of these specific contexts, clinical observation of profound pain relief and improved tolerability relative to orally administered drugs (eg, opioids) has led to widespread adoption of the technique. An ESI typically combines the injection of corticosteroids, often administered with a concomitant local anesthetic, into the epidural space.

ESI is used to maximize local delivery of corticosteroids adjacent to inflamed nerve roots, thereby limiting systemic effects. The therapeutic aim of epidural administration of corticosteroids is alleviation of pain and reduction in pain-related activity limitation. Analgesic benefit from ESI also has diagnostic value for clinicians with respect to localization of the structural etiology of low back pain. Relief of pain favors a radicular localization.[50] Failure to alleviate symptoms after a single or repeated administration may indicate a nonneural structural cause such as paraspinal muscle, articular, or a centrally mediated syndrome.[51] Epidural steroids are used to relieve pain of presumed radicular origin at all spinal segments, but the risk–benefit ratio varies with greater risk

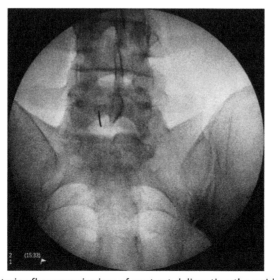

Fig. 1. Anteroposterior fluoroscopic view of contrast delineating the epidural space.

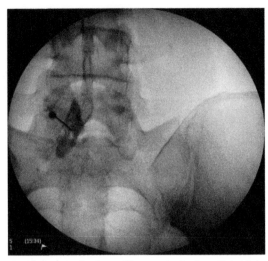

Fig. 2. Anteroposterior fluoroscopic view of intraarticular facet joint injections L4/L5 and L5/S1 segments.

of serious adverse events associated with cervical and thoracic needle placement.[52] There is a range of accepted clinical indications for epidural delivery of steroids.[9] Some of these are defined by structural pathology, such as intervertebral disc herniation or lumbar stenosis characterized by imaging techniques. In many instances, the predominant symptom pattern (eg, lateralization, pattern of radiation) of the low back pain syndrome forms the basis for the clinical indication.[39]

ESIs are moderately invasive and are usually used as a treatment choice when a more conservative treatment is unsuccessful or when a patient is not a candidate for surgery. Imaging, clinical, and neurophysiologic findings are important ancillary

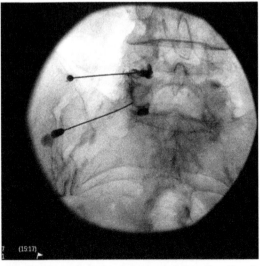

Fig. 3. Anteroposterior fluoroscopic view of contrast delineating the right sacroiliac joint.

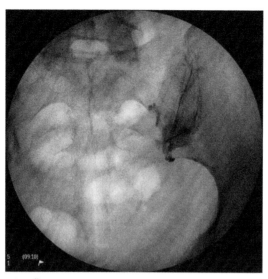

Fig. 4. Anteroposterior fluoroscopic view of contrast delineating left L3 transforaminal epidural space.

tools to target the specific spinal root(s) associated with radicular pain. Most practitioners rely on MRI, computed tomography, or computed tomography myelography to characterize the underlying anatomy and rule out other possible causes of severe pain (eg, tumor, infection, compression fracture). Most practitioners use fluoroscopic guidance with multiple planes of view during the ESI procedure to ensure accurate needle placement and confirm adequate spread of contrast material.[6]

Epidural Steroid Injection: Three Approaches

The optimal method of local intraspinal steroid delivery is a matter of debate. The 3 most common ESI techniques for the injection of corticosteroid into the epidural space are the (1) interlaminar, (2) transforaminal, and (3) caudal approaches. There is conflicting evidence as to the relative analgesic effectiveness of these 3 approaches as well as the rates of adverse events.[53,54] In the commonly occurring clinical scenario in which the culprit radicular segment is indeterminate or there is a presumption of a multisegmental (ie, polyradicular) distribution of pain, there are likely advantages to the interlaminar and caudal approaches.[55,56] The interlaminar approach is an injection into the dorsal epidural space and the caudal approach is an injection into the sacral hiatus.[42] Whereas a focal syndrome owing to lateralized subligamentous disc protrusion at an isolated level may be better targeted with the transforaminal approach. Even with the posterior approaches (ie, interlaminar and caudal), patterns of contrast spread on lateral view confirm that corticosteroid bathes the anterior as well as the posterior epidural space.[52]

A transforaminal injection is a direct deposition to a symptomatic spinal nerve in the intervertebral foramen in close proximity to the root and the ganglion. Because a high concentration of corticosteroid is placed in close proximity to the site of inflammation near the spinal nerve within the lateral epidural space, some practitioners favor this approach.[57] Thomas and colleagues[58] conducted a small, prospective, randomized, double-blind study comparing the effectiveness of transforaminal versus interspinous corticosteroid injections in treating 31 patients for radicular pain. The results showed significantly better pain reduction in the transforaminal group after 30 days. However, there is not an abundance of outcomes evidence favoring 1 particular epidural approach.

Some potential benefits of using a transforaminal approach may include a low risk of dural puncture, more specific and effective delivery of steroid to the site of pathology, increased localized spread into the ventral epidural space, and subsequently a reduced amount of medication necessary to produce the desired effect.[9] However, a transforaminal injection is also associated with higher risks and may be more unpleasant for patients given the soft tissues traversed.[58,59] Rare catastrophic effects can occur with transforaminal epidural injections, presumably owing to intraluminal arterial injection.[60]

Epidural Steroid Injection: Efficacy

Even though ESIs are in widespread use for pain indications of spinal origin owing to repeated demonstration of analgesic signal, there is an ongoing debate about the durability of analgesic and functional benefits. A large, heterogeneous evidence base evaluating the effectiveness of ESI has accumulated over more than 5 decades.[9,39] Practice and resulting study variation extends to almost every technical aspect of ESI, including the type and dose of steroids, volume of injectate, frequency of administration, approaches to identifying the epidural space, and the use of diverse imaging techniques. This lack of standardization reflects the development of a technique and portfolio of corticosteroid formulations antedating the current regulatory approval process. There is no more compelling illustration of this variability than the fact that the range of clinical "success" rates in a review of more than 40 studies[9] was 18% to 90%. Equally important, definition of study populations and assessment methodologies of analgesic efficacy has changed dramatically since the introduction of this technique nearly 70 years ago. The evidence for analgesic effectiveness is at once challenging to interpret and must be considered on a syndrome-specific basis and tailored to the individual patient context.

There is general consensus that ESIs offer short-term analgesic benefits in the treatment of radicular low back pain syndromes with or without a well-correlated compressive structural lesion such as an intervertebral disc protrusion.[28,61,62] The methods of study used make it difficult to determine the extent of benefit attributable to the corticosteroid component, the sodium channel blockade and sympatholytic effects of local anesthetic, or even the focal "washout" of inflammatory mediators with normal saline.[3] The evidence for durable benefit in patients with neurogenic claudication associated with lumbar spinal stenosis is mixed. One recent, randomized, controlled, effectiveness trial conducted by Friedly and colleagues[20] studied 400 subjects with lumbar spinal stenosis to determine the effectiveness of ESIs and found minimal benefit for glucocorticoid plus lidocaine over lidocaine alone. The strengths of this study include the use of a composite of pain, function, and imaging measures to define the study population and blinding of treatment allocation. The study found decreased pain and improved function in both the glucocorticoid plus lidocaine group and in the cohort receiving lidocaine alone at 3 weeks. There was benefit favoring corticosteroid at the 3-week time point but no differences between groups with respect to pain-related functional disability or pain intensity after 6 weeks. Major flaws in the study design complicate interpretation of this study's results. Specifically, 4 different corticosteroid formulations were used (methylprednisolone, betamethasone, triamcinolone, and dexamethasone). The variability introduced by this design weakness was compounded by a wide range of doses, variable number of lumbar segments/sites injected, differing number of injections (n = 1–3), and 2 different injection techniques (interlaminar and transforaminal). One major limitation of such a study design is that it cannot support conclusions about corticosteroid efficacy as an analgesic for the indication of lumbar stenosis.

Epidural Steroid Injection: Dosage

Corticosteroid dosing is an important factor to consider when balancing therapeutic benefit and the risk of systemic side effects. When ESIs are guided fluoroscopically, the steroids are often mixed with inactive carrier fluids. This may dilute the drug, thereby decreasing the amount of steroid reaching the site of pathology and decreasing its effects. Increasing the volume of the injectate may increase the likelihood that the medication reaches the targeted region. It seems likely that administering a larger dose of steroids around the affected nerve root should be more effective than a smaller dose.[9] However, the increased likelihood of adverse effects from larger doses limits the amount of corticosteroid that can be administered. As discussed, the NASS recommends specific limits of corticosteroid doses administered at each ESI session. The NASS also makes the recommendation that no more than 3 ESIs are performed in a 6-month period of time, because an increased number of injections increase the cumulative risk of chronic adverse effects.[10]

Epidural Steroid Injection: Fluoroscopy

Fluoroscopically guided ESIs have gained widespread adoption over the use of surface landmarks and loss-of-resistance techniques (so-called blind approaches) as a technical modification to improve the effectiveness of this common procedure. Fluoroscopy allows for more accurate and rapid needle placement at the suspected site of local inflammation.[6] More important, it may help to reduce the risk of major, but extremely rare, complications such as paraplegia resulting from intraarterial injection (when contrast is injected with continuous imaging methods), injection directly into the spinal cord parenchyma in the cervical region, or inadvertent dural puncture.[63] Fredman and colleagues[64] reported that in nonfluoroscopically guided ESIs, 50% of cases were injected at an incorrect spinal level, with the injectate reaching the area of pathology in only 26% of cases. Although repeated fluoroscopically guided procedures may expose patients to radiation, appropriate precautions can be taken to reduce this exposure risk.[63]

LOCAL INJECTION FOR CHRONIC LOW BACK PAIN SYNDROMES ATTRIBUTED TO THE LUMBAR FACET JOINTS

Chronic, axial-predominant low back pain syndromes are a more difficult diagnostic challenge owing to the many peripheral (eg, articular surfaces, paraspinal muscle, ligament, bone, intervertebral disc) structures that can incite symptoms and the multiple central factors that may contribute to their persistence. The leading cause of axial predominant chronic low back pain is lumbar zygapophyseal (facet) joint degeneration.[65] Several injection techniques, some involving local corticosteroid, target the facet joints as putative sources of chronic low back pain. Degenerative changes typical of osteoarthritis are commonly characterized on imaging studies of the lumbar facet joints, an anatomic structure long considered to play a causative role in acute and chronic low back pain. Lumbar facet joints are synovial joints that are richly innervated with encapsulated, unencapsulated, and free nerve endings, containing substance P, calcitonin gene-related peptide, as well as neuropeptide Y.[65–67] Nerve fibers have also been found in subchondral bone and intraarticular inclusions of lumbar zygapophyseal joints, implying that facet-mediated pain may originate in structures other than the joint capsule.[65] The innervation of these joints has been studied extensively and many strategies have been developed to disrupt nociceptive transmission from this site (eg, radiofrequency ablation).[68]

Intraarticular facet injections as well as local blockade of the medial branches of the posterior ramus of the spinal nerve roots have long been targeted for both diagnostic and therapeutic purposes. When performed as diagnostic blocks, facet injections are used to support an assessment that a specific facet joint or, more likely, group of joints is the source of pain. Intraarticular therapeutic facet joint injections are used to reduce the inflammation and swelling of facet joint tissue much as at other large and small joints throughout the body.[42] Accurate targeting of these small joints requires image guidance with fluoroscopy or computed tomography scanning.[69]

Forty years ago, Mooney and Robertson[70] first described corticosteroid injection into facet joints and claimed it led to significant long-term improvement. Few studies have rigorously studied their efficacy. One important randomized, placebo-controlled trial of 95 patients did not demonstrate long-term analgesic and functional benefits of facet joint injections of methylprednisolone acetate for the treatment of chronic low back pain.[71] Blockade of the innervation of these joints using local anesthetic for short-term relief (sometimes admixed with corticosteroid) remains a widely used procedure.

SACROILIAC JOINT INJECTION
Comment: Area of Overlap – Spinal Injections into Facet/Sacroiliac Joints Related to Discussion in Other Chapters About Intraarticular Injections

SIJ injections of corticosteroids are used to localize and treat pain attributed to the SIJ. Localization of chronic low back and buttock pain to this structure is challenging, because it is defined by symptom report and provocative maneuvers with weak sensitivity and specificity for pain localization. Moreover, pain attributed to the SIJ is not associated typically with findings on examination, such as sensory deficit or reflex asymmetry. Some experts regard injection of local anesthetic into this joint with subsequent provocative testing as the "gold standard" for this problem. Once diagnosed, SIJ injections of corticosteroids can be used in pain therapy.[72] SIJ corticosteroid injections seem to be an effective palliative treatment for some patients with focal SIJ pain, a localization that is more common after instrumented fusion of the lumbar spine. A systematic review by McKenzie-Brown and colleagues[73] showed evidence for accurate diagnosis of SIJ pain by SIJ injections and also showed moderate evidence for therapeutic SIJ injections.

Most patients who are responsive to SIJ steroid injections improve after 1 to 3 injections coupled with physical therapy, but some require frequent injections on a long-term basis. It is anticipated that the role of this injection approach as a diagnostic tool will increase as more devices to fuse the joint are introduced into widespread clinical practice. Fluoroscopically guided SIJ injections have been associated with minimal adverse effects, with the most common being vasovagal reaction.[74]

Complications

Local corticosteroid injection into the epidural space, SIJ, and for the targeting of facet disease is generally safe and well-tolerated, especially relative to public health burden related to oral analgesics (eg, opioids, NSAIDs) for the treatment of spinal pain and the largely irreversible, potentially long-term complications sometimes associated with spine surgery.[30–32] Complications from injectable corticosteroids may be divided broadly into drug related and technique related. The drug-related adverse effects are linked to acute (ie, local and systemic) as well as cumulative exposure. Complications owing to the drug itself can be caused by formulation issues (eg, nonsterile preparation, particle formation) or by target mechanisms. Technical and mechanical complications of the procedure, such as inadvertent dural puncture with low cerebrospinal fluid pressure headache, intravascular injection, and inaccurate needle placement must also be considered to understand the scope of complications that can arise with ESIs.[46]

A prospective evaluation study by Manchikanti and colleagues[63] found that major complications from ESIs are rare but minor side effects are common. There have been rare, isolated case reports of catastrophic adverse effects associated with ESIs, including reports of epidural abscess, meningitis and hypercortisolism.[7] Although there have been reports of incidents in which adverse effects have occurred after an ESI, the etiology of such events and the statistical significance of their frequency is unknown.

SIDE EFFECTS OF THE STEROIDS

Owing to their extensive function in the body, insufficient or chronic supraphysiologic levels of corticosteroids can have severe effects. Many side effects related to the administration of steroids are generally attributed to the pharmacology of the steroids. Despite their common clinical use, there are many well-known adverse effects of exogenous corticosteroids such as suppression of the hypothalamus–pituitary–adrenal axis, Cushing syndrome, osteoporosis, weight gain, fluid retention, hyperglycemia, hypertension, insomnia, mood swings, psychosis, headache, gastrointestinal disturbances, and menstrual disturbances.[63,75] Therefore, administration of exogenous corticosteroids should be carefully monitored and limited. It is important for patients to be aware of the associated side effects and potential risks.

Complications: Dosage

Although there is a relatively low chance of a patient developing adverse systemic effects from one corticosteroid injection, the risk may increase significantly depending on the number and frequency of injections performed. Many patients with a short-term radicular syndrome benefit from a single injection and do not require a repeat injection.[32] In a systematic review of lumbar transforaminal injections, 94% of patients achieved 50% or greater relief of pain after 1 injection.[76] The decision to repeat an injection or perform a series is based on a composite assessment of reduction in pain intensity, improvement in activity tolerance, and durability of benefit. The NASS recommends that, if a patient requires more than 4 injections in 1 year, alternative treatment such as surgical intervention should be considered owing to the possible systemic side effects of multiple corticosteroid injections.[38]

Complications: Steroid Formulation

The formulation of an injected corticosteroid is important when considering its effects and risks. Steroids are usually suspended in polyethylene glycol and a preservative is often added. It has been theorized that preservatives have neurotoxic (eg, demyelinating) properties but concentrations of preservatives in ESIs as used in clinical practice are most likely too low to cause concern.[7] The most commonly used preservative in corticosteroid formulations is benzyl alcohol. Benzyl alcohol is used in methylprednisolone, triamcinolone, and dexamethasone formulations (see **Table 1**).[11]

Acute vascular adverse events after corticosteroid exposure have been associated with the particulate size found in formulations (see **Table 1**). Derby and colleagues[77] showed that nonparticulate dexamethasone has particles that are 10 times smaller than an RBC (7.5–7.8 mm), and have a low tendency to aggregate. In contrast, particulate steroids such as methylprednisolone, betamethasone, and triamcinolone have particles that tend to form aggregates that are often much larger than RBCs. Corticosteroids with particulates or aggregates larger than RBCs have been shown to be more likely to cause damage because they cannot pass through small vessels easily. Rare, catastrophic complications, such as brain and spinal cord embolic infarcts, have been attributed to the injection of particulate corticosteroids.[47] Nonparticulate, water-soluble steroids that do not aggregate or pack densely are generally considered safer than particulate steroid suspensions in the field of chronic pain management and should reduce the risk of embolic infarcts owing to solubility.[77]

Although nonparticulate steroids are associated with reduced risk, there is debate over whether they are as efficacious as particulate steroids. A study by Kennedy and colleagues[78] found that both particulate corticosteroids (triamcinolone) and nonparticulate corticosteroids (dexamethasone) resulted in significant improvements in pain and function for lumbar transforaminal steroid injections. However, dexamethasone required more injections for an equal level of efficacy to triamcinolone.[78] This evidence for the therapeutic equivalency of nonparticulate to particulate steroids supports the idea that nonparticulate steroids should be used as the first-line drug in transforaminal injections.[79]

Complications: Needle Placement

The mechanism of injury from ESIs is often needle placement. Complications arising from direct injection into the spinal cord, vertebral artery, or radicular artery include spinal cord infarct, epidural hematoma, and brainstem hemorrhage.[63] Inaccurate needle placement is more dangerous when particulate steroids are being injected.[78] It has been shown convincingly that fluoroscopic guidance during the administrations of an ESI reduces the risk of harmful injection.[9] In work done by Johnson and colleagues,[80] contrast epidurography was performed during and after 5334 ESIs administered at various spinal levels. Out of the 5334 observed ESIs, only 4 minor complications were reported. Injection of variable amounts of contrast material with epidurography filming provided safe and accurate needle placement.

ORAL STEROIDS

Oral administration of systemic steroids is commonly used for acute radicular pain because imaging is not required (as in the case of ESI), the cost of this treatment is low, and can be readily prescribed by primary care physicians. A study by Goldberg and colleagues[41] tested the effectiveness of oral prednisone in the treatment of acute sciatica compared with a placebo. In this randomized, double-blind, controlled clinical trial, 269 subjects with acute sciatica were assigned randomly either oral prednisone or placebo. The results showed no improvement in radicular pain intensity and only modest improvement in function with a short course of prednisone relative to placebo. There was no significant between-group difference in likelihood of surgery. An improvement of function does not necessarily merit oral steroid use over other types of administration. Because oral steroids do not decrease the likelihood of surgery or improve pain more than placebo, they may be of limited value for some patients.

Contraindications

There are various contraindications for the use of ESIs. Absolute contraindications include hypersensitivity to the administered agents, infection, local malignancy, and concurrent anticoagulant therapy.[6] There are clear guidelines[81] with regard to holding anticoagulation to manage the risk of these common therapies. Relative contraindications for ESIs include congestive heart failure, uncontrolled diabetes mellitus, and immunosuppressed patients, the latter of whom may require antibiotic prophylaxis for the procedure.[6]

REFERENCES

1. Murray CJ, Abraham J, Ali MK, et al. The state of US health, 1990-2010: burden of diseases, injuries, and risk factors. JAMA 2013;310(6):591–606.
2. Andersson GBJ. Epidemiological features of chronic low-back pain. Lancet 1999; 354(9178):581–5.
3. Cohen SP, Hanling S, Bicket MC, et al. Epidural steroid injections compared with gabapentin for lumbosacral radicular pain: multicenter randomized double blind comparative efficacy study. BMJ 2015;350:h1748. Available at: www.bmj.com/content/350/bmj.h1748/rapid-responses. Accessed July 20, 2015.
4. Alangari AA. Genomic and non-genomic actions of glucocorticoids in asthma. Ann Thorac Med 2010;5(3):133–9.
5. Devor M, Govrin-Lippmann R, Raber P. Corticosteroids suppress ectopic neural discharge originating in experimental neuromas. Pain 1985;22(2):127–37.
6. Collighan N, Gupta S. Epidural steroids. Continuing education in anaesthesia, Critical Care & Pain 2010;10(1):1–5.
7. Price C, Arden NK, Coglan L, et al. Cost-effectiveness and safety of epidural steroids in the management of sciatica. Health Technol Assess 2005;9(33):1–58.
8. He Y, Yi W, Suino-Powell K, et al. Structures and mechanism for the design of highly potent glucocorticoids. Cell Res 2014;24(6):713–26.
9. Cluff R, Mehio AK, Cohen SP, et al. The technical aspects of epidural steroid injections: a national survey. Anesth Analg 2002;95(2):403–8.
10. North American Spine Society (NASS). Coverage policy recommendations. Lumbar fusion. NASS 2014. Available at: https://www.spine.org/Documents/PolicyPractice/CoverageRecommendations/LumbarFusion.pdf. Accessed July 20, 2014.
11. MacMahon PJ, Eustace SJ, Kavanagh EC. Injectable corticosteroid and local anesthetic preparations: a review for radiologists 1. Radiology 2009;252(3): 647–61.
12. Mensah-Nyagan AG, Meyer L, Schaeffer V, et al. Evidence for a key role of steroids in the modulation of pain. Psychoneuroendocrinology 2009;34:S169–77.
13. Reina MA, Franco CD, López A, et al. Clinical implications of epidural fat in the spinal canal. A scanning electron microscopic study. Acta Anaesthesiol Belg 2009;60(1):7.
14. Fyneface-Ogan S. Anatomy and clinical importance of the epidural space. Epidural Analgesia-Current Views and Approaches 2012;12:1–12.
15. Hogan QH. Epidural anatomy: new observations. Can J Anaesth 1998;45:R40–8.
16. De Andrés J, Reina MA, Machés F, et al. Epidural fat: considerations for minimally invasive spinal injection and surgical therapies. Issues 2011;1(1):45–53.
17. Oren I, Fleishman SJ, Kessel A, et al. Free diffusion of steroid hormones across biomembranes: a simplex search with implicit solvent model calculations. Biophys J 2004;87(2):768–79.
18. Ciriaco M, Ventrice P, Russo G, et al. Corticosteroid-related central nervous system side effects. J Pharmacol Pharmacother 2013;4(Suppl 11):S94.
19. Fietta P, Fietta P, Delsante G. Central nervous system effects of natural and synthetic glucocorticoids. Psychiatry Clin Neurosci 2009;63(5):613–22.

20. Friedly JL, Comstock BA, Turner JA, et al. A randomized trial of epidural gluco-corticoid injections for spinal stenosis. N Engl J Med 2014;371(1):11–21.
21. Rhen T, Cidlowski JA. Antiinflammatory action of glucocorticoids—new mecha-nisms for old drugs. N Engl J Med 2005;353(16):1711–23.
22. Markman JD, Kress BT, Frazer M, et al. Screening for neuropathic characteristics in failed back surgery syndromes: challenges for guiding treatment. Pain Med 2015;16(3):520–30.
23. De Bosscher K, Vanden Berghe W, Haegeman G. The interplay between the glucocorticoid receptor and nuclear factor-κB or activator protein-1: molecular mechanisms for gene repression. Endocr Rev 2003;24(4):488–522.
24. Takahashi H, Suguro T, Okazima Y, et al. Inflammatory cytokines in the herniated disc of the lumbar spine. Spine 1996;21(2):218–24.
25. Binder DK, Schmidt MH, Weinstein PR. Lumbar spinal stenosis. Semin Neurol 1981–2002;22(2):157–66.
26. Kobayashi S, Baba H, Uchida K, et al. Effect of mechanical compression on the lumbar nerve root: localization and changes of intraradicular inflammatory cyto-kines, nitric oxide, and cyclooxygenase. Spine 2005;30(15):1699–705.
27. U.S. Food and Drug Administration. Slides for the November 24-25, 2014 Meeting of the Anesthetic and Analgesic Drug Products Advisory Committee (AADPAC). 2014. Available at: www.fda.gov/AdvisoryCommittees/CommitteesMeetingMaterials/Drugs/AnestheticAndAnalgesicDrugProductsAdvisoryCommittee/ucm425962.htm. Accessed July 20, 2015.
28. Chou R, Loeser JD, Owens DK, et al. Interventional therapies, surgery, and inter-disciplinary rehabilitation for low back pain: an evidence-based clinical practice guideline from the American Pain Society. Spine 2009;34(10):1066–77.
29. Windsor RE, Storm S, Sugar R, et al. Cervical transforaminal injection: review of the literature, complications, and a suggested technique. Pain Physician 2003; 6:457–65.
30. Swegle JM, Logemann C. Management of common opioid-induced adverse ef-fects. Am Fam Physician 2006;74(8):1347–54.
31. Horlocker TT, Bajwa ZH, Ashraf Z, et al. Risk assessment of hemorrhagic compli-cations associated with nonsteroidal antiinflammatory medications in ambulatory pain clinic patients undergoing epidural steroid injection. Anesth Analg 2002; 95(6):1691–7.
32. Bartleson JD, Maus TP. Diagnostic and therapeutic spinal interventions epidural injections. Neurol Clin Pract 2014;4(4):347–52.
33. Gomes T, Mamdani MM, Dhalla IA, et al. Opioid dose and drug-related mortality in patients with nonmalignant pain. Arch Intern Med 2011;171(7):686–91.
34. Webster BS, Verma SK, Gatchel RJ. Relationship between early opioid prescrib-ing for acute occupational low back pain and disability duration, medical costs, subsequent surgery and late opioid use. Spine 2007;32(19):2127–32.
35. Bhala N, Emberson J, Merhi A, et al. Vascular and upper gastrointestinal effects of non-steroidal anti-inflammatory drugs: meta-analyses of individual participant data from randomised trials. Lancet 2013;382(9894):769–79.
36. Markman JD, Frazer ME, Rast SA, et al. Double-blind, randomized, controlled, crossover trial of pregabalin for neurogenic claudication. Neurology 2015;84(3): 265–72.
37. Markman JD, Gewandter JS, Chowdhry AK, et al. A randomized, double-blind, placebo-controlled crossover trial of oxymorphone hydrochloride and propoxy-phene/acetaminophen combination for the treatment of neurogenic claudication associated with lumbar spinal stenosis. Spine 2015;40(10):684–91.

38. North American Spine Society. Lumbar transforaminal epidural steroid injections review and recommendation statement. NASS 2013. Available at: www.spine.org/Documents/ResearchClinicalCare/LTFESIReviewRecStatement.pdf. Accessed July 20, 2015.

39. Pinto RZ, Maher CG, Ferreira ML, et al. Epidural corticosteroid injections in the management of sciatica: a systematic review and meta-analysis. Ann Intern Med 2012;157(12):865–77.

40. White AH, Derby R, Wynne G. Epidural injections for the diagnosis and treatment of low-back pain. Spine 1979;5(1):78–86.

41. Goldberg H, Firtch W, Tyburski M, et al. Oral steroids for acute radiculopathy due to a herniated lumbar disk: a randomized clinical trial. JAMA 2015;313(19):1915–23.

42. Chou R, Hashimoto R, Friedly J, et al. Pain management injection therapies for low back pain. Rockville (MD): Technology assessment report prepared for Agency for Healthcare Research and Quality (AHRQ). Project ID: ESIB0813. 2014.

43. Bjarnason I, Hayllar J, Macpherson AJ, et al. Side effects of nonsteroidal anti-inflammatory drugs on the small and large intestine in humans. Gastroenterology 1993;104(6):1832–47.

44. Rosen DS, O'Toole JE, Eichholz KM, et al. Minimally invasive lumbar spinal decompression in the elderly: outcomes of 50 patients aged 75 years and older. Neurosurgery 2007;60(3):503–10.

45. McLachlan AJ, Bath S, Naganathan V, et al. Clinical pharmacology of analgesic medicines in older people: impact of frailty and cognitive impairment. Br J Clin Pharmacol 2011;71(3):351–64.

46. Manchikanti L, Boswell MV, Singh V, et al. Comprehensive evidence-based guidelines for interventional techniques in the management of chronic spinal pain. Pain Physician 2009;12:699–802.

47. Gazelka HM, Burgher AH, Huntoon MA, et al. Determination of the particulate size and aggregation of clonidine and corticosteroids for epidural steroid injection. Pain Physician 2012;15:87–93.

48. Lievre JA, Bloch-Michel H, Pean G, et al. L'hydrocortisone en injection locale. Rev Rhum 1953;20:310–1.

49. Osterman MJ, Martin JA. Epidural and spinal anesthesia use during labor: 27-state reporting area, 2008. Natl Vital Stat Rep 2011;59(5):1–13.

50. Ghahreman A, Bogduk N. Predictors of a favorable response to transforaminal injection of steroids in patients with lumbar radicular pain due to disc herniation. Pain Med 2011;12(6):871–9.

51. Novak S, Nemeth WC. The basis for recommending repeating epidural steroid injections for radicular low back pain: a literature review. Arch Phys Med Rehabil 2008;89(3):543–52.

52. Derby R, Lee S, Kim B, et al. Complications following cervical epidural steroid injections by expert interventionalists in 2003. Pain Physician 2004;7:445–50.

53. Cohen SP, Bicket MC, Jamison D, et al. Epidural steroids: a comprehensive, evidence-based review. Reg Anesth Pain Med 2013;38(3):175–200.

54. Kozlov N, Benzon HT, Malik K. Epidural steroid injections: update on efficacy, safety, and newer medications for injection. Minerva Anestesiol 2014;81(8):901–9.

55. Singh V, Manchikanti L. Role of caudal epidural injections in the management of chronic low back pain. Pain Physician 2002;5(2):133–48.

56. Rathmell JP. The argument for use of epidural steroid injections in management of acute radicular pain. Perm J 2007;11(4):54.

57. Thomas E, Cyteval C, Abiad L, et al. Efficacy of transforaminal versus interspinous corticosteroid injections in discal radiculalgia–a prospective, randomized, double-blind study. Clin Rheumatol 2003;22:299–304.
58. Kennedy DJ, Dreyfuss P, Aprill CN, et al. Paraplegia following image-guided transforaminal lumbar spine epidural steroid injection: two case reports. Pain Med 2009;10(8):1389–94.
59. Salahadin A, Datta S, Andrea MT. Epidural steroids in the management of chronic spinal pain: a systematic review. Pain Physician 2007;10:185–212.
60. Scanlon GC, Moeller-Bertram T, Romanowsky SM, et al. Cervical transforaminal epidural steroid injections: more dangerous than we think? Spine 2007;32(11): 1249–56.
61. Barré L, Lutz GE, Southern D, et al. Fluoroscopically guided caudal epidural steroid injections for lumbar spinal stenosis: a retrospective evaluation of long-term efficacy. Pain Physician 2004;7(2):187–93.
62. American Society of Anesthesiologists Task Force on Chronic Pain Management. Practice guidelines for chronic pain management: an updated report by the American Society of Anesthesiologists Task Force on Chronic Pain Management and the American Society of Regional Anesthesia and Pain Medicine. Anesthesiology 2010;112(4):810.
63. Manchikanti L, Malla Y, Wargo BW, et al. A prospective evaluation of complications of 10,000 fluoroscopically directed epidural injections. Pain Physician 2012;15(2):131–40.
64. Fredman B, Nun BN, Zohar E, et al. Epidural steroids for treating "failed back surgery syndrome": is fluoroscopy really necessary? Anesth Analg 1999;88(2): 367–72.
65. Cohen SP, Raja SN. Pathogenesis, diagnosis, and treatment of lumbar zygapophysial (facet) joint pain. Anesthesiology 2007;106(3):591–614.
66. Cavanaugh JM, Ozaktay AC, Yamashita HT, et al. Lumbar facet pain: biomechanics, neuroanatomy and neurophysiology. J Biomech 1996;29(9):1117–29.
67. Ashton IK, Ashton BA, Gibson SJ, et al. Morphological basis for back pain: the demonstration of nerve fibers and neuropeptides in the lumbar facet joint capsule but not in ligamentum flavum. J Orthop Res 1992;10(1):72–8.
68. Carragee EJ. Persistent low back pain. N Engl J Med 2005;352(18):1891–8.
69. Murtagh FR. Computed tomography and fluoroscopy guided anesthesia and steroid injection in facet syndrome. Spine 1988;13(6):686–9.
70. Mooney V, Robertson J. The facet syndrome. Clin Orthop Relat Res 1976;115: 149–57.
71. Carette S, Marcoux S, Truchon R, et al. A controlled trial of corticosteroid injections into facet joints for chronic low back pain. N Engl J Med 1991;325(14): 1002–7.
72. Dussault RG, Kaplan PA, Anderson MW. Fluoroscopy-guided sacroiliac joint injections 1. Radiology 2000;214(1):273–7.
73. McKenzie-Brown AM, Shah RV, Sehgal N, et al. A systematic review of sacroiliac joint interventions. Pain Physician 2005;8(1):115–25.
74. Plastaras CT, Joshi AB, Garvan C, et al. Adverse events associated with fluoroscopically guided sacroiliac joint injections. PM R 2012;4(7):473–8.
75. Bellini M, Barbieri M. Systemic effects of epidural steroid injections. Anaesthesiol Intensive Ther 2013;45(2):93–8.
76. MacVicar J, King W, Landers MH, et al. The effectiveness of lumbar transforaminal injection of steroids: a comprehensive review with systematic analysis of the published data. Pain Med 2013;14:14–28.

77. Derby R, Lee S, Lee J, et al. Size and aggregation of corticosteroids used for epidural injections. Pain Med 2008;9(2):227–34.
78. Kennedy DJ, Plastaras C, Casey E, et al. Comparative effectiveness of lumbar transforaminal epidural steroid injections with particulate versus nonparticulate corticosteroids for lumbar radicular pain due to intervertebral disc herniation: a prospective, randomized, double-blind trial. Pain Med 2014;15(4):548–55.
79. El-Yahchouchi C, Geske JR, Carter RE, et al. The noninferiority of the nonparticulate steroid dexamethasone vs the particulate steroids betamethasone and triamcinolone in lumbar transforaminal epidural steroid injections. Pain Med 2013; 14(11):1650–7.
80. Johnson BA, Schellhas KP, Pollei SR. Epidurography and therapeutic epidural injections: technical considerations and experience with 5334 cases. AJNR Am J Neuroradiol 1999;20(4):697–705.
81. Horlocker TT. Regional anaesthesia in the patient receiving antithrombotic and antiplatelet therapy. Br J Anaesth 2011;107(Suppl 1):i96–106.

Infection Risk and Safety of Corticosteroid Use

Jameel Youssef, MD*, Shannon A. Novosad, MD, Kevin L. Winthrop, MD, MPH

KEYWORDS

- Corticosteroids • Bacterial infections • Rheumatic diseases
- Opportunistic infections

KEY POINTS

- The risk of serious bacterial infections is higher in patients with rheumatic diseases who are taking corticosteroids.
- The risk of certain opportunistic infections (OIs), such as *Pneumocystis jiroveci* pneumonia (PJP), herpes zoster (HZ), and tuberculosis (TB), has also been shown higher.
- Vaccination and screening strategies should be used to decrease the risk for these and other infections in patients with rheumatic diseases who are starting corticosteroids.

INTRODUCTION

Because of their potent anti-inflammatory properties, corticosteroids have been used for decades to treat many diseases, including rheumatic diseases. They are frequently used in chronic fashion for rheumatoid arthritis (RA), and several randomized controlled trials (RCTs) have established their efficacy. They have been shown to reduce radiographic disease progression and improve disease activity.[1,2] The dosages used in RA are often lower than for other rheumatic diseases, such as vasculitis or systemic lupus erythematosus (SLE).[3]

Because of their known efficacy in RA, corticosteroids are likely to be used frequently as monotherapy or in combination with biologic or nonbiologic disease-modifying antirheumatic drugs (DMARDs), and it is important for clinicians to know the risks associated with this therapy. There are several well-established risks,

Disclosures: J. Youssef has no financial disclosures. S.A. Novosad has no financial disclosures. K.L. Winthrop has no relevant disclosures.
Funding: S.A. Novosad's work on this article was in part supported by a National Institutes of Health training grant (2T32HL083808-06).
Oregon Health & Science University, 3181 Southwest Sam Jackson Park Road, Portland, OR 97239, USA
* Corresponding author. OHSU Rheumatology, 3181 Southwest Sam Jackson Park Road, Mail Code OP09, Portland, OR 97239.
E-mail address: youssefj@ohsu.edu

including osteoporosis, avascular necrosis, glaucoma, diabetes mellitus, and cardio-vascular disease.[4–9] Although an increased risk of infection is also well established, controversy remains regarding the dose and duration of corticosteroids necessary to substantially raise risk. In addition, there are questions regarding which specific types of infections have an increased risk. The prevention and surveillance for infection among patients with rheumatic diseases taking corticosteroids also vary widely and are often provider dependent.

There are multiple anti-inflammatory and immunosuppressive effects of glucocorticoids. They affect virtually all immune cells, and their precise effects depend on the differentiation and activation state of the cell.[10] They antagonize macrophage differentiation as well as suppress macrophage production of interleukin 1, interleukin 6, tumor necrosis factor, and the proinflammatory prostaglandins and leukotrienes. Glucocorticoids also suppress the tumoricidal and microbicidal activities of activated macrophages.[11] These agents also suppress neutrophil adhesion to endothelial cells and impair their lysosomal enzyme release, respiratory burst, and chemotaxis to the inflamed site.[11] Glucocorticoids can cause marked lymphopenia involving all lymphocyte subpopulations; they inhibit T-cell activation by inhibiting interleukins 2, 3, 4, and 6.[11] The maturity of double-positive T lymphocytes ($CD4^+$ $CD8^+$), which are the majority of the thymocyte population, can be impaired by glucocorticoids because these cells are highly sensitive to glucocorticoid induced apoptosis.[12] Glucocorticoids also have immunosuppressive effects on maturation and function of dendritic cells (antigen-presenting cells that can interact with naïve T cells to instruct the adaptive immune response).[12,13]

INFECTION IN RHEUMATIC DISEASES AND CORTICOSTEROIDS

At baseline, patients with rheumatic diseases have an increased risk of infection over the general population, and this has been particularly well documented in RA. Smitten and colleagues[14] evaluated 24,530 patients with RA from the PharMetrics claims database in the United States and 500,000 non-RA controls. They documented age-adjusted and gender-adjusted incidence of hospitalized infections of 4.4 and 2.2 per 100 person-years in RA and non-RA cohorts, respectively. A population-based study in Minnesota identified hospitalized infection incidence of 9 of 100 person-years among patients with RA compared with 5 of 100 in those without RA. After controlling for age, gender, smoking, corticosteroid use, and other factors, they found that patients with RA still had a higher risk of infection (hazard ratio [HR] 1.83; 95% CI, 1.52–2.21).[15] This increased infection risk is likely multifactorial and in part due to the immunodysregulation and mechanical joint/organ damage associated with the disease.[15,16] Other rheumatic diseases, such as SLE, are also well documented as having higher infection rates likely in part due to impaired cellular and humoral immunity.[17–19]

The current evidence base detailing the risk of infections with corticosteroids is largely derived from RCTs and observational studies (both population-based and single/multicenter). In general, individual RCTs have reported few infections. Observational studies, however, have consistently shown increased risks with corticosteroids. In general, most of these studies have divided daily prednisone dosages into low-dose, moderate-dose, and high-dose categories. Although this is somewhat arbitrary, most studies consider low-dose therapy as less than 5 mg daily, or by some studies less than or equal to 7.5 mg, of prednisone or equivalent daily. The duration of therapy is also important but perhaps is less well defined in terms of associated infectious risk. The exact doses and duration that substantially change the benefit-risk equation for corticosteroids likely vary by individual and underlying risk factors for infection.

RANDOMIZED CONTROLLED TRIALS

Several trials evaluating the efficacy and/or safety of corticosteroids have been conducted in RA (**Table 1**). In most RCTs, the prednisone dose and the duration of therapy were clearly defined; however, the low number of patients enrolled in the trials and the lack of a standardized way of reporting adverse events in these publications make interpretation difficult. For example, few RCTs clearly reported the number of serious bacterial infections in each treatment arm. Dixon and colleagues[20] recently performed a meta-analysis of RCTs published through January 2010 (see **Table 1**). They included 21 RCTs of patients with RA or undifferentiated inflammatory polyarthritis, treated with corticosteroids in one arm and no corticosteroids in the other arm through January 2010. The prednisone dose varied between the trials but was mostly less than 10 mg daily. A few trials included pulse doses of steroids and others included step-down prednisone regimens. The duration of treatment was short compared with the observational studies and did not exceed 3.5 years. No significant increased risk of infection was noted in the corticosteroid arms in most of the trials. Overall, they found 5.8% and 5.4% of the corticosteroid-treated and noncorticosteroid-treated groups had infections, respectively. There was no significant difference between the 2 groups, with a relative risk (RR) of infection associated with corticosteroid therapy of 0.97 (95% CI, 0.69–1.36). RCTs published since this meta-analysis are similar in both the dose of prednisone used and infections reported.

OBSERVATIONAL STUDIES

Observational studies have consistently demonstrated an increased risk of serious infections (generally defined as infections requiring hospitalization or intravenous [IV] antibiotics or resulting in disability or death), sometimes even with prednisone equivalent (PEQ) doses of 5 mg or less daily. A national collaboration of observational databases (Safety Assessment of Biologic Therapy [SABER]) in the United States found that in patients with RA, systemic corticosteroid use was significantly associated with increased risk of serious bacterial infections, with a stepwise increase in risk of infection with higher steroid doses, with an adjusted HR (aHR) of 1.32 (95% CI, 1.10–1.58) for PEQ less than 5 mg/d, 1.78 (95% CI, 1.47–2.15) for 5 to 10 mg/d, and 2.95 (95% CI, 2.41–3.61) for doses greater than 10 mg/d.[30] Dixon and colleagues[31] performed a nested case-control analysis of 16,207 patients aged greater than or equal to 65 years with RA in Quebec, Canada, between 1985 and 2003. After adjusting for disease severity, other DMARDs, and comorbidities, they found an increased risk of serious bacterial infections with as low as 5 mg PEQ for 1 week as well as a dose-dependent and duration-dependent stepwise increase in the risk of serious bacterial infections. In this study, the adjusted odds ratios (ORs) of serious bacterial infections were 1.03 (95% CI, 1.02–1.11) and 2.0 (95% CI, 1.69–2.26) in current users of 5 mg of prednisone daily for the past 7 days and 5 mg daily for the past 3 years, respectively.

Other studies have reiterated the idea that even low-dose steroids may pose a hazard for patients. In another population-based study in patients with RA, Wolfe and colleagues[32] identified an increased risk for hospitalized pneumonia for prednisone dose of 5 mg/d (HR 1.4; 95% CI, 1.1–1.6), with a higher risk at doses greater than 10 mg daily [HR 2.3 (95% CI, 1.6–3.2)]. Smitten and colleagues[14] found that doses less than or equal to 5 mg daily were associated with an increased risk of hospitalized infections (RR 1.32; 95% CI, 1.06–1.63). An analysis of Medicare beneficiaries with RA found that compared with methotrexate alone, glucocorticoid use doubled the rate of serious bacterial infections. This increased risk was dose dependent, with an RR of 1.53 (95% CI, 0.95–2.48) for doses between 6 mg and 9 mg up to 5.48 (95% CI,

Table 1
Recent randomized controlled trials in patients with rheumatoid arthritis treated with systemic corticosteroids[a]

Author, Year, Country, Duration	Population	Arms of Study	Type of Infection/Outcome	Outcome (Percentage of Infections in Each Treatment Arm)
Capell et al,[21] 2004, UK, 2 y	RA patients not on DMARDs, n = 167	1. SSZ plus prednisone 7 mg 2. SSZ plus placebo	• Infections leading to discontinuation	• None reported
Choy et al,[22] 2008, UK, 2 y	Early RA patients on MTX within 2 y of diagnosis, n = 467	1. MTX 2. MTX plus cyclosporine 3. MTX plus step-down prednisolone 4. MTX plus cyclosporine and prednisolone	• Serious infections • Respiratory tract infections	• 5.9%, 2.5%, 3.4%, and 1.7% serious infections in the 4 arms, respectively • 46.1%, 42.8%, 42.6%, and 47.4% respiratory tract infections in the 4 arms, respectively
Durez et al,[23] 2007, Belgium, 46 wk	Early RA patients, n = 44	1. MTX 2. MTX plus 1 g IV methylprednisolone 3. MTX plus infliximab infusions at wk 0, 2, and 6, then every 8 wk	• Serious infections • Nonserious infections	• No serious infections • 100%, 80%, and 80% nonserious infections in the 3 respective arms
Gerlag et al,[24] 2004, the Netherlands, 2 wk	RA patients on DMARDs, n = 21	1. Prednisolone, 60 mg week 1; prednisolone, 40 mg week 2 2. Placebo	• Adverse events	• 9% Skin infections in the placebo arm
Kirwan et al,[25] 2004, Belgium and Sweden, UK, 12 wk	Patients with RA, n = 143	1. Budesonide, 3 mg 2. Budesonide, 9 mg 3. Prednisolone, 7.5 mg 4. Placebo	• Viral infection • Respiratory infection	• 10.8%, 2.7%, 0%, and 0% viral infections in the 4 respective arms • 18.9%, 11.1%, 15.3%, and 3.2% respiratory infections in the 4 respective arms
Sheldon,[26] 2003, UK, 4 wk	Patients with RA, n = 26	1. Budesonide 2. Placebo with usual DMARDs	• Adverse events	• 7.1% Influenza infections in the budesonide arm • 8.3% Influenza infections in the placebo arm

Study	Population	Groups	Outcome	Results
Svensson et al,[1] 2005, Sweden, 2 y	Early RA patients on DMARDs, n = 250	1. DMARD plus prednisolone 7.5 mg 2. DMARD, no prednisolone	• Withdrawal due to adverse events	• 0.7% Infections in the nonprednisolone arm (1 abscess) • No discontinuations due to infection in the prednisolone arm
van Everdingen et al,[27] 2002, the Netherlands, 2 y	Previously untreated patients with early RA, n = 81	1. Prednisolone, 10 mg 2. Placebo	• Infections treated with antibiotics	• 42.5% Infections in the prednisolone arm • 53.6% Infections in the placebo arm
Wassenberg et al,[2] 2005, Germany, Austria, and Switzerland, 2 y	Patients with RA of <2 y duration, n = 192	1. Prednisolone, 5 mg, plus DMARD therapy 2. Placebo plus DMARD therapy	• Adverse events	• 3.1% Bronchitis infections and 1% influenza infections in the prednisolone arm • 3% Influenza infections in the placebo arm
Buttgereit et al,[28] 2013, Europe and US, 12 wk	Patients with RA on DMARDs, n = 350	1. MR prednisone plus DMARDs 2. Placebo plus DMARDs	• Incidence of infection, nasopharyngitis, and bronchitis	• Incidence of infection in the prednisone group 13% vs 12% in the placebo • Incidence of pharyngitis 4.8% in the prednisone group vs 3.4% in the placebo • Incidence of bronchitis 1.3% in the Prednisone groups vs 4.2% in the placebo
Bakker et al,[29] 2012, the Netherlands, 2 y	Patients with RA, DMARDs naive, n = 239	1. MTX plus prednisone, 10 mg daily 2. MTX plus placebo	• Infections treated with antibiotics	• 0.8% Infections in the prednisone group • No infections in the placebo group

Abbreviations: MR, modified-release; MTX, methotrexate; SSZ, sulfasalazine.

[a] Inclusion and exclusion criteria of the RCTs after 2010 were based on Dixon and colleagues' meta-analysis.[20]

Adapted from Dixon WG, Suissa S, Hudson M. The association between systemic glucocorticoid therapy and the risk of infection in patients with rheumatoid arthritis: systematic review and meta-analyses. Arthritis Res Ther 2011;13(4):R139; with permission.

3.29–9.11) for doses greater than or equal to 20 mg/d.[33] Among 86,039 patients with RA aged greater than or equal to 66 years in Ontario, Canada, the OR of serious bacterial infections was the highest for current exposure to corticosteroids compared with other DMARDs. For those using less than 5 mg daily, the OR was 3.96 (95% CI, 3.67–4.27) and for those using greater than 20 mg/d it was 7.57 (95% CI, 6.87–8.34).[34]

On the other hand, other studies have found an increased risk only with higher doses of corticosteroids. In a retrospective analysis of 5326 patients with RA, the risk of serious bacterial infection was only elevated in patients on a PEQ dose of more than 10 mg daily with an aHR of 1.85 (95% CI, 1.21–2.85), with no increased risk of infection at lower doses.[35]

Dixon and colleagues[20] performed a meta-analysis of 42 observational studies (case-control or cohort studies in patients with RA or inflammatory polyarthritis that reported an RR or rate ratio for the association between systemic corticosteroid therapy and infection). The use of systemic corticosteroid therapy was associated with an increased risk of infection, with an RR of 1.67 (95% CI, 1.49–1.87). There was a higher RR reported from case-control studies compared with cohort studies, with RRs of 1.95 (95% CI, 1.61–2.36) and 1.55 (95% CI, 1.35–1.79), respectively. Overall, no matter the study type, the risk of infection was found dose related: studies with average PEQ less than 5 mg/d had an RR of 1.37 (95% CI, 1.18–1.58), whereas studies with average PEQ 5 to 10 mg/d had an RR of 1.93 (95% CI, 1.67–2.23), and only 1 study reported an RR for a PEQ dose of 10 to 20 mg/d (RR 2.97; 95% CI, 1.89–4.67).

Lastly, work from Strangfeld and colleagues[36] suggested that for patients with RA, the risk of serious infections decreased over time in biologic users because the use of biologic agents allowed for decreased prednisone utilization and/or dosage over time (**Table 2**).

OPPORTUNISTIC INFECTIONS

In addition to serious bacterial infections, the risk of OIs (infections generally thought to occur in those with weakened immune systems) is increased with corticosteroids. There is a well-documented risk with some infections, such as PJP, HZ, and TB. The risk with other OIs, such as aspergillosis, nontuberculous mycobacterial disease,[41] candidiasis, and cryptococcosis, has been suggested but the evidence base is less robust.[42–44] With some OIs, such as TB and PJP that are endemic in certain parts of the world, the country being studied must be kept in mind when comparing incidence rates from different regions.

PNEUMOCYSTIS JIROVECI PNEUMONIA

The current evidence base regarding the association between PJP and corticosteroids is largely derived from case series and single-center studies. A study from the Mayo Clinic of 116 patients with PJP (without HIV) from 1985 to 1991 found that 105 patients (91%) had received corticosteroids for a variety of indications within 1 month of PJP diagnosis; the median PEQ dose of patients with PJP was 30 mg/d.[45] A case-control study of 15 patients with SLE and PJP and 60 matched SLE patients without PJP revealed a high daily dose of prednisone (49 vs 20 mg/d; $P<.01$) to be associated with PJP infection.[46] In another case series at the Mayo Clinic, 7 patients with giant cell arteritis and PJP infection were identified. All were taking prednisone (median dose 50 mg [range 30–80 mg] daily).[47] In an institutional case series conducted within a Singapore hospital, the risk of developing PJP among patients with autoimmune disease was increased in those treated with high-dose

Table 2
Recent observational studies evaluating risk of infections in patients with rheumatoid arthritis treated with systemic corticosteroids

Author, Year, Country, Duration, Study Type	Population	Prednisone or Prednisone Equivalent Dose	Infections	Results	Risk Ratios[a]
Wolfe et al,[32] 2006, US, 2001–2004, prospective	RA, n = 16,788	PEQ ≤5 PEQ 5–10 PEQ >10	Pneumonia requiring hospitalization	Increased risk of infection; dose dependent	HR of hospitalization for pneumonia: • Any PEQ, HR 1.7 (95% CI, 1.5–2) • PEQ ≤5, HR 1.4 (95% CI, 1.1–1.6) • PEQ 5–10, HR 2.1 (95% CI, 1.7–2.7) • PEQ >10, HR 2.3 (95% CI, 1.6–3.2)
Curtis et al,[35] 2007, US, 5/1998–12/ 2003, retrospective	Patients with RA: n = 2393 on TNF, n = 2933 on MTX	PEQ ≤5 PEQ 5–10 PEQ >10	Hospitalization with confirmed bacterial infection	Increased risk of infection in patients on PEQ >10 mg daily	Adj HR of confirmed infections: • PEQ ≤5, HR 1.49 (95% CI, 0.82–2.72) • PEQ 5–10, HR 1.46 (95% CI, 0.84–2.54) • PEQ >10, HR 1.85 (95% CI, 1.21–2.85)
Franklin et al,[37] 2007, NOAR, 1990–1999, prospective	Patients with inflammatory polyarthritis, n = 2108	Ever use	SBI	Increase risk of SBI	RR of SBI in patient on CS: • Univariate analysis, RR 2.3 (95% CI, 1.6–3.5) • Multivariate analysis, RR 2.2 (95% CI, 1.5–3.4)
Schneeweiss et al,[33] 2007, US, 1/1995– 12/2003, prospective	RA >65 y old, n = 15,597	PEQ ≤5 PEQ 6–9 PEQ 10–19 PEQ ≥20	SBI	Increased risk of infection; dose dependent	ARR of SBI as per PEQ: • PEQ ≤5 mg, ARR 1.34 (95% CI, 0.85–2.13) • PEQ 6–9, ARR 1.53 (95% CI, 0.95–2.48) • PEQ 10–19, ARR 2.97 (95% CI, 1.89–4.68) • PEQ ≥20, ARR 5.48 (95% CI, 3.29–9.11)

(continued on next page)

Table 2
(continued)

Author, Year, Country, Duration, Study Type	Population	Prednisone or Prednisone Equivalent Dose	Infections	Results	Risk Ratios[a]
Smitten et al,[14] 2008, US, 1/1999–7/2006, retrospective	RA patients (n = 24,530) compared with 500,000 non-RA patients	PEQ ≤5 6–10 >10	Any infection requiring hospitalization	Increased risk of infection; dose dependent	RR of hospitalization for infection risk as per PEQ: • PEQ ≤5, RR 1.32 (95% CI, 1.06–1.63) • PEQ = 6–10, RR 1.94 (95% CI, 1.53–2.46) • PEQ >10, RR 2.98 (95% CI, 2.41–3.69)
Greenberg et al,[38] 2010, US, CORRONA, 10/2001–9/2006, prospective	Patients with RA on DMARDs, n = 7971	PEQ <10 PEQ >10	Overall infections (includes both Opportunistic and non-OIs)	Increased risk of overall infections with PEQ >10	IRR of overall infections as per PEQ: • Any dose, IRR 1.05 (95% CI, 0.97–1.15) • PEQ >10, IRR 1.30 (95% CI, 1.11–1.53) IRR of OIs: Any CS dose, IRR 1.63 (95% CI, 1.20–2.21)
Dixon et al,[31] 2012, Quebec, 1985–2003, nested case-control	RA >65 y old, n = 16,207	PEQ <5 PEQ 5–9.9 PEQ 10–14.9 PEQ 15–19.9 PEQ ≥20	Nonserious infections	Increased risk of nonserious infections if PEQ >5; dose dependent	ARR of nonserious infections: • PEQ <5, RR 1.1 (95% CI, 0.99–1.22) • PEQ 5–9.9, RR 1.1 (95% CI, 1.04–1.16) • PEQ 10–14.9, RR 1.25 (95% CI, 1.17–1.34) • PEQ 15–19.9, RR 1.26 (95% CI, 1.12–1.42) • PEQ ≥20, RR 1.85 (95% CI, 1.68–2.05)
Dixon et al,[20] 2011, N/A, up to 1/2010, meta-analysis	21 RCTs 42 Observational studies	Any dose	Any Infection	CS therapy was associated with increased risk of infection in observational studies, not in RCTs	RR of increased infection risk as per PEQ: • In RCTs, RR 0.97 (95% CI, 0.69–1.36) • In observational studies, RR 1.67 (95% CI, 1.49–1.87)

Study	Population	Dose	Infection type	Result	HR/OR of serious infection risk

Grijalva et al,[30] 2011, US, 1998–2007, retrospective	1—RA, n = 10,484, 2—Pso or SpA, n = 3215	Any dose	Infection requiring hospitalization In patients on DMARDs	Increased risk of infection; dose dependent in RA group and Pso/SpA group	HR of serious infection risk as per PEQ:
					• RA group:
					  PEQ 0–<5, HR 1.32 (95% CI, 1.10–1.58)
					  PEQ 5–10, HR 1.78 (95% CI, 1.47–2.15)
					  PEQ >10, HR 2.95 (95% CI, 2.41–3.61)
					• Pso and SpA group:
					  0–<5, 1.15 (0.75–1.77)
					  5–10, 2.01 (1.08–3.73)
					  >10, 2.77 (1.44–5.32)

Xie et al,[39] 2012, China, 1/2009–2/2011, retrospective	RA, n = 2452	Any dose	Nosocomial infections	Increased risk of infection	OR of nosocomial infections by multivariate analysis: 1.02 (95% CI, 1.01–1.03)
van Dartel et al,[40] 2013, DREAM, 2005–2010, prospective	Patients with RA, n = 2044	Any dose	SBI	Increased risk of infection	• HR of SBI by multivariate analysis: HR 1.54 (95% CI, 1.08–2.20) • HR of SBI by univariate analysis: HR 1.78 (95% CI, 1.26–2.53)
Widdifield et al,[34] 2013, Ontario, 1992–2010, nested case control	RA ≥66 Y/O, n = 86,039	PEQ ≤5, PEQ 6–9, PEQ 10–19, PEQ ≥20	Serious infections	Increased risk of infection; dose dependent	Adj OR of serious infections as per PEQ: • PEQ ≤5, OR 3.96 (95% CI, 3.67–4.27) • PEQ 6–9, OR 4.28 (95% CI, 3.70–4.96) • PEQ 10–19, OR 5.98 (95% CI, 5.42–6.59) • PEQ ≥20, OR 7.57 (95% CI, 6.87–8.34)

Abbreviations: adj, adjusted; ARR, adjusted rate ratio; CS, corticosteroids; DREAM, Dutch Rheumatoid Arthritis Monitoring Registry; IRR, incidence rate ratio; MTX, methotrexate; N/A, not applicable; NOAR, Norfolk Arthritis Register; PEQ, PEQ dose measured by mg/d; Pso, psoriasis; SBI, serious bacterial infections; SpA, spondyloarthritis; TNF, tumor necrosis factor inhibitors; Y/O, years old.

[a] HR, OR, and IRR where indicated.

corticosteroids ($\geq$30 mg/d oral prednisolone or equivalent) compared with those on a dose less than 30 mg/d of oral prednisone (RR 19; 95% CI, 2–183).[48]

There is increased colonization with PJP in patients with autoimmune disease on systemic corticosteroids.[49] In a prospective analysis, Fritzsche and colleagues[50] induced sputum in 102 patients with autoimmune disease on corticosteroids (for more than 1 week) and 117 healthy controls and performed PCR testing for PJP. In 29 (28.5%) patients with autoimmune disease and 3 (2.6%) healthy controls; they found evidence of PJP colonization (OR 15.10; 95% CI, 4.43–51.38). These patients were also on other DMARDs, however, and the median prednisone dose did not differ between carriers and noncarriers. The significance of PJP colonization is unclear, although in those who develop disease, it is presumed colonization serves as the source of their disease.

Early observational studies in patients with antineutrophilic cytoplasmic antibody (ANCA)–associated vasculitis, notably granulomatosis with polyangiitis (GPA), showed that they are at increased risk of PJP.[51,52] Treatment with methotrexate, cyclophosphamide, and prednisone was associated with this risk.[53–55] In a study by Godeau and colleagues,[56] a group of 12 patients with GPA and PJP was compared with 32 GPA patients without PJP by multivariate analysis. A low pretreatment lymphocyte count at a cutoff of 800/mm^3 (P = .018) and lymphocyte count at month 3 at a cutoff of 600/mm^3 were independently and significantly associated with PJP.

Herpes Zoster

Several large population-based studies have found an association between corticosteroid use and HZ infection in those with rheumatic diseases, in particular RA. A study from Olmsted County, Minnesota, using an inception cohort of 813 newly diagnosed RA patients between 1980 and 2007 and a similar group without RA found the use of systemic steroids was significantly associated with HZ (HR 1.78; 95% CI, 1.14–2.76).[57] In another large population-based study, 10,614 RA patients and 1721 patients with noninflammatory musculoskeletal diseases (osteoarthritis, mechanical back pain, and so forth) without prior HZ were followed for 33,825 patient-years. The annualized incidence rate per 1000 patient-years was 13.2 in RA and 14.6 in musculoskeletal disease patients and did not differ significantly after adjustment for age and gender. Prednisone use was found significantly associated with HZ in patients with RA (HR 1.5; 95% CI, 1.2–1.8). There was no difference between doses less than 5 mg and doses higher than 5 mg daily.[58]

Other studies have evaluated the relationship between corticosteroid dose and incidence of HZ. In the German biologics registry, Rheumatoid Arthritis: Observation of Biologic Therapy,[59] risk factors for HZ episodes after the initiation of TNF inhibitors or conventional DMARDs were evaluated in 5040 patients. After adjusting for age and disease severity score, treatment with systemic corticosteroids of 10 mg daily or more was associated with an increased risk of HZ (aHR 2.52; 95% CI, 1.12–5.65). No increased risk was noted with a lower corticosteroid dose of 1 to 9 mg daily. In the SABER collaboration, a baseline use of 10 mg/d or more was associated with an increased risk of HZ among rheumatic disease patients compared with no baseline steroid use (aHR 2.13; 95% CI, 1.64–2.75).[60] In the Consortium of Rheumatology Researchers of North America registry (CORRONA) registry, a prednisone dose of at least 7.5 mg/d was associated with increased risk of HZ among RA patients (HR 1.78; 95% CI, 1.20–2.63) compared with no glucocorticoid use.[61]

In addition, in diseases other than RA, such as psoriasis and dermatomyositis, the risk of HZ has been shown increased with the use of corticosteroids.[62,63]

Strongyloidiasis

Strongyloidiasis is a chronic parasitic infection, usually acquired through direct contact with contaminated soil. An estimated 30 to 100 million people are infected worldwide and the prevalence is higher in tropical and subtropical regions. Immunosuppressed patients might be at risk for hyperinfection syndrome and disseminated strongyloidiasis, which has a high mortality rate; however, there is no population-based study to evaluate this risk.

Buonfrate and colleagues[64] conducted a systematic review of case reports/case series published from January 1991 to April 2011 in the general population. They found 213 articles with a total of 244 cases. In the areas of low/no endemicity, approximately half of the patients were immigrants and 3% were veterans; 67% of all patients were on corticosteroid treatment and, of those patients, 5.5% were being treated for lupus, 2.4% for RA, and 1.2% for sarcoidosis. The mortality rate was high 153/244 (62.7%).

Tuberculosis

The baseline rate of TB is increased in those with rheumatic diseases compared with the general population. In Canada, the incidence rate of TB in patients with RA was 45.8 per 100,000 person-years compared with a baseline rate of 4.2 per 100,000 in the general population.[65] In a US cohort identified using an integrated claims database, the incidence rate of TB in the RA population was 21.33 per 100,000 compared with 9.48 per 100,000 in age-matched and gender-matched controls without RA.[14] A study out of the United States using data from Kaiser Permanente Northern California (a large health maintenance organization) found the rate of TB in the RA population was 8.7 per 100,000 compared with 2.8 per 100,000 in the general population and 5.2 per 100,000 in the general population 50 years and older.[66] This incidence rate varies according to the baseline rate in the population being studied. For example, among patients with SLE in Hong Kong, the rate of TB was 700 per 100,000 compared with 110 per 100,000 in the general population.[67] A record linkage study in the United Kingdom found an RR of 9.4 (95% CI, 7.9–11.1) in those patients with SLE and 8.0 (95% CI, 4.9–12.2) in polymyositis for developing TB.[68]

The increased risk for TB within these disease states is presumably due to both the diseases and the immunosuppressive therapies used to treat them, although surprisingly few observational studies have evaluated the risk of TB with corticosteroid use. A retrospective case-control study in the United Kingdom (not limited to those with rheumatic diseases) found that among 497 new cases of TB and 1966 age-matched and gender-matched controls the adjusted OR for TB was 2.8 (95% CI, 1.0–7.9) for PEQ doses less than 15 mg/d and 7.7 (95% CI, 2.8–21.4) for doses greater than 15 mg/d.[69] Among 269 patients with rheumatic diseases treated for 1035 corticosteroid years of therapy, the incidence rate of TB was 2000 per 100,000, and cumulative and mean daily steroid doses and history of steroid pulse therapy were identified as risk factors.[70] Among a cohort of 24,282 patients with RA in Quebec, 18% of those with TB were current glucocorticoid users compared with 8% for controls (P = .03). The RR of TB was 2.4 (95% CI, 1.1–5.4) with use of corticosteroids.[71] Tam and colleagues[67] found the cumulative dose of prednisone and the presence of nephritis were independent risk factors for developing TB and that patients with TB were more likely to have received IV pulse-dose methylprednisolone. Increasing the prednisolone dose by 1 g was associated with a 23% increased risk of developing TB.

VACCINATION AND OTHER PREVENTION STRATEGIES
Pneumocystis jiroveci Pneumonia

The dose and duration of prednisone use necessary to trigger PJP prophylaxis have not been rigorously established. The current practice of starting PJP prophylaxis in patients with PEQ doses of greater than 16 mg daily for more than 8 weeks is largely based on the aforementioned study from the Mayo Clinic in 1996 that included patients with a confirmed diagnosis of PJP between 1985 and 1991 (HIV negative); 90% had used systemic corticosteroids in the month preceding infection. The median PEQ dose of patients with PJP was 30 mg/d, and the median duration of treatment prior to development of PJP was 12 weeks; 25% of these patients were receiving as little as 16 mg of PEQ and 25% developed PJP in 8 weeks or less. The major limitations of this study, however, were the inability to calculate the absolute risk, the number needed to be treated, and the small number of patients with rheumatic diseases who were enrolled in the study. Only 22.4% of patients enrolled in this study had inflammatory diseases, whereas the remainder had hematologic malignancies, organ transplants, and/or miscellaneous conditions that were not classified.[45]

Katsuyama and colleagues[72] evaluated 702 patients with RA on biologic therapies. Nine patients (1.28%) developed PJP; 8 of them (88.9%) were on corticosteroids at a mean dose (±SD) of 8.83 mg ± 14.9 mg. In the first phase of the study, they identified 3 risk factors for developing PCP: age greater than or equal to 65 years, coexistence of pulmonary disease, and corticosteroids. In the second phase of the study, they enrolled 214 patients with RA who were also on biologic therapy. They started 94 patients with at least 2 risk factors on prophylaxis with trimethoprim (TMP)/sulfamethoxazole (SMX) or inhaled aerosolized pentamidine; 49 (22.9%) of the 214 study subjects were taking glucocorticoids, with a mean dose of 6.28 mg ± 6.46 mg prednisolone equivalent. There were no cases of PJP in the second phase of the study. They calculated that the incidence of PJP decreased from 0.93/100 patient-years in the first phase of the study to 0/100 patient-years in the second phase of the study.

European League Against Rheumatism (EULAR)-based recommendations encourage prophylaxis against *Pneumocystis jirovecii* with TMP-SMX in all patients with ANCA-associated vasculitis being treated with cyclophosphamide.[73] There are multiple reports of PJP developing in patients treated with rituximab for hematological malignancies, solid organ transplantation, and autoimmune diseases.[52,55] Therefore, there is also a suggestion for prophylaxis in patients with ANCA-associated vasculitis who are treated with rituximab.[52,55] There is no clear recommendation regarding duration of treatment, or if this treatment should be discontinued after induction therapy once maintenance treatment is introduced.

TMP-SMX should be prescribed as prophylaxis for either daily intake of 1 single-strength tablet (80 mg TMP and 400 mg SMX) or 1 double-strength tablet 3 times weekly, with dose reduction in cases of chronic kidney disease (1 tablet 3 times weekly when glomerular filtration rate is 15–30 mL/min).[52] For patients who exhibit either intolerance or contraindication (ie, glomerular filtration rate below 15 mL/min) to TMP-SMX, alternative therapy with atovaquone, (1500 mg daily), dapsone (100 mg daily), or nebulized pentamidine (once-monthly 300 mg) can be pursued.[52]

In patients on methotrexate, TMP-SMX can increase the toxicity of methotrexate and should be used with caution.[74] Other strategies, such as atovaquone, dapsone, or pentamidine, may be considered in these cases because interactions with TMP-SMX could result in fatality.[52]

Herpes Zoster

Centers for Disease Control and Prevention (CDC) guidelines recommend a single dose of the shingles vaccine (zoster vaccine live [Zostavax]) for all persons ages greater than or equal to 60 years who have no contraindications, including persons who report a previous episode of zoster.[75] The efficacy of the shingles vaccine was evaluated in a double-blind, randomized, placebo-controlled trial involving 38,546 healthy adults aged greater than or equal to 60 years who had a history of varicella or at least 30 years of residence in the continental United States. The vaccine reduced the risk for developing HZ by 51.3% and postherpetic neuralgia by 66.5%.[76]

Furthermore, the CDC recommends vaccination in immunocompetent patients ages greater than or equal to 60 years in whom immunosuppressive treatments are anticipated or who have diseases that might lead to immunodeficiency. Such patients should receive 1 dose of the shingles vaccine at least 14 days before initiation of immunosuppressive therapy. A study of patients with various autoimmune diseases that compared 2 cohorts of patients, 1 with diabetes and the other 1 with healthy controls, showed that the age-specific rates of HZ for patients with RA or SLE greater than or equal to 40 years of age were greater than the corresponding rates in healthy individuals greater than 60 years old.[77] Given these elevated rates at baseline and that the vaccine is licensed for use in those ages 50 and older,[78] the authors advocate administration of the vaccine in all patients with rheumatic diseases once they reach the age of 50 as long as no contraindications are present.

According to American College of Rheumatology guidelines, the shingles vaccine is contraindicated in patients taking biologic agents.[79] According to CDC guidelines, high-dose corticosteroids (>20 mg/d of PEQ) lasting 2 or more weeks, methotrexate (>0.4 mg/kg/wk), azathioprine (>3.0 mg/kg/d), 6-mercaptopurine (>1.5 mg/kg/d), or biologic DMARDs are contraindicated for shingles vaccine and vaccination should be deferred for at least 1 month after discontinuation of such therapy.[80]

Tuberculosis

Currently, to the authors' knowledge, no rheumatic disease guidelines explicitly recommend screening for latent TB prior to initiation of corticosteroids, although the CDC guidelines on latent TB recommend screening in those who may need long-term immunosuppression, including long-term prednisone use.[81] Given that studies have shown increased risk for development of TB in those with rheumatic diseases in general and further increased risk with moderate-dose to high-dose steroids, the authors recommend screening for latent TB prior to initiating chronic therapy with corticosteroids. The dosage of prednisone (or PEQ) that would put someone at risk is not clear. The CDC's latent TB guidelines speculate that the dose of prednisone (or PEQ) that might increase risk is 15 mg for 2 to 4 weeks because this dose has been shown to suppress tuberculin reactivity,[81] although the work discussed previously suggests increased risk for chronic use of lower doses.[69]

Furthermore, interpretation of tests for latent TB, either tuberculin skin tests (TSTs) or interferon gamma release assays (IGRAs), such as QuantiFERON (QIAGEN Inc, USA) or T-SPOT (Oxford Immunotec Inc, USA). TB may be difficult in those already taking corticosteroids. In a study of 724 patients from Korea with rheumatic diseases, corticosteroid use was associated with discordant results between TSTs and QuantiFERON tests, with an OR of 2.44 (95% CI, 1.24–4.82).[82] In patients with SLE, the use of corticosteroids adversely affected the results of TSTs whereas for the T-SPOT.TB it did not.[83] Similarly, Matulis and colleagues[84] found that corticosteroids did not

Table 3
Prevention strategies

Disease	Prevention Strategies
Influenza	Annual vaccination in those with rheumatic diseases[88]
HZ	Vaccine in all patients with rheumatic diseases ages ≥50[75,77,78]
Pneumococcal pneumonia	In patients without prior vaccination, 1 dose of PCV13 in those on chronic steroid therapy should be given followed by PPSV23 ≥8 wk later. A second dose of PPSV23 is indicated 5 y after first dose.[88]
PJP	Treat with TMP/SMX (160 mg/800 mg) 3 times a week if on PEQ >16 mg daily for more than 8 wk.[45]
TB	Screen for latent TB using either TSTs or IGRAs[a] in those anticipated to start long-term corticosteroid therapy (10 mg for at least 1 mo) and treat for latent TB if positive.[81] If already on chronic steroid therapy, screen with IGRA and be aware of risk of false-negative results with TSTs or IGRAs.

Abbreviations: PCV13, 13-valent pneumococcal conjugate vaccine; PPSV23, 23-valent pneumococcal polysaccharide vaccine.
[a] IGRA is preferred if patient has a history of bacille Calmette-Guérin vaccine.

significantly affect IGRAs and that a positive IGRA response was associated with increased number of prognostically relevant risk factors for latent TB. Vassilopoulos and colleagues[85] found that the T-SPOT.TB was more sensitive than the TST in patients taking prednisone. Calabrese and colleagues[86] evaluated the rate of indeterminate QuantiFERON testing in those with chronic inflammatory diseases compared with the general hospital population as well as a healthy reference group and found indeterminate results in 5.3%, 1.9%, and 1.5%, respectively. In addition, they found in those patients with chronic inflammatory diseases, steroids significantly increased the likelihood of an indeterminate test (adjusted risk ratio 1.4; 95% CI, 1.02–2.0). The use of corticosteroids has been associated with decreased performance of both TSTs and IGRAs, increasing the risk of false-negative results in patients currently taking corticosteroids.[87] Based on the totality of data published in this setting, the authors recommend using IGRAs for screening if patients are already taking corticosteroids. Any interpretation (of either a TST or IGRA), however, must take into account a patient's a priori risk of TB and the fact that the predictive values of the tests are also influenced by the patient's level of immunosuppression (**Table 3**).

SUMMARY

Although RCTs of corticosteroid use in rheumatic diseases have not reported an increased risk of infection, observational studies have found a consistently elevated risk of infections (both serious and opportunistic). Given this, the risk-benefit ratio must be kept in mind whenever long-term steroid therapy is considered.

The current EULAR recommendation for the use of corticosteroids in RA patients is to use low-dose steroids for a limited time period during initial therapy for RA. Given the risks of such therapy, however, this recommendation should be individualized so that certain patients with existing risk factors for infection (eg, elderly, diabetes, and other comorbidities) might avoid such therapy or use it only in a limited fashion. Proper patient selection, vaccination, and screening can limit the infection risks and should, therefore, be pursued in any patient taking corticosteroid therapy.

REFERENCES

1. Svensson B, Boonen A, Albertsson K, et al. Low-dose prednisolone in addition to the initial disease-modifying antirheumatic drug in patients with early active rheumatoid arthritis reduces joint destruction and increases the remission rate: a two-year randomized trial. Arthritis Rheum 2005;52(11):3360–70.
2. Wassenberg S, Rau R, Steinfeld P, et al. Very low-dose prednisolone in early rheumatoid arthritis retards radiographic progression over two years: a multicenter, double-blind, placebo-controlled trial. Arthritis Rheum 2005;52(11):3371–80.
3. Duru N, van der Goes MC, Jacobs JW, et al. EULAR evidence-based and consensus-based recommendations on the management of medium to high-dose glucocorticoid therapy in rheumatic diseases. Ann Rheum Dis 2013; 72(12):1905–13.
4. Lukert BP, Raisz LG. Glucocorticoid-induced osteoporosis: pathogenesis and management. Ann Intern Med 1990;112(5):352–64.
5. Clore JN, Thurby-Hay L. Glucocorticoid-induced hyperglycemia. Endocr Pract 2009;15(5):469–74.
6. Kersey JP, Broadway DC. Corticosteroid-induced glaucoma: a review of the literature. Eye (Lond) 2006;20(4):407–16.
7. Walker BR. Glucocorticoids and cardiovascular disease. Eur J Endocrinol 2007; 157(5):545–59.
8. Powell C, Chang C, Naguwa SM, et al. Steroid induced osteonecrosis: an analysis of steroid dosing risk. Autoimmun Rev 2010;9(11):721–43.
9. Weinstein RS. Glucocorticoid-induced osteonecrosis. Endocrine 2012;41(2): 183–90.
10. McEwen BS, Biron CA, Brunson KW, et al. The role of adrenocorticoids as modulators of immune function in health and disease: neural, endocrine and immune interactions. Brain Res Brain Res Rev 1997;23(1–2):79–133.
11. Boumpas DT, Chrousos GP, Wilder RL, et al. Glucocorticoid therapy for immune-mediated diseases: basic and clinical correlates. Ann Intern Med 1993;119(12): 1198–208.
12. Coutinho AE, Chapman KE. The anti-inflammatory and immunosuppressive effects of glucocorticoids, recent developments and mechanistic insights. Mol Cell Endocrinol 2011;335(1):2–13.
13. Purton JF, Monk JA, Liddicoat DR, et al. Expression of the glucocorticoid receptor from the 1A promoter correlates with T lymphocyte sensitivity to glucocorticoid-induced cell death. J Immunol 2004;173(6):3816–24.
14. Smitten AL, Choi HK, Hochberg MC, et al. The risk of hospitalized infection in patients with rheumatoid arthritis. J Rheumatol 2008;35(3):387–93.
15. Doran MF, Crowson CS, Pond GR, et al. Frequency of infection in patients with rheumatoid arthritis compared with controls: a population-based study. Arthritis Rheum 2002;46(9):2287–93.
16. Goldenberg DL. Infectious arthritis complicating rheumatoid arthritis and other chronic rheumatic disorders. Arthritis Rheum 1989;32(4):496–502.
17. Bermas BL, Petri M, Goldman D, et al. T helper cell dysfunction in systemic lupus erythematosus (SLE): relation to disease activity. J Clin Immunol 1994;14(3): 169–77.
18. Marquart HV, Svendsen A, Rasmussen JM, et al. Complement receptor expression and activation of the complement cascade on B lymphocytes from patients with systemic lupus erythematosus (SLE). Clin Exp Immunol 1995;101(1):60–5.

19. Tektonidou MG, Wang Z, Dasgupta A, et al. Burden of serious infections in adults with systemic lupus erythematosus. A national population-based study, 1996-2011. Arthritis Care Res (Hoboken) 2015;67(8):1078–85.

20. Dixon WG, Suissa S, Hudson M. The association between systemic glucocorticoid therapy and the risk of infection in patients with rheumatoid arthritis: systematic review and meta-analyses. Arthritis Res Ther 2011;13(4):R139.

21. Capell HA, Madhok R, Hunter JA, et al. Lack of radiological and clinical benefit over two years of low dose prednisolone for rheumatoid arthritis: results of a randomised controlled trial. Ann Rheum Dis 2004;63(7):797–803.

22. Choy EH, Smith CM, Farewell V, et al, CARDERA (Combination Anti-Rheumatic Drugs in Early Rheumatoid Arhritis) Trial Group. Factorial randomised controlled trial of glucocorticoids and combination disease modifying drugs in early rheumatoid arthritis. Ann Rheum Dis 2008;67(5):656–63.

23. Durez P, Malghem J, Nzeusseu Toukap A, et al. Treatment of early rheumatoid arthritis: a randomized magnetic resonance imaging study comparing the effects of methotrexate alone, methotrexate in combination with infliximab, and methotrexate in combination with intravenous pulse methylprednisolone. Arthritis Rheum 2007;56(12):3919–27.

24. Gerlag DM, Haringman JJ, Smeets TJ, et al. Effects of oral prednisolone on biomarkers in synovial tissue and clinical improvement in rheumatoid arthritis. Arthritis Rheum 2004;50(12):3783–91.

25. Kirwan JR, Hallgren R, Mielants H, et al. A randomised placebo controlled 12 week trial of budesonide and prednisolone in rheumatoid arthritis. Ann Rheum Dis 2004;63(6):688–95.

26. Sheldon P. Ileum-targeted steroid therapy in rheumatoid arthritis: double-blind, placebo-controlled trial of controlled-release budesonide. Rheumatol Int 2003;23(4):154–8.

27. van Everdingen AA, Jacobs JW, Siewertsz Van Reesema DR, et al. Low-dose prednisone therapy for patients with early active rheumatoid arthritis: clinical efficacy, disease-modifying properties, and side effects: a randomized, double-blind, placebo-controlled clinical trial. Ann Intern Med 2002;136(1):1–12.

28. Buttgereit F, Mehta D, Kirwan J, et al. Low-dose prednisone chronotherapy for rheumatoid arthritis: a randomised clinical trial (CAPRA-2). Ann Rheum Dis 2013;72(2):204–10.

29. Bakker MF, Jacobs JW, Welsing PM, et al. Low-dose prednisone inclusion in a methotrexate-based, tight control strategy for early rheumatoid arthritis: a randomized trial. Ann Intern Med 2012;156(5):329–39.

30. Grijalva CG, Chen L, Delzell E, et al. Initiation of tumor necrosis factor-alpha antagonists and the risk of hospitalization for infection in patients with autoimmune diseases. JAMA 2011;306(21):2331–9.

31. Dixon WG, Abrahamowicz M, Beauchamp ME, et al. Immediate and delayed impact of oral glucocorticoid therapy on risk of serious infection in older patients with rheumatoid arthritis: a nested case-control analysis. Ann Rheum Dis 2012;71(7):1128–33.

32. Wolfe F, Caplan L, Michaud K. Treatment for rheumatoid arthritis and the risk of hospitalization for pneumonia: associations with prednisone, disease-modifying antirheumatic drugs, and anti-tumor necrosis factor therapy. Arthritis Rheum 2006;54(2):628–34.

33. Schneeweiss S, Setoguchi S, Weinblatt ME, et al. Anti-tumor necrosis factor alpha therapy and the risk of serious bacterial infections in elderly patients with rheumatoid arthritis. Arthritis Rheum 2007;56(6):1754–64.

34. Widdifield J, Bernatsky S, Paterson JM, et al. Serious infections in a population-based cohort of 86,039 seniors with rheumatoid arthritis. Arthritis Care Res (Hoboken) 2013;65(3):353–61.

35. Curtis JR, Patkar N, Xie A, et al. Risk of serious bacterial infections among rheumatoid arthritis patients exposed to tumor necrosis factor alpha antagonists. Arthritis Rheum 2007;56(4):1125–33.

36. Strangfeld A, Eveslage M, Schneider M, et al. Treatment benefit or survival of the fittest: what drives the time-dependent decrease in serious infection rates under TNF inhibition and what does this imply for the individual patient? Ann Rheum Dis 2011;70(11):1914–20.

37. Franklin J, Lunt M, Bunn D, et al. Risk and predictors of infection leading to hospitalisation in a large primary-care-derived cohort of patients with inflammatory polyarthritis. Ann Rheum Dis 2007;66(3):308–12.

38. Greenberg JD, Reed G, Kremer JM, et al, CORRONA Investigators. Association of methotrexate and tumour necrosis factor antagonists with risk of infectious outcomes including opportunistic infections in the CORRONA registry. Ann Rheum Dis 2010;69(2):380–6.

39. Xie WL, Li ZL, Xu Z, et al. The risk factors for nosocomial infection in chinese patients with active rheumatoid arthritis in shanghai. ISRN Rheumatol 2012;2012:215692.

40. van Dartel SA, Fransen J, Kievit W, et al. Predictors for the 5-year risk of serious infections in patients with rheumatoid arthritis treated with anti-tumour necrosis factor therapy: a cohort study in the dutch rheumatoid arthritis monitoring (DREAM) registry. Rheumatology (Oxford) 2013;52(6):1052–7.

41. Dirac MA, Horan KL, Doody DR, et al. Environment or host?: a case-control study of risk factors for mycobacterium avium complex lung disease. Am J Respir Crit Care Med 2012;186(7):684–91.

42. MacDougall L, Fyfe M, Romney M, et al. Risk factors for cryptococcus gattii infection, british columbia, canada. Emerg Infect Dis 2011;17(2):193–9.

43. Garnacho-Montero J, Amaya-Villar R, Ortiz-Leyba C, et al. Isolation of aspergillus spp. from the respiratory tract in critically ill patients: risk factors, clinical presentation and outcome. Crit Care 2005;9(3):R191–9.

44. Dimopoulos G, Ntziora F, Rachiotis G, et al. Candida albicans versus non-albicans intensive care unit-acquired bloodstream infections: differences in risk factors and outcome. Anesth Analg 2008;106(2):523–9.

45. Yale SH, Limper AH. Pneumocystis carinii pneumonia in patients without acquired immunodeficiency syndrome: associated illness and prior corticosteroid therapy. Mayo Clin Proc 1996;71(1):5–13.

46. Lertnawapan R, Totemchokchyakarn K, Nantiruj K, et al. Risk factors of pneumocystis jeroveci pneumonia in patients with systemic lupus erythematosus. Rheumatol Int 2009;29(5):491–6.

47. Kermani TA, Ytterberg SR, Warrington KJ. Pneumocystis jiroveci pneumonia in giant cell arteritis: a case series. Arthritis Care Res (Hoboken) 2011;63(5):761–5.

48. Chew LC, Maceda-Galang LM, Tan YK, et al. Pneumocystis jirovecii pneumonia in patients with autoimmune disease on high-dose glucocorticoid. J Clin Rheumatol 2015;21(2):72–5.

49. Mekinian A, Durand-Joly I, Hatron PY, et al. Pneumocystis jirovecii colonization in patients with systemic autoimmune diseases: prevalence, risk factors of colonization and outcome. Rheumatology (Oxford) 2011;50(3):569–77.

50. Fritzsche C, Riebold D, Munk-Hartig A, et al. High prevalence of pneumocystis jirovecii colonization among patients with autoimmune inflammatory diseases and corticosteroid therapy. Scand J Rheumatol 2012;41(3):208–13.

51. Jarrousse B, Guillevin L, Bindi P, et al. Increased risk of pneumocystis carinii pneumonia in patients with wegener's granulomatosis. Clin Exp Rheumatol 1993;11(6):615–21.
52. Kronbichler A, Jayne DR, Mayer G. Frequency, risk factors and prophylaxis of infection in ANCA-associated vasculitis. Eur J Clin Invest 2015;45(3):346–68.
53. Ognibene FP, Shelhamer JH, Hoffman GS, et al. Pneumocystis carinii pneumonia: a major complication of immunosuppressive therapy in patients with wegener's granulomatosis. Am J Respir Crit Care Med 1995;151(3 Pt 1):795–9.
54. Guillevin L, Cordier JF, Lhote F, et al. A prospective, multicenter, randomized trial comparing steroids and pulse cyclophosphamide versus steroids and oral cyclophosphamide in the treatment of generalized wegener's granulomatosis. Arthritis Rheum 1997;40(12):2187–98.
55. Besada E, Nossent JC. Should pneumocystis jiroveci prophylaxis be recommended with rituximab treatment in ANCA-associated vasculitis? Clin Rheumatol 2013;32(11):1677–81.
56. Godeau B, Mainardi JL, Roudot-Thoraval F, et al. Factors associated with pneumocystis carinii pneumonia in wegener's granulomatosis. Ann Rheum Dis 1995; 54(12):991–4.
57. Veetil BM, Myasoedova E, Matteson EL, et al. Incidence and time trends of herpes zoster in rheumatoid arthritis: a population-based cohort study. Arthritis Care Res (Hoboken) 2013;65(6):854–61.
58. Wolfe F, Michaud K, Chakravarty EF. Rates and predictors of herpes zoster in patients with rheumatoid arthritis and non-inflammatory musculoskeletal disorders. Rheumatology (Oxford) 2006;45(11):1370–5.
59. Strangfeld A, Listing J, Herzer P, et al. Risk of herpes zoster in patients with rheumatoid arthritis treated with anti-TNF-alpha agents. JAMA 2009;301(7):737–44.
60. Winthrop KL, Baddley JW, Chen L, et al. Association between the initiation of anti-tumor necrosis factor therapy and the risk of herpes zoster. JAMA 2013;309(9): 887–95.
61. Pappas DA, Hooper MM, Kremer JM, et al. Herpes zoster reactivation in patients with rheumatoid arthritis: analysis of disease characteristics and disease modifying anti-rheumatic drugs. Arthritis Care Res (Hoboken) 2015. [Epub ahead of print].
62. Zisman D, Bitterman H, Shalom G, et al. Psoriatic arthritis treatment and the risk of herpes zoster. Ann Rheum Dis 2014. [Epub ahead of print].
63. Fardet L, Rybojad M, Gain M, et al. Incidence, risk factors, and severity of herpesvirus infections in a cohort of 121 patients with primary dermatomyositis and dermatomyositis associated with a malignant neoplasm. Arch Dermatol 2009;145(8):889–93.
64. Buonfrate D, Requena-Mendez A, Angheben A, et al. Severe strongyloidiasis: a systematic review of case reports. BMC Infect Dis 2013;13:78.
65. Brassard P, Kezouh A, Suissa S. Antirheumatic drugs and the risk of tuberculosis. Clin Infect Dis 2006;43(6):717–22.
66. Winthrop KL, Baxter R, Liu L, et al. Mycobacterial diseases and antitumour necrosis factor therapy in USA. Ann Rheum Dis 2013;72(1):37–42.
67. Tam LS, Li EK, Wong SM, et al. Risk factors and clinical features for tuberculosis among patients with systemic lupus erythematosus in hong kong. Scand J Rheumatol 2002;31(5):296–300.
68. Ramagopalan SV, Goldacre R, Skingsley A, et al. Associations between selected immune-mediated diseases and tuberculosis: record-linkage studies. BMC Med 2013;11:97.

69. Jick SS, Lieberman ES, Rahman MU, et al. Glucocorticoid use, other associated factors, and the risk of tuberculosis. Arthritis Rheum 2006;55(1):19–26.
70. Kim HA, Yoo CD, Baek HJ, et al. Mycobacterium tuberculosis infection in a corticosteroid-treated rheumatic disease patient population. Clin Exp Rheumatol 1998;16(1):9–13.
71. Brassard P, Lowe AM, Bernatsky S, et al. Rheumatoid arthritis, its treatments, and the risk of tuberculosis in quebec, canada. Arthritis Rheum 2009;61(3): 300–4.
72. Katsuyama T, Saito K, Kubo S, et al. Prophylaxis for pneumocystis pneumonia in patients with rheumatoid arthritis treated with biologics, based on risk factors found in a retrospective study. Arthritis Res Ther 2014;16(1):R43.
73. Mukhtyar C, Guillevin L, Cid MC, et al. EULAR recommendations for the management of primary small and medium vessel vasculitis. Ann Rheum Dis 2009;68(3): 310–7.
74. Davis SA, Krowchuk DP, Feldman SR. Prescriptions for a toxic combination: use of methotrexate plus trimethoprim-sulfamethoxazole in the united states. Southampt Med J 2014;107(5):292–3.
75. Shingles (Herpes Zoster). Centers for Disease Control and Prevention. 2014. Available at: http://www.cdc.gov/vaccines/vpd-vac/shingles/hcp-vaccination. htm. Accessed June 12, 2015.
76. Oxman MN, Levin MJ, Johnson GR, et al. A vaccine to prevent herpes zoster and postherpetic neuralgia in older adults. N Engl J Med 2005;352(22):2271–84.
77. Curtis J, Yang S, Chen L, et al. Herpes zoster infection across auto-immune and inflammatory diseases: implications for vaccination. Ann Rheum Dis 2014; 73(Suppl 2):452.
78. ZOSTAVAX Zoster Vaccine Live Product Information. Available at: MerckVaccines.com. Accessed June 12, 2015.
79. Singh JA, Furst DE, Bharat A, et al. 2012 update of the 2008 american college of rheumatology recommendations for the use of disease-modifying antirheumatic drugs and biologic agents in the treatment of rheumatoid arthritis. Arthritis Care Res (Hoboken) 2012;64(5):625–39.
80. Contraindications and Precautions to Commonly Used Vaccines in Adults. Centers for Disease Control and Prevention. 2015. Available at: http://www.cdc. gov/vaccines/schedules/hcp/imz/adult-contraindications.html. Accessed June 12, 2015.
81. Targeted tuberculin testing and treatment of latent tuberculosis infection. American thoracic society. MMWR Recomm Rep 2000;49(RR-6):1–51.
82. Kim JH, Cho SK, Han M, et al. Factors influencing discrepancies between the QuantiFERON-TB gold in tube test and the tuberculin skin test in korean patients with rheumatic diseases. Semin Arthritis Rheum 2013;42(4):424–32.
83. Arenas Miras Mdel M, Hidalgo-Tenorio C, Jimenez-Gamiz P, et al. Diagnosis of latent tuberculosis in patients with systemic lupus erythematosus: T.SPOT.TB versus tuberculin skin test. Biomed Res Int 2014;2014:291031.
84. Matulis G, Juni P, Villiger PM, et al. Detection of latent tuberculosis in immunosuppressed patients with autoimmune diseases: performance of a mycobacterium tuberculosis antigen-specific interferon gamma assay. Ann Rheum Dis 2008; 67(1):84–90.
85. Vassilopoulos D, Stamoulis N, Hadziyannis E, et al. Usefulness of enzyme-linked immunospot assay (elispot) compared to tuberculin skin testing for latent tuberculosis screening in rheumatic patients scheduled for anti-tumor necrosis factor treatment. J Rheumatol 2008;35(7):1271–6.

86. Calabrese C, Overman RA, Dusetzina SB, et al. Indeterminate QuantiFERON-TB gold in-tube results in patients with chronic inflammatory diseases on immunosuppressive therapy. Arthritis Care Res (Hoboken) 2014;67(8): 1063–9.
87. Bartalesi F, Vicidomini S, Goletti D, et al. QuantiFERON-TB gold and the TST are both useful for latent tuberculosis infection screening in autoimmune diseases. Eur Respir J 2009;33(3):586–93.
88. Recommended Adult Immunization Schedule–United States - 2015. Centers for Disease Control and Prevention. Available at: http://www.cdc.gov/vaccines/schedules/hcp/adult.html. Accessed June 12, 2015.

Glucocorticoid-induced Osteoporosis

Xena Whittier, MD[a], Kenneth G. Saag, MD, MSc[b],*

KEYWORDS

- Glucocorticoids • Osteoporosis • Fracture risk • Prevention

KEY POINTS

- Glucocorticoid-induced osteoporosis (GIOP) is one of the most common and serious adverse effects associated with glucocorticoid use.
- GIOP is associated with significant morbidity secondary to resultant fractures, and despite GIOP being a well-characterized problem, it remains undertreated, and prevention strategies are underused.
- This article highlights GIOP pathophysiology, epidemiologic associations, effective treatment, and lifestyle modifications that can reduce fracture risk for long-term glucocorticoid users and additionally emphasizes the importance of early intervention.

INTRODUCTION

Glucocorticoid-induced osteoporosis (GIOP) is one of the most common and serious adverse effects associated with glucocorticoid use. GIOP, the most common secondary form of osteoporosis, is associated with significant morbidity secondary to resultant fractures. Despite GIOP being a well-characterized problem that can occur rapidly, within the first few months of glucocorticoid use, it remains undertreated, and prevention strategies are underused. This article highlights GIOP pathophysiology, epidemiologic associations, effective treatment, and lifestyle modifications that can reduce fracture risk for long-term glucocorticoid users and additionally emphasizes the importance of early intervention.

Conflict of Interest: Consultant with Amgen, Lilly Merck. Research/Grant with Amgen, Lilly, Merck (Dr K.G. Saag).

[a] Division of Clinical Immunology and Rheumatology, 851 Faculty Office Tower, 510 20th Street South, Birmingham, AL 35294, USA; [b] Division of Clinical Immunology and Rheumatology, Department of Medicine, Center for Education and Research on Therapeutics (CERTs), Center for Outcomes, Effectiveness Research and Education (COERE), Center of Research Translation (CORT) in Gout and Hyperuricemia, University of Alabama at Birmingham, 820 Faculty Office Tower, 510 20th Street South, Birmingham, AL 35294, USA
* Corresponding author.
E-mail address: ksaag@uab.edu

Rheum Dis Clin N Am 42 (2016) 177–189
http://dx.doi.org/10.1016/j.rdc.2015.08.005   rheumatic.theclinics.com
0889-857X/16/$ – see front matter © 2016 Elsevier Inc. All rights reserved.

GLUCOCORTICOID EFFECTS ON BONE

Glucocorticoids lead to decreased bone formation and increased bone resorption (**Fig. 1**). The effects on osteoblasts, which are essential for bone formation, include decreased differentiation and maturation leading to their decreased number and function.[1,2] In addition, excess glucocorticoid results in osteoblast apoptosis, further contributing to reduced bone formation.[1-3] Osteocytes also undergo apoptosis and, because they are involved in repair of microdamage to bone, this leads to a decrease in bone quality.[1] Glucocorticoids increase the expression of cytokines, including receptor of activator of NF-kappa β ligand (RANKL), that are involved in differentiation of osteoclasts and conversely decrease those involved in inhibition of osteoclasts, with the net effect of increased bone resorption.[1] Indirect effects of glucocorticoids contribute to bone loss as well, such as decreases in calcium resorption, suppression of sex hormones and growth hormones, and alteration of parathyroid hormone pulsatility.[1] However, subclinical secondary hyperparathyroidism leading to bone resorption is considered a more minor pathway for bone loss in GIOP. Areas of exploration include determining whether there are genetic factors that may make an individual more susceptible to adverse effects from glucocorticoids. A polymorphism in the glucocorticoid receptor gene has been identified that is associated with increased sensitivity to glucocorticoids with regard to cortisol suppression and insulin response, and although lower bone mineral density (BMD) in the spine was also found compared with controls, this did not reach statistical significance.[4] To date, genetic testing has not found a role in risk stratification for GIOP.

EPIDEMIOLOGY

Up to 40% of persons receiving glucocorticoids develop bone loss over time.[5] Bone loss secondary to glucocorticoids occurs early in their course of use; most

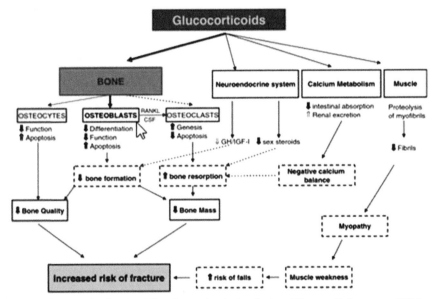

Fig. 1. Pathogenesis of GIOP. CSF, colony-stimulating factor; GH, growth hormone; IGF, insulinlike growth factor; RANKL, receptor activator of nuclear factor kappa-B ligand. (*Adapted from* Canalis E, Mazziotti G, Giustina A, et al. Glucocorticoid-induced osteoporosis: pathophysiology and therapy. Osteoporos Int 2007;18(10):1319–28; with permission.)

significantly in the first 6 months. The initial rate of bone loss is rapid at up to 12% in the first year and then averages 2% to 3% a year.[6] It is trabecular bone that is first affected, leading to an increased risk for fractures, particularly of the vertebrae.[1] Later effects on cortical bone include the femoral neck of the hip. Among patients at risk for GIOP, age plays a major role, with postmenopausal women and older men at greatest fracture risk.[7] Other risk factors that independently increase the risk for glucocorticoid-induced fractures are the same as those associated with traditional osteoporosis, except for glucocorticoid dose and mechanism of administration.[8] Dose and duration of glucocorticoid use have a significant impact on fracture risk. The average daily dose of glucocorticoids seems more predictive of fracture than the cumulative dose.[9] Doses as low as 2.5 mg of prednisone oral daily are associated with increased fracture risk, but at doses greater than 7.5 mg (the approximate physiologic amount of glucocorticoid produced endogenously) this risk increases 5-fold.[9] This increase leads to the debate of whether there is a threshold dose that would confer a greater risk of fracture. A meta-analysis suggests that using more than 5 mg of prednisolone or equivalent daily leads to a decrease in BMD and increase in fracture risk.[10] Cessation of glucocorticoid use results in decline in fracture risk, although not back to baseline.[9] Supporting the premise that there is likely not a completely safe dose, it seems that even inhaled corticosteroids and intra-articular steroids can increase risk, therefore no route of administration and perhaps no dose is completely innocuous.[11,12] In addition to the use of glucocorticoids themselves, many of the diseases that they are used to treat, such as rheumatoid arthritis (RA) and chronic obstructive pulmonary disease, are associated with bone loss, independent of glucocorticoid use.[1,9] Proinflammatory cytokines involved in the pathophysiology of these conditions affect changes in bone formation and bone resorption.[1] As an example, in RA several cytokines, such as tumor necrosis alpha and interleukin (IL)-1, IL-6, IL-11, and IL-17, increase expression of RANKL leading to increased bone resorption.[13–15] Based on an understanding of this pathophysiology, there has been debate about whether low-dose glucocorticoids could be protective to bone in RA.[16–19] Randomized trials of lower dose prednisone in RA have failed to consistently show an increased fracture risk. However, these studies are of insufficient size or duration to identify fracture signals adequately.[20–24]

DIAGNOSIS/IDENTIFYING PATIENTS AT RISK
Bone Mineral Density Measurement

BMD measurement does not have the same utility in glucocorticoid-exposed patients as it does in postmenopausal osteoporosis. Comparison of fractures between these two groups at similar BMD measurements shows higher fracture risk in the glucocorticoid users.[25] Thus, fracture risk for GIOP is partially independent of BMD and may relate to the direct toxic effect of glucocorticoids on osteoblasts and osteocytes.[26] Despite these limitations, BMD measurement can still be used as a tool to help risk stratify patients with GIOP for treatment decisions and to follow patients over time, particularly in response to bone-specific therapies.

FRAX

The FRAX tool (https://www.Shef.ac.uk/FRAX/) developed by the World Health Organization provides the 10-year probabilities of hip fracture and a major osteoporotic fracture (fractures of the hip, spine, forearm, and humerus). It incorporates numerous osteoporosis risk factors, including the use of glucocorticoids. In assessing glucocorticoid users, there are some restrictions associated with FRAX. This tool does not input specific glucocorticoid doses or duration[8] but relies on an average dose of 7.5 mg of prednisolone per day. In addition, only the femoral neck BMD is incorporated into the calculation and patients with GIOP may lose bone mass in the spine or the hip trochanter earlier, thereby underestimating risk.[8] There is an adjustment for FRAX that can be applied and takes into account the dose of glucocorticoids (**Table 1**).[27]

Other Testing Strategies

Patients on glucocorticoids who present with low bone mass or fractures should also be initially evaluated for other secondary causes of bone loss. Hyperparathyroidism, osteomalacia (most commonly caused by vitamin D deficiency or relative insufficiency), and more rarely other metabolic bone disorders may coincidentally be detected and require alternate therapeutic approaches. Beyond routine blood chemistries and a complete blood count, selective biochemical tests, including a 25-hydroxy (OH) vitamin D, parathyroid hormone, serum phosphorus, and occasionally a serum immunoelectrophoresis (looking for a paraproteinemia), may be prudent. For patients who have an intermediate risk based on dual-energy x-ray absorptiometry (DXA) or FRAX, lateral vertebral imaging by conventional radiography or using the DXA machine to obtain a vertebral fracture assessment is appropriate to exclude vertebral compression fractures. The trabecular bone score (TBS) is an additional technique that may be used to assess bone as an adjunct to DXA. It has the benefit of analyzing skeletal microarchitecture, and can be extrapolated from data obtained from a DXA scan. The higher the TBS, the better the bone microarchitecture. TBS has been shown in primary osteoporosis to predict current and future fragility fractures and has been used to assess treatment effect. TBS may be decreased in patients on glucocorticoids compared with normal controls, even when there is no significant change in BMD.[28] Larger studies are needed to ascertain whether TBS provides added value in this clinical setting, but TBS could prove to be another tool to aid in the prevention and treatment of GIOP.

PREVENTION AND TREATMENT
Lifestyle Measures and Assessment

Despite most of the evidence being consensus opinion extrapolated from data in other forms of osteoporosis, these measures should not be minimized and patients should be educated on how to make these modifications (**Box 1**). Regrettably, lifestyle

Table 1
Adjustments to 10-year FRAX by glucocorticoid dose

Fracture Site and Dose	Glucocorticoid Dose (Prednisolone Equivalent mg/dL)	Average Percentage Adjustment for All Ages
Hip Fracture		
Low	<2.5	−35
Medium	2.5–7.5	No adjustment
High	≥7.5	+20
Major Osteoporotic		
Low	<2.5	−20
Medium	2.5–7.5	No adjustment
High	≥7.5	+15

Box 1
American College of Rheumatology (ACR) recommendations on counseling for lifestyle modification and assessment of patients starting on glucocorticoids at any dose with an anticipated duration greater than or equal to 3 months

Assessments

Fall risk assessment

Baseline dual x-ray absorptiometry

Serum 25-hydroxyvitamin vitamin D level

Baseline height

Assessment of prevalent fragility fractures

Consider radiographic imaging of the spine or vertebral fracture assessment for patients initiating or currently receiving prednisone greater than or equal to 5 mg/d or its equivalent

Recommendations

Weight-bearing activities

Smoking cessation

Avoidance of excessive alcohol intake (>2 drinks per day)

Nutritional counseling on calcium and vitamin D intake

Calcium intake (supplement plus oral intake) 1200–1500 mg/d

Vitamin D supplementation

modifications are difficult for most patients to implement and the overall magnitude of their benefit is limited.

Calcium and Vitamin D

Calcium and vitamin D combined are effective in decreasing bone loss among glucocorticoid users compared with calcium or placebo.[29–32] A meta-analysis focused on lumbar spine BMD outcome revealed a 3.2% positive difference in the percentage change in BMD in those patients taking calcium plus vitamin D.[31] Despite calcium's benefits as an essential bone building block and the role of vitamin D in maximizing calcium absorption and minimizing its losses, calcium and vitamin D have not been shown to independently reduce fracture risk in GIOP. Thus, for most persons on chronic glucocorticoids, calcium and vitamin D are necessary but not sufficient. International guidelines for the treatment of GIOP all recognize the need for adequate calcium and vitamin D supplementation, although they vary slightly in dosing and target groups. Consistent with the Institute of Medicine recommendations,[33] we recommend at least 1200 mg of elemental calcium per day, acquired preferentially from diet rather than supplements. Calcium is best consumed with food to promote an acid environment and older adults on proton pump inhibitors may absorb more calcium citrate than other forms of calcium. Vitamin D can be administered through daily multivitamins or through calcium supplements to achieve at least 600 IU of vitamin D per day. For patients who have 25-OH vitamin D levels less than 20 ng/mL a short course (typically 50,000 IUs 2 times per week for 2 months) of ergocalciferol (vitamin D_2) is appropriate to replete the fat-soluble vitamin D stores. There is growing concern that too much calcium and too much vitamin D are neither necessary nor perhaps safe. Hypercalcemia, nephrolithiasis, and potentially a heightened risk of cardiovascular adverse events have been associated with overzealous use of calcium supplements and/or vitamin D in some, but not in all, studies.

Bisphosphonates

Bisphosphonates constitute the first-line therapy for the treatment of GIOP. They inhibit osteoclast activity and therefore result in decreased bone resorption. At present, alendronate, risedronate, and zoledronic acid are approved by the US Food and Drug Administration (FDA) for the treatment of GIOP. Risedronate and zoledronic acid are also approved for prevention. Off-label use of ibandronate, pamidronate, and etidronate is supported by some clinical trial data showing efficacy on BMD end points as well as an open-label study that showed lower fracture risk on ibandronate.[34] All bisphosphonates are poorly absorbed orally. They should be taken on an empty stomach with a full 240-mL (8 ounce) glass of water and nothing eaten for at least 30 minutes afterward to maximize their absorption. It is also necessary to remain upright afterward for at least 30 minutes after ingestion. Dyspepsia and, less commonly, esophagitis are the most frequently reported adverse events. Arthralgias can occur and can often be distinguished from other causes with a dechallenge-rechallenge strategy. A particular issue with all bisphosphonates in GIOP is that some of the potential recipients are premenopausal women of childbearing potential. There is no compelling evidence of concerns to the fetus after prolonged use of a bisphosphonate by the mother, albeit based on very limited data. There is no clear evidence of serious risk to the unborn child (as long as the drug is not actively onboard at the time of delivery, when fetal hypocalcemia might be expected).[35–38] It is still best to avoid these drugs in young women and in children, except among those at greatest risk and those who have already experienced fragility fractures associated with their glucocorticoid use.

There are also concerns regarding longer term safety of bisphosphonates in GIOP. Because a low-turnover bone state follows prolonged use of glucocorticoids, bisphosphonates may be limited in their long-term effectiveness and theoretically could contribute to an oversuppression of bone turnover, which likely represents the mechanism for the very rare side effects of osteonecrosis of the jaw and atypical femoral fractures.[39] Despite these theoretic concerns, some expert groups, such as the UK National Osteoporosis Guidelines Group, recommend continued bisphosphonate use as long as supraphysiologic glucocorticoids are still being used.[40] Counseling on proper use and potential side effects should be performed for every patient to ensure a full understanding of benefits and risks and to maximize compliance, which is low long term.

- Alendronate
  - In a randomized, double-blind, placebo-controlled study by Saag and colleagues[41] and its extension study by Adachi and colleagues,[42] alendronate significantly increased BMD at the spine and trochanter, while maintaining BMD at the femoral neck in patients receiving glucocorticoids. There was also a significant reduction in vertebral fractures in the extension study. A meta-analysis of oral bisphosphonates overall showed similar vertebral fracture risk reduction to that seen in postmenopausal osteoporosis.[43]
  - Recommended dose for treatment: 10 mg daily or 70 mg weekly orally in postmenopausal women and men with osteoporosis and 35 mg weekly in premenopausal women.
- Risedronate
  - Prevents bone loss in the lumbar spine, femoral neck, and trochanter in patients taking glucocorticoids as shown in randomized trials by both Cohen

and colleagues[44] for new users and Reid and colleagues[45] for prevalent users. Significant risk reduction by 70% of new vertebral fractures was also observed in a post hoc analysis that combined these two studies.[46]

o Recommended dose for prevention or treatment: 5 mg daily or 35 mg weekly orally.

- Zoledronic acid
  o A randomized controlled, noninferiority trial of zoledronic acid versus risedronate for prevention and treatment of GIOP showed that zoledronic acid was noninferior and was more efficacious in increasing BMD than risedronate.[47] Despite this being the largest bisphosphonate GIOP study to date, BMD was not a part of the inclusion criteria and patients on average had lower fracture risk than in other studies. There was no significant fracture risk reduction seen comparing zoledronic acid with risedronate. Zoledronic acid can cause an acute phase reaction leading to arthralgias/myalgias, low-grade fevers, and less commonly flulike symptoms in about 10% of patients given an intravenous infusion.
  o Recommended dose for prevention or treatment: 5 mg once a year intravenously in persons with adequate renal function (glomerular filtration rate >35 mL/min).

Teriparatide

A bone anabolic agent, teriparatide is a recombinant human parathyroid hormone.[1–34] Because the pathogenesis of GIOP includes decreased osteoblast differentiation and maturation leading to decreased bone formation,[1] anabolic agents such as teriparatide might counteract this by direct effects on osteoblasts that include increasing the number of osteoblast precursors, promoting differentiation into mature cells, and increasing survival with the combined effect of increasing bone formation.[48,49] In a study comparing teriparatide with alendronate for GIOP, there were greater increases in BMD in the spine and hip with teriparatide.[50] The study was not statistically powered for fracture risk reduction, but even so there were also fewer morphometrically assessed vertebral fractures in the teriparatide group compared with alendronate, although no significant difference was found for nonvertebral fractures.[50] Teriparatide is FDA approved for GIOP and is given as 20 μg subcutaneously daily. The main side effect of teriparatide is a mild hypercalcemia (on average 1 mg/dL). In the initial development of teriparatide a Fisher rat model developed osteosarcoma. A black-box warning in the product circular cautions about this finding, although to date the postmarket rate of this outcome has mirrored the background rate of osteosarcoma in general populations.[51] It is recommended that teriparatide not be given to children or young adults with open epiphyses or those who have received past radiation therapy. Patients with bone malignancy are likely also not good teriparatide candidates. A finite anabolic window further limits therapy to a 24-month maximum. Teriparatide may be cost-effective compared with alendronate in glucocorticoid users with incident vertebral fractures.[52]

Denosumab

Denosumab is a fully human monoclonal antibody against RANKL. After binding to RANKL, it prevents RANKL from binding to receptor of activator of NF-kappa β, which is necessary for the formation and function of osteoclasts, and therefore inhibits osteoclast activity and thereby bone resorption.[53] Denosumab has been shown to decrease the risk of vertebral, nonvertebral, and hip fracture in postmenopausal women with osteoporosis and is approved by the FDA for treatment in this group.[53]

It has not yet been approved for GIOP and is currently undergoing phase III clinical trials comparing its effect on BMD with risedronate. During a study testing its efficacy in RA, some of the patients receiving it were on glucocorticoids. The relative improvement in bone mass seen with denosumab (particularly at the standard dose of 60 mg every 6 months) compared with placebo seemed to be qualitatively similar between patients receiving and not receiving glucocorticoids.[54]

Raloxifene

Raloxifene is a selective estrogen receptor modulator, shown in postmenopausal osteoporosis to reduce vertebral fracture risk. A small randomized controlled trial showed preservation to slight gain of bone mass at the spine with raloxifene compared with placebo.[55] Although it is not approved for GIOP, it may represent another therapeutic option for women who are not at heightened risk for venous thromboembolic disease.

Percutaneous Vertebroplasty

As discussed earlier, there is considerable evidence in support of medical management to prevent vertebral fractures in patients with GIOP. Some studies suggest that percutaneous vertebroplasty (PVP) and percutaneous kyphoplasty (PKP) may address pain and improve postfracture mobility in postmenopausal women. Case reports not controlled for underlying vertebral fracture risk suggest that patients with GIOP were at increased risk for vertebral refracture (at time of initial PVP) at vertebral sites above and below the vertebral level treated, compared with those with primary osteoporosis.[56] A cluster phenomenon of multiple vertebral refractures occurred within a short time of the initial procedure, requiring additional procedures. PVP and PKP should therefore be used with caution in patients with GIOP until their safety and comparative effectiveness are better delineated in this patient population.

International Guidelines for Glucocorticoid-induced Osteoporosis

Postmenopausal women and men greater than or equal to 50 years of age
There are numerous international guidelines for the management of GIOP. In general, it is agreed that lifestyle modifications, as noted previously, should be implemented and attempts should be made to minimize exposure to glucocorticoids whether by reducing the dose or initiating a steroid-sparing agent whenever possible. The threshold for intervention with bone-specific pharmacologic agents varies between countries and is related to cost and access. **Table 2** provides a comparison of the guidelines between the American College of Rheumatology (ACR) and the International Osteoporosis Foundation and the European Calcified Tissue Society.[8,57]

Premenopausal women and men aged less than 50
There are limited data for fracture risk and treatment in these younger women and men; however, the ACR has provided limited guidance.[8] If the patient had not had a fragility fracture there was not enough evidence for an expert panel to recommend treatment. In the presence of fragility fracture, if glucocorticoids have been taken for 3 months or more, then any of the FDA-approved drugs for GIOP should be considered for treatment.[8] If glucocorticoid use is less than 3 months and the dose greater than or equal to 5 mg/d, treatment should include alendronate or risedronate; if the dose is greater than or equal to 7.5 mg/d, zoledronic acid can be offered.[8] In women of childbearing age who have not experienced a fracture, there was no consensus on treatment of patients with glucocorticoid use of less than 3 months or for those with greater than 3 months of use at doses less than 7.5 mg/d. However, in this group, if

Table 2
Comparison of guidelines for prevention and treatment of GIOP for postmenopausal women and men more than 50 years of age

	ACR[8]	IOF-ECTS[57]
Bone density and/or FRAX score requiring treatment	Determination made based on FRAX and overall clinical risk incorporating BMD	BMD T-score and FRAX with country-specific thresholds
Minimum glucocorticoid dose and duration requiring treatment	Low risk: ≥7.5 mg/d for at least 3 mo[a] Medium risk: any dose for at least 3 mo use[b] High risk: any dose for at least 1 mo use[c]	≥7.5 mg/d for ≥3 mo
Other indications for treatment	—	Previous fracture Age ≥70 y
Calcium and vitamin D supplementation	Calcium 1200–1500 mg/d Vitamin D 800–000 IU/d	Recommended but doses not specified
Pharmacotherapy	Alendronate or risedronate for all low-risk, medium-risk, and high-risk patients Zoledronic acid for low-risk and medium-risk patients taking ≥7.5 mg/d and all high-risk patients Teriparatide for high-risk patients taking ≥5 mg/d for ≤1 mo or any dose used for >1 mo	Alendronate, etidronate, risedronate, zoledronic acid, and teriparatide all options

Abbreviations: ACR, American College of Rheumatology; IOF-ECTS, International Osteoporosis Foundation and the European Calcified Tissue Society.
[a] Low risk: FRAX less than 10% for 10-year major osteoporotic fracture.
[b] Medium risk: FRAX 10% to 20% for 10-year major osteoporotic fracture.
[c] High risk: FRAX greater than 20% for 10-year major osteoporotic fracture.

exposed to greater than or equal to 3 months of use and greater than or equal to 7.5 mg/d, then alendronate, risedronate, or teriparatide is recommended.[8] Despite these guidelines and the notable limitations for certain age and sex groups, treatment of younger patients must be highly individualized based on other risk factors and with patient preference considerations. Even younger patients, such as those with systemic lupus erythematosus, are at higher risk of fracturing while on prolonged glucocorticoids.[58]

SUMMARY

GIOP is a well-established entity that is associated with significant morbidity and mortality caused by fractures. Preventative treatment and lifestyle modifications can effectively reduce bone loss. Despite international guidelines, many patients, even among those at greatest risk, receive neither testing nor treatment.[59] Among those who start therapy, less than half are still taking an oral bisphosphonate a year later.[60] Rheumatologists and other health care providers focused on bone health are well poised to internationally address this persistent issue and reduce the risk of this unnecessary comorbidity among patients with inflammatory disease who require chronic glucocorticoid treatment.

ACKNOWLEDGMENTS

Special thanks to Josh Melnick, MPH, for assistance with article preparation.

REFERENCES

1. Canalis E, Mazziotti G, Giustina A, et al. Glucocorticoid-induced osteoporosis: pathophysiology and therapy. Osteoporos Int 2007;18(10):1319–28.
2. Weinstein RS, Jilka RL, Parfitt AM, et al. Inhibition of osteoblastogenesis and promotion of apoptosis of osteoblasts and osteocytes by glucocorticoids. Potential mechanisms of their deleterious effects on bone. J Clin Invest 1998;102(2): 274–82.
3. Manolagas SC, Weinstein RS. New developments in the pathogenesis and treatment of steroid-induced osteoporosis. J Bone Miner Res 1999;14(7): 1061–6.
4. Huizenga NA, Koper JW, De Lange P, et al. A polymorphism in the glucocorticoid receptor gene may be associated with an increased sensitivity to glucocorticoids in vivo. J Clin Endocrinol Metab 1998;83(1):144–51.
5. Dykman TR, Gluck OS, Murphy WA, et al. Evaluation of factors associated with glucocorticoid-induced osteopenia in patients with rheumatic diseases. Arthritis Rheum 1985;28(4):361–8.
6. LoCascio V, Bonucci E, Imbimbo B, et al. Bone loss in response to long-term glucocorticoid therapy. Bone Miner 1990;8(1):39–51.
7. Tatsuno I, Sugiyama T, Suzuki S, et al. Age dependence of early symptomatic vertebral fracture with high-dose glucocorticoid treatment for collagen vascular diseases. J Clin Endocrinol Metab 2009;94(5):1671–7.
8. Grossman JM, Gordon R, Ranganath VK, et al. American College of Rheumatology 2010 recommendations for the prevention and treatment of glucocorticoid-induced osteoporosis. Arthritis Care Res (Hoboken) 2010; 62(11):1515–26.
9. van Staa TP, Leufkens HG, Abenhaim L, et al. Oral corticosteroids and fracture risk: relationship to daily and cumulative doses. Rheumatology (Oxford) 2000; 39(12):1383–9.
10. van Staa TP, Leufkens HG, Cooper C. The epidemiology of corticosteroid-induced osteoporosis: a meta-analysis. Osteoporos Int 2002;13(10):777–87.
11. Briot K, Cortet B, Roux C, et al. 2014 update of recommendations on the prevention and treatment of glucocorticoid-induced osteoporosis. Joint Bone Spine 2014;81(6):493–501.
12. Emkey RD, Lindsay R, Lyssy J, et al. The systemic effect of intraarticular administration of corticosteroid on markers of bone formation and bone resorption in patients with rheumatoid arthritis. Arthritis Rheum 1996;39(2):277–82.
13. Peel NF, Moore DJ, Barrington NA, et al. Risk of vertebral fracture and relationship to bone mineral density in steroid treated rheumatoid arthritis. Ann Rheum Dis 1995;54(10):801–6.
14. Gough AK, Lilley J, Eyre S, et al. Generalised bone loss in patients with early rheumatoid arthritis. Lancet 1994;344(8914):23–7.
15. Hofbauer LC, Gori F, Riggs BL, et al. Stimulation of osteoprotegerin ligand and inhibition of osteoprotegerin production by glucocorticoids in human osteoblastic lineage cells: potential paracrine mechanisms of glucocorticoid-induced osteoporosis. Endocrinology 1999;140(10):4382–9.
16. Sambrook PN, Eisman JA, Yeates MG, et al. Osteoporosis in rheumatoid arthritis: safety of low dose corticosteroids. Ann Rheum Dis 1986;45(11):950–3.

17. Verhoeven AC, Boers M. Limited bone loss due to corticosteroids; a systematic review of prospective studies in rheumatoid arthritis and other diseases. J Rheumatol 1997;24(8):1495–503.

18. Verstraeten A, Dequeker J. Vertebral and peripheral bone mineral content and fracture incidence in postmenopausal patients with rheumatoid arthritis: effect of low dose corticosteroids. Ann Rheum Dis 1986;45(10):852–7.

19. Lodder M, Lems W, Kostense P. Bone loss due to glucocorticoids: update of a systematic review of prospective studies in rheumatoid arthritis and other diseases. Ann Rheum Dis 2003;62(Suppl 1):94.

20. Kirwan JR. The effect of glucocorticoids on joint destruction in rheumatoid arthritis. The Arthritis and Rheumatism Council Low-Dose Glucocorticoid Study Group. N Engl J Med 1995;333(3):142–6.

21. Svensson B, Boonen A, Albertsson K, et al. Low-dose prednisolone in addition to the initial disease-modifying antirheumatic drug in patients with early active rheumatoid arthritis reduces joint destruction and increases the remission rate: a two-year randomized trial. Arthritis Rheum 2005;52(11):3360–70.

22. Wassenberg S, Rau R, Steinfeld P, et al. Very low-dose prednisolone in early rheumatoid arthritis retards radiographic progression over two years: a multicenter, double-blind, placebo-controlled trial. Arthritis Rheum 2005;52(11):3371–80.

23. Capell HA, Madhok R, Hunter JA, et al. Lack of radiological and clinical benefit over two years of low dose prednisolone for rheumatoid arthritis: results of a randomised controlled trial. Ann Rheum Dis 2004;63(7):797–803.

24. van Everdingen AA, Jacobs JW, Siewertsz Van Reesema DR, et al. Low-dose prednisone therapy for patients with early active rheumatoid arthritis: clinical efficacy, disease-modifying properties, and side effects: a randomized, double-blind, placebo-controlled clinical trial. Ann Intern Med 2002;136(1):1–12.

25. van Staa TP, Laan RF, Barton IP, et al. Bone density threshold and other predictors of vertebral fracture in patients receiving oral glucocorticoid therapy. Arthritis Rheum 2003;48(11):3224–9.

26. Kanis JA, Johansson H, Oden A, et al. A meta-analysis of prior corticosteroid use and fracture risk. J Bone Miner Res 2004;19(6):893–9.

27. Kanis JA, Johansson H, Oden A, et al. Guidance for the adjustment of FRAX according to the dose of glucocorticoids. Osteoporos Int 2011;22(3):809–16.

28. Ulivieri FM, Silva BC, Sardanelli F, et al. Utility of the trabecular bone score (TBS) in secondary osteoporosis. Endocrine 2014;47(2):435–48.

29. Buckley LM, Leib ES, Cartularo KS, et al. Calcium and vitamin D3 supplementation prevents bone loss in the spine secondary to low-dose corticosteroids in patients with rheumatoid arthritis. A randomized, double-blind, placebo-controlled trial. Ann Intern Med 1996;125(12):961–8.

30. Sambrook P, Birmingham J, Kelly P, et al. Prevention of corticosteroid osteoporosis. A comparison of calcium, calcitriol, and calcitonin. N Engl J Med 1993;328(24):1747–52.

31. Amin S, LaValley MP, Simms RW, et al. The role of vitamin D in corticosteroid-induced osteoporosis: a meta-analytic approach. Arthritis Rheum 1999;42(8):1740–51.

32. Homik J, Suarez-Almazor ME, Shea B, et al. Calcium and vitamin D for corticosteroid-induced osteoporosis. Cochrane Database Syst Rev 2000;(2):CD000952.

33. Institute of Medicine. Dietary reference intakes for calcium, phosphorus, magnesium, vitamin D, and fluoride. Institute of Medicine; 1997.

34. Ringe JD, Dorst A, Faber H, et al. Intermittent intravenous ibandronate injections reduce vertebral fracture risk in corticosteroid-induced osteoporosis: results from a long-term comparative study. Osteoporos Int 2003;14(10):801–7.

35. Levy S, Fayez I, Taguchi N, et al. Pregnancy outcome following in utero exposure to bisphosphonates. Bone 2009;44(3):428–30.

36. Biswas PN, Wilton LV, Shakir SA. Pharmacovigilance study of alendronate in England. Osteoporos Int 2003;14(6):507–14.

37. Rutgers-Verhage AR, deVries TW, Torringa MJ. No effects of bisphosphonates on the human fetus. Birth Defects Res A Clin Mol Teratol 2003;67(3):203–4.

38. Ornoy A, Wajnberg R, Diav-Citrin O. The outcome of pregnancy following pre-pregnancy or early pregnancy alendronate treatment. Reprod Toxicol 2006; 22(4):578–9.

39. Teitelbaum SL, Seton MP, Saag KG. Should bisphosphonates be used for long-term treatment of glucocorticoid-induced osteoporosis? Arthritis Rheum 2011; 63(2):325–8.

40. Compston J, Bowring C, Cooper A, et al. Diagnosis and management of osteoporosis in postmenopausal women and older men in the UK: National Osteoporosis Guideline Group (NOGG) update 2013. Maturitas 2013;75(4):392–6.

41. Saag KG, Emkey R, Schnitzer TJ, et al. Alendronate for the prevention and treatment of glucocorticoid-induced osteoporosis. Glucocorticoid-Induced Osteoporosis Intervention Study Group. N Engl J Med 1998;339(5):292–9.

42. Adachi JD, Saag KG, Delmas PD, et al. Two-year effects of alendronate on bone mineral density and vertebral fracture in patients receiving glucocorticoids: a randomized, double-blind, placebo-controlled extension trial. Arthritis Rheum 2001; 44(1):202–11.

43. Kanis JA, Stevenson M, McCloskey EV, et al. Glucocorticoid-induced osteoporosis: a systematic review and cost-utility analysis. Health Technol Assess 2007;11(7):iii–iv, ix–xi, 1–231.

44. Cohen S, Levy RM, Keller M, et al. Risedronate therapy prevents corticosteroid-induced bone loss: a twelve-month, multicenter, randomized, double-blind, placebo-controlled, parallel-group study. Arthritis Rheum 1999; 42(11):2309–18.

45. Reid DM, Hughes RA, Laan RF, et al. Efficacy and safety of daily risedronate in the treatment of corticosteroid-induced osteoporosis in men and women: a randomized trial. European Corticosteroid-Induced Osteoporosis Treatment Study. J Bone Miner Res 2000;15(6):1006–13.

46. Wallach S, Cohen S, Reid DM, et al. Effects of risedronate treatment on bone density and vertebral fracture in patients on corticosteroid therapy. Calcif Tissue Int 2000;67(4):277–85.

47. Reid DM, Devogelaer JP, Saag K, et al. Zoledronic acid and risedronate in the prevention and treatment of glucocorticoid-induced osteoporosis (HORIZON): a multicentre, double-blind, double-dummy, randomised controlled trial. Lancet 2009;373(9671):1253–63.

48. Canalis E, Giustina A, Bilezikian JP. Mechanisms of anabolic therapies for osteoporosis. N Engl J Med 2007;357(9):905–16.

49. Lane N, Sanchez S, Modin G, et al. Bone mass continues to increase at the hip after parathyroid hormone treatment is discontinued in glucocorticoid induced osteoporosis: results of a randomized controlled clinical trial. J Bone Miner Res 2000;15(5):944–51.

50. Saag KG, Shane E, Boonen S, et al. Teriparatide or alendronate in glucocorticoid-induced osteoporosis. N Engl J Med 2007;357(20):2028–39.

51. Krohn K, Kellier N, Masica D, et al. Post-marketing case series study of adult osteosarcoma and for(s)teo: study findings from the first 9 years. Osteoporos Int 2014;25(Suppl 1):S61.
52. Murphy DR, Smolen LJ, Klein TM, et al. The cost effectiveness of teriparatide as a first-line treatment for glucocorticoid-induced and postmenopausal osteoporosis patients in Sweden. BMC Musculoskelet Disord 2012;13:213.
53. Cummings SR, San Martin J, McClung MR, et al. Denosumab for prevention of fractures in postmenopausal women with osteoporosis. N Engl J Med 2009; 361(8):756–65.
54. Dore RK, Cohen SB, Lane NE, et al. Effects of denosumab on bone mineral density and bone turnover in patients with rheumatoid arthritis receiving concurrent glucocorticoids or bisphosphonates. Ann Rheum Dis 2010;69(5):872–5.
55. Mok CC, Ying KY, To CH, et al. Raloxifene for prevention of glucocorticoid-induced bone loss: a 12-month randomised double-blinded placebo-controlled trial. Ann Rheum Dis 2011;70(5):778–84.
56. Sun H, Sharma S, Li C. Cluster phenomenon of vertebral refractures after percutaneous vertebroplasty in a patient with glucocorticosteroid-induced osteoporosis: case report and review of the literature. Spine (Phila Pa 1976) 2013; 38(25):E1628–32.
57. Lekamwasam S, Adachi JD, Agnusdei D, et al. A framework for the development of guidelines for the management of glucocorticoid-induced osteoporosis. Osteoporos Int 2012;23(9):2257–76.
58. Bultink IE, Harvey NC, Lalmohamed A, et al. Elevated risk of clinical fractures and associated risk factors in patients with systemic lupus erythematosus versus matched controls: a population-based study in the United Kingdom. Osteoporos Int 2014;25(4):1275–83.
59. Curtis JR, Westfall AO, Allison JJ, et al. Longitudinal patterns in the prevention of osteoporosis in glucocorticoid-treated patients. Arthritis Rheum 2005;52(8): 2485–94.
60. Curtis JR, Westfall AO, Allison JJ, et al. Channeling and adherence with alendronate and risedronate among chronic glucocorticoid users. Osteoporos Int 2006;17(8):1268–74.

Index

Note: Page numbers of article titles are in **boldface** type.

Rheum Dis Clin N Am 42 (2016) 191–203
http://dx.doi.org/10.1016/S0889-857X(15)00105-2
0889-857X/16/$ – see front matter © 2016 Elsevier Inc. All rights reserved.

rheumatic.theclinics.com

Moving?

Make sure your subscription moves with you!

To notify us of your new address, find your **Clinics Account Number** (located on your mailing label above your name), and contact customer service at:

Email: journalscustomerservice-usa@elsevier.com

800-654-2452 (subscribers in the U.S. & Canada)
314-447-8871 (subscribers outside of the U.S. & Canada)

Fax number: 314-447-8029

Elsevier Health Sciences Division
Subscription Customer Service
3251 Riverport Lane
Maryland Heights, MO 63043

*To ensure uninterrupted delivery of your subscription, please notify us at least 4 weeks in advance of move.

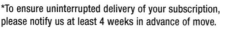

Printed and bound by CPI Group (UK) Ltd, Croydon, CR0 4YY

03/10/2024

01040497-0003